Contemporary Topics in Immunobiology

Volume 10

CONTEMPORARY TOPICS IN IMMUNOBIOLOGY

A Continuation Order Plan is available for this series. A continuation order will bring delivery of each new volume immediately upon publication. Volumes are billed only upon actual shipment. For further information please contact the publisher.

CONTEMPORARY TOPICS IN IMMUNOBIOLOGY

VOLUME 10

In Situ Expression of Tumor Immunity

EDITED BY

ISAAC P. WITZ

Department of Microbiology
The George S. Wise Faculty of Life Sciences
Tel Aviv University
Tel Aviv, Israel

and

M. G. HANNA, JR.

Frederick Cancer Research Center
Frederick, Maryland

Springer Science+Business Media, LLC

The Library of Congress cataloged the first volume in this series as follows:

Contemporary topics in immunobiology. v. 1-
  1972—
  New York, Plenum Press.
    v. illus. 24cm. annual.

  1. Immunology—Periodicals.
  QR180.C632   574.2'9'05   79-179761
  ISSN 0093—4054   rev   MARC—S
  Library of Congress   72 [r74c2]

ISBN 978-1-4684-3679-2   ISBN 978-1-4684-3677-8 (eBook)
DOI 10.1007/978-1-4684-3677-8

© 1980 Springer Science+Business Media New York
Originally published by Plenum Press, New York in 1980
Softcover reprint of the hardcover 1st edition 1980

Contributors

Ora Amitai

Department of Microbiology
The George S. Wise Faculty of Life Sciences
Tel Aviv University
Tel Aviv, Israel

Gideon Berke

Deparment of Cell Biology
The Weizmann Institute of Science
Rehovot, Israel

C. D. Bucana

Cancer Biology Program
NCI Frederick Cancer Research Center
Frederick, Maryland 21701

Robert Evans

The Jackson Laboratory
Bar Harbor, Maine 04609

M. Fopp

Department of Tumor Biology
Karolinska Institute
Radiumhemmet, Karolinska Sjukhuset
S-104 01 Stockholm 60, Sweden
Present address: Department of Oncology and Hematology
Clinic of Medicine
Kanton Spital
CH-9007 St. Gallen, Switzerland

P. Frost

Department of Immunology and Microbiology
Wayne State University
Detroit, Michigan 48201

U. Galili

Department of Tumor Biology
Karolinska Institute
Radiumhemmet, Karolinska Sjukhuset
S-104 01 Stockholm 60, Sweden

James Gerson

Laboratories of Immunodiagnosis and Immunobiology
National Cancer Institute
Bethesda, Maryland 20205

G. Yancey Gillespie

Department of Pathology and The Cancer Research Center
University of North Carolina School of Medicine
Chapel Hill, North Carolina 27514

M. G. Hanna, Jr.

Cancer Biology Program
NCI Frederick Cancer Research Center
Frederick, Maryland 21701

J. Stephen Haskill
Medical University of South Carolina
Charleston, South Carolina 29401

Ronald B. Herberman
Laboratories of Immunodiagnosis and Immunobiology
National Cancer Institute
Bethesda, Maryland 20205

Howard T. Holden
Laboratories of Immunodiagnosis and Immunobiology
National Cancer Institute
Bethesda, Maryland 20205

C. Huet
Institut de Recherches Scientifiques sur le Cancer
Villejuif, France

Harry L. Ioachim
Department of Pathology
Lenox Hill Hospital
New York, New York 10021 and
Department of Pathology
College of Physicians and Surgeons
Columbia University
New York, New York 10032

Yona Keisari
Laboratories of Immunodiagnosis and Immunobiology
National Cancer Institute
Bethesda, Maryland 20205

R. S. Kerbel
National Cancer Institute of Canada Research Group
Division of Cancer Research
Department of Pathology
Queen's University
Kingston, Ontario, Canada K7L 3N6

M. King
Institut de Recherches Scientifiques sur le Cancer
Villejuif, France

Holger Kirchner
Laboratories of Immunodiagnosis and Immunobiology
National Cancer Institute
Bethesda, Maryland 20205

E. Klein
Department of Tumor Biology
Karolinska Institute
Radiumhemmet, Karolinska Sjukhuset
S-104 01 Stockholm 60, Sweden

H. Robson MacDonald
Unit of Human Cancer Immunology
Lausanne Branch
Ludwig Institute for Cancer Research
and Department of Immunology
Swiss Institute for Experimental Cancer Research
1066 Epalinges-sur-Lausanne, Switzerland

R. Matre
Broegelmann Research Laboratory for Microbiology
and Department of Microbiology
The Gade Institute
University of Bergen
Bergen, Norway

K. Moore
Paterson Laboratories
Christie Hospital and Holt Radium Institute
Manchester M20 9BX, England

Present address: Department of Bacteriology
University of Edinburgh Medical School
Teviot Place
Edinburgh, Scotland

M. Moore   *Paterson Laboratories*
Christie Hospital and Holt Radium Institute
Manchester M20 9BX, England

Judith L. Pace   *Department of Pathology and The Cancer Research Center*
University of North Carolina School of Medicine
Chapel Hill, North Carolina 27514

V. A. Pollack   *Cancer Biology Program*
NCI Frederick Cancer Research Center
Frederick, Maryland 21701

Theresa P. Pretlow   *Department of Pathology*
University of Alabama in Birmingham
Birmingham, Alabama 35294

Thomas G. Pretlow II   *Department of Pathology*
University of Alabama in Birmingham
Birmingham, Alabama 35294

Paolo Puccetti   *Laboratories of Immunodiagnosis and Immunobiology*
National Cancer Institute
Bethesda, Maryland 20205

Maya Ran   *Department of Microbiology*
The George S. Wise Faculty of Life Sciences
Tel Aviv University
Tel Aviv, Israel

Stephen W. Russell   *Department of Pathology and The Cancer Research Center*
University of North Carolina School of Medicine
Chapel Hill, North Carolina 27514

Barbara Schick   *Department of Cell Biology*
The Weizmann Institute of Science
Rehovot, Israel

Bernard Sordat   *Unit of Human Cancer Immunology*
Lausanne Branch
Ludwig Institute for Cancer Research
and Department of Immunology
Swiss Institute for Experimental Cancer Research
1066 Epalinges-sur-Lausanne, Switzerland

Tadayoshi Taniyama   *Laboratories of Immunodiagnosis and Immunobiology*
National Cancer Institute
Bethesda, Maryland 20205

O. Tønder   *Broegelmann Research Laboratory for Microbiology*
and Department of Microbiology
The Gade Institute
University of Bergen
Bergen, Norway

R. R. Twiddy   *National Cancer Institute of Canada Research Group*
                        Division of Cancer Research
                        Department of Pathology
                        Queen's University
                        Kingston, Ontario, Canada K7L 3N6

F. Vánky   *Department of Tumor Biology*
                        Karolinska Institute
                        Radiumhemmet, Karolinska Sjukhuset
                        S-104 01 Stockholm 60, Sweden

Luigi Varesio   *Laboratories of Immunodiagnosis and Immunobiology*
                        National Cancer Institute
                        Bethesda, Maryland 20205

S. von Kleist   *Institute of Tumor Immunology*
                        University of Freiburg
                        Freiburg im Breisgau, Germany

B. M. Vose   *Department of Tumor Biology*
                        Karolinska Institute
                        Radiumhemmet, Karolinska Sjukhuset
                        S-104 01 Stockholm 60, Sweden
                        Present address: Department of Immunology
                        Paterson Laboratories
                        Christie Hospital and Holt Radium Institute
                        Manchester M20 9BX, England

F. Wesenberg   *Broegelmann Research Laboratory for Microbiology*
                        and Department of Microbiology
                        The Gade Institute
                        University of Bergen
                        Bergen, Norway

Sandra White   *Laboratories of Immunodiagnosis and Immunobiology*
                        National Cancer Institute
                        Bethesda, Maryland 20205

Isaac P. Witz   *Department of Microbiology*
                        The George S. Wise Faculty of Life Sciences
                        Tel Aviv University
                        Tel Aviv, Israel

Margalit Yaakubowicz   *Department of Microbiology*
                        The George S. Wise Faculty of Life Sciences
                        Tel Aviv University
                        Tel Aviv, Israel

Preface

Because of several valid (and some invalid) reasons, the research field of tumor immunology has been declining in popularity. The simplistic dogmas, articles of faith, and theories of the late 1960s and early 1970s on the immunological mechanisms of the host-tumor interrelationships have frequently been refuted by some of the new developments in cancer biology, cancer biochemistry, and immunology. Furthermore, some of the conventional assays used to monitor "tumor-host immune relations" did not always reflect the host's true clinical situation or his prognosis. Several approaches to immunological intervention were less successful than expected. In addition, the concept of "immune surveillance," which was basic to many researchers in the field of cancer immunology, seemed to fall apart. Much of the criticism was based on results from solid, well-performed, and well-controlled experiments, but there was also unjust criticism based on ill-conceived and badly performed studies, and on misinterpretations of experimental data.

There are many misconceptions about the tumor-host relationship. It is very often assumed that tumor immunity, as expressed systemically, is truly reflected at the tumor site. Several studies reported in this volume and elsewhere indicate that such is not always the case. Certain immune effectors may be selectively prevented from reaching the tumor site or the close vicinity of the tumor cells because of mechanical or chemical barriers, whereas others may be selectively attracted to the site by chemotaxis or other mechanisms. A selected subpopulation of immune effector components at the tumor site may bring about completely different biological effects from those generated by the more heterogeneous population of peripheral immune components. Thus, a comprehensive understanding of tumor-host relations requires a detailed analysis of immune components found in association with tumors and their functions, as well as of antitumor effector mechanisms operating systemically.

In order to review and critically analyze data obtained from studies of *in situ* tumor immunity performed independently by several groups, a workshop dedicated to this topic was held in Tel Aviv in June 1978. Many researchers active in this field and most of the contributors to this volume attended the workshop. We wish to thank all the authors for their endeavors.

The studies presented in this volume deal mainly with three topics: (1) The general methodology used to identify, isolate, and assay the functions of tumor-derived immune components. This includes some novel approaches and relevant model systems. (2) The biological functions of tumor-associated immune components and their regulation. (3) *In situ* expressions of immunity in human cancer (which also takes into account the other two topics). In Chapter 1, Drs. Ronald Herberman, Steven Russell, and one of us (I. P. W.) provide a comprehensive introduction to the subsequent chapters by reviewing the main findings, focusing on the unsolved problems, and identifying open questions pertaining to all three topics. We are grateful to them and all the authors for their contributions to this important subject.

Isaac P. Witz
M. G. Hanna, Jr.

Contents

Chapter 5

**Intratumor Host Cells of Experimental Rat Neoplasms:
Characterization and Effector Function**

M. Moore and K. Moore

Chapter 6

Evidence for Mononuclear Phagocytes in Solid Neoplasms and Appraisal of Their Nonspecific Cytotoxic Capabilities

Stephen W. Russell, G. Yancey Gillespie, and Judith L. Pace

Chapter 7

Mononuclear Cells and IgG Associated with Human Malignant Tissue

O. Tønder, R. Matre, and F. Wesenberg

Chapter 8

**Evidence for Membrane-Bound Antibodies Directed against
Antigens Expressed on Tumors**

    S. von Kleist, M. King, and C. Huet

Chapter 9

Tumor-Localizing Lymphocytotoxic Antibodies

    Maya Ran, Margalit Yaakubowicz, Ora Amitai, and Isaac P. Witz

Chapter 10

Correlations between Tumor Antigenicity, Malignant Potential, and Local Host Immune Response

Harry L. Ioachim

Chapter 11

Host Cell Analysis of a Rapidly Metastasizing Mouse Tumor and Derived Low-Metastatic Variant Lines

R. S. Kerbel, R. R. Twiddy, and P. Frost

Chapter 12

Cellular Basis for Regulation of Tumor Growth

Robert Evans

Chapter 13

Immunological Stimulation *in Situ:* The Acute and Chronic Inflammatory Responses in the Induction of Tumor Immunity

M. G. Hanna, Jr., C. D. Bucana, and V. A. Pollack

Chapter 14

Tumor Immunity in the Peritoneal Cavity

   Gideon Berke and Barbara Schick

Chapter 15

The Multicellular Tumor Spheroid: A Quantitative Model for Studies of *in Situ* Immunity

   H. Robson MacDonald and Bernard Sordat

Chapter 1

A Review of Data, Problems, and Open Questions Pertaining to in Situ Tumor Immunity

Stephen W. Russell*

Department of Pathology and The Cancer Research Center
University of North Carolina School of Medicine
Chapel Hill, North Carolina 27514

Isaac P. Witz†

Department of Microbiology
The George S. Wise Faculty of Life Sciences
Tel Aviv University
Tel Aviv, Israel

and

Ronald B. Herberman‡

Laboratories of Immunodiagnosis and Immunobiology
National Cancer Institute
Bethesda, Maryland 20205

I. PROBLEMS (TECHNICAL AND INTERPRETIVE) ASSOCIATED WITH THE ISOLATION OF IMMUNE EFFECTOR CELLS FROM TUMORS

A. Introduction

Isolation of cellular and humoral immune components from solid neoplasms is a relatively new approach to the study of a host's response to its tumor. While

---

*Contributor of Section I.
† Contributor of Section II.
‡Contributor of Section III.

1

this line of research has the potential for providing a great deal of new information about antitumor immunity, as might be expected it is an approach that is fraught with technical problems. The objectives of this chapter are to call attention to these problems and, when possible, to suggest solutions to them. By including such information in this monograph it is hoped that new investigators in the field will be provided with a starting point from which to launch their research that is technically more sound than would otherwise have been the case. Emphasis has been given to the recovery of inflammatory cells from tumors, in view of the comprehensive review of intratumoral immunoglobulin recently published by Witz (1977).

B. Morphologic Examination of Tumors

Dispersing a tumor by some means is usually necessary to recover immune effector elements from it. Before this procedure is undertaken it often is advisable to sample the neoplasm for morphologic studies. The objectives in doing so are twofold: (1) to determine the distribution of inflammatory cells in the neoplasm, and (2) to assess the extent to which microscopic foci of necrosis are present. An additional use for morphologic studies will be discussed under Section C.6 below.

Contact or close proximity between target and host cells is a requirement for the efficient expression of many effector cell functions, especially of cytotoxicity. Understanding how inflammatory cells relate to the biology of a neoplasm may be more complete, therefore, if it is known how they were distributed in the lesion. Were they relegated to the periphery of the tumor (Lauder *et al.*, 1977; Russell and Gillespie, 1977), to bands of connective tissue that separated lobules of neoplastic cells (Abraham and Barbolt, 1978), or were they uniformly distributed and in intimate contact with tumor cells (Lauder *et al.*, 1977; Russell and Gillespie, 1977)? Conventional light microscopy can be used to make such assessments; however, the likelihood of overlooking many inflammatory cells, especially macrophages, in tissue sections and the problem of subjectivity in making cell identifications based purely on morphologic criteria limit the usefulness of this approach. It may, therefore, be necessary to couple light microscopy with other techniques, such as immune hemadsorption (Tønder *et al.*, 1975; Russell *et al.*, this volume), histochemistry (Monis and Weinberg, 1961; Lauder *et al.*, 1977; Woods and Papadimitriou, 1977; Abraham and Barbolt, 1978), or fluorescence microscopy (Wood and Gollahon, 1978) before inflammatory cells can be localized accurately in tumors. To ensure representative sampling in all of these approaches, multiple sections taken from as many locations in the tumor as is practicable should be studied.

Necrosis in tumors usually can be identified grossly if it is extensive. These areas should be excised and discarded from the specimen that is taken for disaggregation. The residual "viable" tissue may additionally contain microscopic foci of necrosis. This is not a problem restricted to tumors with areas of grossly identifiable necrosis, as even small tumors that appear by eye to consist entirely of viable tissue may contain microscopic foci of necrosis. If the frequency of such necrotic foci is not appreciated, results of later analyses may be misinterpreted. For example, as will be seen in Section C.5, if necrosis is extensive estimation of percent recovery by DNA, analysis is likely to be spuriously low. An estimate of the extent of necrosis is also of value when considering whether or not a portion (or all) of the inflammatory cells recovered from a tumor could have been there because of nonspecific reaction against dead tissue.

C. Tumor Disaggregation

1. Obtaining a Representative Sample

Because inflammatory cells may be distributed uniformly throughout tumors (Russell and Gillespie, 1977) the taking of tissue for disaggregation from a single area in a neoplasm may seriously bias results. Ideally, all grossly viable tissue should be processed. If it is not practicable to do so because of the size of a tumor, the largest amount of neoplasm that can be handled, consisting of portions from many different sites, should be minced. After fragments are well mixed, a representative sample can be taken for disaggregation.

2. Mechanical vs. Enzymatic Means of Tumor Disaggregation

At this point the investigator must decide whether to disperse a tumor mechanically or by enzymatic digestion. Each approach has advantages, and it is clear that each type of neoplasm must be considered as a separate entity in making this choice. For these reasons it is impossible to generalize, and one must usually make the determination of which approach to use by trying each of them in pilot studies. There are some important general points to remember, however. For example, the most important source of damage to cells during tissue disaggregation is mechanical injury (Rinaldini, 1958; Boeryd et al., 1965; Wiepjes and Prop, 1970; Russell et al., 1976). Enzymatic approaches to disaggregation generally are the most efficient, therefore, because they minimize mechanical trauma. The result is usually higher cell recoveries than can be expected from purely mechanical means. The enhanced disaggregation efficiency obtainable with enzymes must be weighed, however, against possible alterations in intratumoral components that may be produced by them.

In studies of intratumoral immunoglobulin the choice of a mechanical approach to disaggregation is particularly apropos because most proteolytic enzymes will cause some degradation of these proteins. As a consequence, the specific binding activity of antibody that is recovered may be markedly reduced.

Many techniques have been used to disrupt tumors mechanically, including vigorous and repeated trituration of small fragments, grinding, homogenization, rubbing of fragments through wire mesh, etc. To my knowledge none of these has been accepted as best, and all tend to cause extensive cell injury. If proteolytic activity has the potential for affecting results adversely, it is advisable to include appropriate inhibitors during mechanical disaggregation procedures in order to inactivate proteases that are likely to be released from broken cells.

Enzymatic digestion is something of a misnomer because in almost all instances this approach includes a mechanical means of gently dispersing the cells from enzyme-treated fragments. The most common approach is to stir fragments in a solution containing enzymes. After cells have been well loosened in their stroma, the rate of disaggregation can sometimes be speeded if, in addition to stirring, fragments are gently run up and down at intervals in a plastic pipette that has been reamed out to enlarge the diameter of its bore.

While gentle, controlled mechanical force is needed to disperse the cells in enzyme-treated fragments, that which is present above this minimum level usually is harmful and, therefore, to be avoided as a potential cause of cell injury. Mechanical injury can be minimized in enzyme-based disaggregation procedures if conscious effort is made to avoid its sources. In our own work (Russell *et al.*, 1976) contributing sources have included, for example, crushing of cells during mincing of the tumor, either through use of a dull blade, by chopping rather than slicing the tissue, or by excessive mincing (we have found that fragments 2-3 mm in their greatest dimension are best); allowing the stirring bar in a digestion flask to rest on the bottom of the flask rather than having it suspended; and stirring for too long a time or at too great a speed (either of these presumably increases exposure of cells to shearing forces).

3. Choice of Enzymes for Use in Tumor Disaggregation

There is no single best choice of enzyme for use in tumor disaggregation and selection, therefore, should be based on trials of various enzymes, alone and in combination. Some generalizations are possible, however, and knowledge of these should speed the selection process.

If possible, the markers and functions that will be used in the study of recovered cells should be known before selection of enzymes is undertaken. Preservation of these properties to the greatest extent possible should be the principal consideration in seeking an enzyme mixture that is efficacious. If a given mixture is effective in all other regards, but damages properties of cells that are of interest, it has no utility and other combinations should be sought.

Mixtures of enzymes usually are more effective at disaggregating tissue than are single enzymes used alone. This usually is due to synergism between enzymes, the most relevant example of such interaction being the combination of collagenase and a number of other proteolytic enzymes that have broader substrate specificities (Russell *et al.*, 1976). When such synergism is found, the concentration of each of the interacting enzymes often can be reduced markedly without experiencing any loss in disaggregation efficiency.

Crudely purified enzymes, compared to those that have been highly refined, are not only much less expensive but are generally more effective in causing rapid disaggregation of tumors. Such increased efficiency of disaggregation is probably due to synergism between the principal enzymatic activity and various other activities that contaminate it. A complication that may attend the use of crudely purified enzymes is that different results may be obtained with the same enzyme provided by different suppliers (presumably because of differences in contaminating activities), or even batch-to-batch from the same supplier. For these reasons, if many tumor disaggregations are projected, purchase of large amounts (consistent with shelf life) of each enzyme in lots known to be efficacious from pilot studies is usually advisable.

It may be necessary to include DNase in the enzyme mixture used for disaggregation because, no matter how careful one is, some cell injury always will be sustained. Nucleic acid gels formed in the absence of DNase can be an important source of decreased cell recovery.

4. Minimizing the Effects of Enzymes on Cells Recovered from Tumors

In all cases where enzymes are used, the effects produced are dependent principally on the duration of exposure and the concentration of enzymes employed in the disaggregation mixture. Deleterious effects usually can be minimized if both enzyme concentration and time of exposure are decreased to the greatest degree that is consistent with maintaining disaggregation efficiency. Disaggregation efficiency is reflected by the slope of the cumulative cell yield plot (Russell *et al.*, 1976): the steeper the slope, the more efficient the disaggregation mixture. The ideal amount of enzyme is that which will give near maximum steepness of the slope, without any component of the mixture being in excess. Time of exposure can be shortened by the simple maneuver of harvesting supernates from digestion flasks at 20- to 30-min intervals. Fresh enzyme solution is added to the residual fragments after each harvest. Fetal bovine serum (FBS) can be added immediately to the harvested supernate, provided that it will not interfere with the performance or interpretation of later tests, in order to neutralize proteolytic activity. The cells are then removed by centrifugation. After resuspending the pellet in cold medium containing 10% FBS, the cells can be held on ice in polypropylene or siliconized glass tubes (the combination of cold and polypropylene or siliconization minimizes loss of adherent cells) until a pool of cells sufficient in size for that particular experiment is obtained.

5. Estimations of Cell Yield and Percent Recovery

When tumors are dispersed into individual cell suspensions by mechanical or enzymatic means, values for cell yield and percent recovery should be determined. These figures are of importance because they are the only means available by which one can assess and report the efficiency with which disaggregation was effected. The percentage of viable cells cannot be used for this purpose because proteolytic enzymes will remove dead and injured cells, thereby giving a misleadingly high level of viability in the final cell suspension.

Cell yield should be reported as cells obtained per gram of tumor. When possible, yield and percent recovery—the latter being the percentage of available cells that was actually recovered—should be reported together. Unfortunately, I am not aware of any method that will permit precise quantification of percent recovery from tumors. Percent recovery values must be regarded, therefore, as estimates. But they are essential estimates, for without them there is the potential for misinterpretation of results. For example, a tumor consisting of a great deal of fibrous connective tissue and few cells will give a figure for cell yield that is low, but in fact such a low number in this case may reflect an excellent percent recovery.

Two approaches to the estimation of percent cell recovery, and the difficulties inherent in each, will be discussed. The first of these is based on DNA recovery. Here, the amount of DNA in the final cell suspension is compared to the amount of DNA per weight of tumor fragments that was used to generate the cell suspension. This approach has been utilized in the analysis of normal tissue (Amsterdam and Jamieson, 1974) and of tumors (Russell *et al.*, 1976). In its application to tumors, the DNA approach suffers from inability to distinguish between DNA that is in viable cells and that which is contained in necrotic areas. This, coupled with inability to exclude microscopic foci of necrosis from fragments selected for disaggregation, tends to skew results toward overestimation of the DNA content of viable tumor material and, thus, toward underestimation of cell (DNA) recovery. The problem is compounded if dead cells are present within the cell suspension produced by dispersion of the tumor. This latter difficulty is circumvented if proteolytic enzymes and DNase are used to effect disaggregation.

The second approach, which is practicable only for tumors in experimental animals, is a modification of the procedure described by Boeryd *et al.* (1965) and depends on *in vivo* radiolabeling of the cells within a tumor. Radioactivity in recovered cells is compared to the amount that was contained in the tumor fragments that were used to produce the cell suspension. To avoid the problem of quenching, a gamma-emitting radioisotope can be used. The principal difficulty with this approach is that not all cells in the neoplasm will take up label, and those that do will do so at different rates and to different degrees. In view of these facts, should selective loss of one or more cell types occur during disaggregation, the results obtained will be biased according to the amount of radioactivity that was associated with the lost cell type(s).

6. *Establishing That Recovered Cells Reflect the Composition of the Intact Tumor*

The importance of verifying that a cell suspension is representative of the tumor from which it was derived, both in terms of cells types and their relative frequencies, cannot be overemphasized. Without such verification quantitative studies may be, at best, meaningless and, at worst, misleading and irreproducible. Technical problems that can contribute to the production of inaccuracy due to selective cell loss have been discussed (Kerbel *et al.*, 1975; Wood *et al.*, 1975; Pross and Kerbel, 1976; Russell *et al.*, 1976; K. Moore and Moore, 1977; Wood and Gollahon, 1977; Normann and Cornelius, 1978) and, therefore, will not be repeated here. Suffice it to say that avoidance of these sources of artifact is one important, indirect means of increasing the likelihood that cell suspensions are representative of the cellular composition of the intact tumor.

Continuing to refine the technique of tumor disaggregation until the highest possible values for cell yield and percent recovery are obtained on a consistent basis is a second, indirect means of helping to assure that cells of all types are recovered. While this is helpful it does not, of course, preclude the possibility of selective cell loss.

The only direct approach to estimating whether or not selective cell loss has occurred during disaggregation involves the microscopic counting of cells of an identifiable type in thinly cut sections of tumor. This figure, expressed as a percentage of total cells counted, can then be compared to the percentage of this same cell type in the suspension that is produced by disaggregation. Many nuclei must be counted in tissue sections, and the tumor must be sampled in many different locations before nuclear counts can be accepted as representative for the tumor. It will be readily apparent that this approach is not comprehensive, as it is clearly impossible to consider all cell types. However, evidence that one or more cell types are being recovered efficiently increases the likelihood that others in the tumor are not being lost to an inordinate degree in the course of disaggregation.

If counts are to be made using sections stained with hematoxylin and eosin, for several reasons the cell type of choice for counting (if present in sufficient numbers) is the polymorphonuclear leukocyte (PMN). Cells of this class can be identified with reasonable accuracy in thinly cut tissue sections because of the distinctive appearance of their nuclei. About the only danger here is in overlooking multilobed nuclei that have been cut in exact cross section, as these will be misinterpreted as small, nonlobed nuclei. Another reason to choose to count PMN is that, due to their relatively great fragility, these cells are a sensitive indicator of selective loss that may have occurred during tumor disaggregation. If it is not practicable to count PMN, one may have to resort to histochemistry or immunofluorescence to identify and count cells of another type accurately.

D. Selective Enrichment of Cell Types Recovered from Tumors

It is not within the scope of this section to discuss the many approaches that have been taken to the separation of the different kinds of cells that may be found in tumors. Instead, a few general points that are applicable to all such approaches will be made.

Cell yield and percent recovery, as well as the degree of purity, should be reported whenever crude cell suspensions are processed for the purpose of isolating a given cell type. Without such information it is impossible for the investigator to determine whether or not substantial loss of the cell type of interest was experienced during the separation procedure, with the possible introduction of selective bias into subsequent functional studies as a consequence. For example, when separations based on size are employed, only cells that are small or large may be recovered in a relatively pure state if cells of that particular type are polydisperse with regard to size. The others may be "lost" because they are grossly contaminated due to overlap with other cell types of similar size.

Anything that reduces the handling of cells *in vitro* will be likely to help preserve the functional activity of recovered cells. In a number of instances, particularly those that have involved the enrichment of intratumoral lymphocytes, we have had the experience of recovering what appeared to be viable lymphocytes, only to find that these cells were completely unable to mediate cytolytic activity *in vitro*. Gentler approaches to the purification of these cells preserved high levels of lytic activity.

With regard to characterizing functions of inflammatory cells isolated from tumors, testing of mixtures of selectivity enriched populations may be instructive and allow the demonstration of functions that otherwise would go unnoticed. In a similar vein, testing of Fc-receptor-bearing inflammatory cells with humoral immune components, i.e., immunoglobulin eluted from tumors or serum from tumor-bearing animals, may have the same result.

An especially important point that needs to be made in this section concerns the assay of antigen-specific killing mediated by effector cells that have been selectively enriched from tumors. Here, the problem of cold target inhibition can be a great one. Even a small level, i.e., 1 or 2%, of contamination by tumor cells co-purified with effector cells will interfere markedly with results obtained. Similarly, when tumor cells isolated from a neoplasm are employed as targets in killing assays rather than cells of established tissue culture lines, it must be ensured that the population used is truly a neoplastic one. Normal stromal cells that also are in the tumor can grossly contaminate such preparations. A marker of some sort that will allow specific identification of tumor cells is essential if one is to be certain that this potential source of error has been excluded.

E. Concluding Remarks

Components of the immune system that will either retard or enhance the growth of a given tumor will most likely be localized and concentrated within that neoplasm. To gain a better understanding of such intratumoral host–tumor cell interactions the various components involved must be separated and subjected to critical examination. Analyses of this kind performed to date have unquestionably shown the feasibility of this approach and have begun to contribute a new dimension to our understanding of the biology of cancer. As will be seen from reading the rest of this monograph, the potential for gain from the study of *in situ* expressions of antitumor immunity is clearly there and can only increase as the technical problems and uncertainties described in this brief chapter are overcome. Let me, therefore, encourage those of you who may be considering this area of research and invite your critical participation in this promising new branch of tumor immunology.

ACKNOWLEDGMENTS

The participants in the International Cancer Research Workshop on In-Situ Expressions of Anti-Tumor Immunity are thanked for critically discussing this topic during the course of their meeting. In particular, appreciation is expressed to those who also offered criticism of the manuscript during its preparation, including Drs. Robert Evans, Ronald B. Herberman, Harry L. Ioachim, Robert S. Kerbel, H. Robson MacDonald, Keith Moore, Thomas G. Pretlow, II, Maya Ran, Olav Tønder, Sabine von Kleist, and Isaac P. Witz. It should be understood that despite this "group effort," responsibility for any omissions or inaccuracies rests solely with the author. Preparation of this manuscript was supported, in part, by United States Public Health Service Research Grant CA23686 and Research Career Development Award CA00497.

II. THE BIOLOGICAL SIGNIFICANCE OF TUMOR-ASSOCIATED IMMUME COMPONENTS

A. Review

There are several categories of questions related to the biological significance of tumor-associated immune components. Although some studies published in this volume provide partial answers to these questions, this volume by and large offers no comprehensive answer to any of them.

One set of questions concerns the selectivity of the tumor localizing components and their functional specificity. This question can be dealt with at several levels.

Can one identify cellular or humoral components that are selectively present within autochthonous or syngeneic tumors but not within the site of allografts or within a lesion of a benign inflammation? Alternatively, can one recognize any elements normally present within the site of inflammation or allografts but selectively excluded from tumor sites? Studies pertaining to this and other related questions were reviewed recently by Haskill *et al.* (1978). From this review and from the studies of Evans, Herberman, Klein, Russell, Moore, Berke, and their co-workers (this volume) it seems that the major cellular elements known to be present in inflammation and allograft sites are also identifiable in primary and in syngeneically transplanted tumors. Important differences between these benign and malignant sites may exist, nonetheless.

Selective qualitative or quantitative inclusion or exclusion of immune components in the tumor compartment can also be approached by comparing the distribution of a certain component in distant locations and in close physical association with the tumor cells. It seems that most types of cellular immune components are qualitatively represented within tumors (Evans, 1977). However, there are several reports on the selective quantitative localization of certain immunocytes within human and experimental tumors compared to the distribution of the same immunocytes in the blood or in lymphatic tissues such as the spleen. For instance, Fc-receptor-positive cells comprise the major population of some murine tumor-infiltrating immunocytes whereas in the spleen they are represented in smaller percentages (Haskill *et al.*, 1975; Kerbel and Pross, 1976). The results of Klein and co-workers (this volume) indicate that in some types of cancer in man the proportion of T cells in the tumor-infiltrating lymphocyte population exceeds that of T cells in the circulating lymphocyte population. A similar situation may exist with humoral immunity. A selective localization of some immunoglobulin classes or subclasses was reported in several cases (Witz, 1977). Similarly, antibodies not readily detectable in the circulation were found to bind *in vivo* to tumor cells. Jacquemin *et al.* (1978) showed that peripheral leukocytes of acute or of chronic myelogenous leukemia patients at blast crisis were coated with IgG antibodies that neutralized the catalytic activity of reverse transcriptase from certain retroviruses. A similar antibody could not be detected in the circulation of such patients. Ran *et al.* (1978, and this volume) demonstrated a selective binding, in some tumor bearers, of lymphocytotoxic antibodies onto cells residing in the tumor. Similar antibodies were hardly detected in the serum.

Differences in the functional state of peripheral immune components and tumor-associated ones were also indicated. Klein and co-workers (this volume) presented data suggesting that some tumor-infiltrating lymphocytes, in contrast to those derived from blood, were in the activated state. Antibody-dependent cellular cytotoxicity (ADCC) mediated by tumor-seeking K cells was higher than ADCC medicated by splenocytes (Tracey *et al.*, 1975). Immune complex binding capacity of tumor-infiltrating immunocytes was higher than that of splenocytes (Braslawsky *et al.*, 1976). Moav and Witz (1978) reported that tumor-associated antitumor antibodies show a significantly higher binding constant to the corresponding syngeneic mouse tumor cells than circulating antibodies. The former antibodies were also appreciably more efficient in mediating complement-dependent lysis. These few examples demonstrate that the tumor compartment may contain a different representation of immune effector components than that in lymphatic tissues or in blood.

Another important aspect of selectivity of tumor localization of immune components is the expression of a distinct and reproducible disease-associated pattern of intratumor localization of immune components. Ioachim *et al.* (1976, and this volume) made the important observation that different histologic types of lung carcinoma had different but characteristic patterns of immunocyte infiltration both in terms of quantities of immunocytes that invaded the tumor tissue and in terms of the immunocyte class involved.

The target specificity of tumor-associated immune components is an important question approached by several of the contributors to this volume. Although this question remains largely open it is not unlikely that a certain proportion of these components, varying from tumor to tumor, has no apparent specificity toward known tumor-associated determinants (e.g., Braslawsky *et al.*, 1976). Identifying the target specificities of tumor-associated immune components requires a substantially increased effort by all of those working in local tumor immunity since the importance of this issue reaches far beyond the problem of tumor–host relations.

Another category of questions concerns the direct or indirect roles played by tumor-associated immune components in resistance to tumor growth or as direct stimulators of tumor progression, propagation, and spread (Prehn, 1977). The fact that tumor-associated immune components express *in vitro* antitumor effector functions has been known for some time (Haskill *et al.*, 1978; Witz, 1977). This and the question of whether they are more or less efficient than those derived from lymphatic organs or from blood was dealt with by many contributors to this volume. *In vivo* experiments are rather scarce, however, and the need for additional *in vivo* studies can hardly be overemphasized.

Obviously it would be of utmost importance to find out whether or not tumor-seeking naturally occurring immune mechanisms are involved in reactivity directed against nascent tumor cells. One approach to this problem is to answer the question of whether or not naturally occurring immune effectors such as natural killer (NK) cells are detectable within growing neoplasms. Although such effectors were shown within murine sarcoma virus (MSV)-induced mouse tumors or rat tumors (Becker and Klein, 1977; Herberman *et al.*, this volume; M. Moore and Moore, this volume) the notable absence of such cells from human tumors was noted (Vose *et al.*, 1977; Klein *et al.*, this volume; Herberman *et al.*, this volume). The work of Wolosin and Greenberg (1979) demonstrating the rapid uptake of naturally occurring antibodies by implanted tumor cells suggests that naturally occurring immune effectors may recognize antigenic determinants on tumor cells and thus be involved in antitumor reactivities right from the onset of tumor progression. If this were indeed the case, what then is the reason for the ultimate failure of these immume components? It seems, inevitably, that the search for "escape mechanisms" focusing on tumor-associated immune components may commence soon.

Do some of the tumor-associated immune components act as adversaries to the tumor-bearing host or as direct stimulators of tumor progression as suggested by Prehn (1977) and shown by Evans (this volume) or by Mantovani (1978)? Can specific or nonspecific suppressor cells be detected within tumors? Although some insight to this problem was provided by contributors to this volume, the problem remains, by and large, open. As to the role of tumor-associated antibodies as antagonists of antitumor resistance very little new data is available beyond the early reports of Sjögren *et al.* (1972), Bansal *et al.* (1972), Ran and Witz (1972), Izsak *et al.* (1974), and Vanky *et al.* (1975). An antihost reactivity mediated by tumor-associated antibodies which might indirectly enhance tumor growth was demonstrated by Ran *et al.* (1978, and this volume). These authors reported on the occurrence of lymphocytotoxic autoantibodies in tumor bearers and on the localization of such antibodies on tumor cell populations.

It seems that both antitumor effector functions as well as immune suppressive activities reside in tumors. What are the mechanisms controlling the influx of these factors into the tumor? Is the antigenicity of the tumor cells a contributing factor in this respect? These questions are approached by Evans, by Ioachim, and by Moore and Moore in this volume.

Do immune components infiltrating the site of the primary local tumor influence metastasis formation? Some information on correlation between the contents of intratumor macrophages and metastasis is available (Eccles and Alexander, 1974; Wood and Gillespie, 1975; Mantovani, 1978), but very little is known about such a relationship regarding lymphocytes (Kerbel, this volume) and no published data exist concerning a possible relationship between tumor-associated antibodies and metastasis formation. Early immune–histopathological data, most of which were provided by Black and his colleagues (e.g., Black and Leis, 1971) suggested rather strongly that immunocyte (mainly monocyte) infiltration into malignant tumors is positively related to favorable prognosis. It is very important that similar clinical studies also be performed with humoral components as the major correlative parameter.

Provided with information on correlations between the intratumor contents and functionality of immune components, the malignant (or benign) behavior of the tumor, and with knowledge and understanding of mechanisms controlling and regulating the traffic of immune components into and from the tumor, one could presumably attempt to manipulate the qualitative or quantitative representation of tumor-associated immune components for the benefit of the tumor-bearer. Immune modulators with known overall *in vivo* activities would be a convenient departure point for such endeavors. Relevant information on this aspect is contained in the contributions of Evans and of Hanna (this volume). Therapeutic trials using experimental systems and involving the passive or adoptive transfer of tumor-associated immune components into tumor-bearers should also be considered. Results of preliminary experiments involving the passive transfer of antitumor antibodies eluted from a mouse tumor showed a promising trend (Ran *et al.*, 1979).

B. Concluding Remarks

From this short review it is clear that very little direct and unambiguous evidence is actually available to show that the types, quantities, or functions of immune components residing within tumors or in the close vicinity of tumor cells have any positive or negative role in tumor growth. In fact, the possibility has not yet been completely ruled out that tumor-seeking immune components are random passengers or bystanders in this compartment. The vast majority of information has yet to be provided.

III. DIFFICULTIES AND SIGNIFICANCE OF CLINICAL STUDIES ON *IN SITU* TUMOR IMMUNITY

A. Introduction

Over the past 15 years, humoral and cell-mediated immunity against a variety of human tumors have been extensively studied (Herberman, 1977). Substantial evidence has been provided for immune reactivity of many cancer patients against tumor-associated antigens. However, the observed reactivity has not been clearly related to extent of disease or prognosis and there is at present no good support for the content:on that *in vitro* assays of tumor immunity reflect important events in resistance of the host against progressive tumor growth. One major problem has been that the immune responses to tumors are quite complex, with possible involvement by several different types of humoral and cell-mediated effector mechanisms. Even with a particular effector mechanism, there is considerable evidence for heterogeneity, with some reactions directed against tumor-associated antigens and others directed against normal tissue antigens or other antigens. In addition, normal individuals as well as cancer patients have been found to have cell-mediated and humoral reactivity with tumor materials and such natural immunity often needs to be distinguised from more restricted and tumor-associated reactivity of cancer patients.

Most studies of clinical tumor immunology have been done with sera or peripheral blood mononuclear cells. One possible solution to some of the complexities mentioned above is to focus attention on the immune components which are present at the site of tumor growth. One would anticipate that the host cells and humoral factors in the tumor would reflect some selection of reactive materials. Tumor-associated immune components might be concentrated *in situ* and less specific materials might be absent or at least in relatively low concentrations. Furthermore, the effector elements present within the tumor would be more likely candidates for having a role in resistance against tumor growth. Lymphoid cells and humoral factors which do not enter the tumor site might be irrelevant to host defenses against the tumor. Alternatively, inhibition of entry of effector elements into, or retention within, the tumor might be an important part of the usual failure of the immune response to reject tumors. Clues to such processes, with consequent studies on the mechanisms for observed differences, would only come from performing parallel studies on immune reactivity *in situ* and in the blood or other peripheral lymphoid cells. Therefore, the pertinent question does not seem to be whether studies on *in situ* immunity or on systemic immunity are more important or valid. Rather, *in situ* studies may be considered useful and valuable adjuncts to the usual clinical studies of tumor immunity and may bring us closer to an understanding of the role of the immune response in cancer patients.

Since a substantial amount of information has already been obtained on *in situ* tumor immunity in animal tumor systems, these may serve as helpful models for pursuing clinical studies along the same lines. However, it has been very difficult to overcome the special logistical and technical problems associated with human tumors, and progress in this area has been slow. Some laboratories are just now beginning to gather pertinent information and much more effort and ingenuity must be expended. In the following discussion, some of the major issues and available data concerning technical problems in performing studies on human tumors, the types of cells and humoral factors present, and their immunologic reactivities will be discussed.

B. Separation of Tumor Cells from Lymphoid Cells

For adequate enumeration and functional studies of lymphoid cells and neoplastic cells within the tumor mass, it is very important to be able to achieve rather complete separation of the populations. By various sedimentation procedures on gradients, it is frequently possible to achieve good separation of lymphocytes from most of the tumor cells and macrophages. However, a major problem has been to adequately separate macrophages from tumor cells, since they are usually overlapping in size and have other similar properties. At best, by gradient separations, one can get fractions relatively enriched for one population or the other. Other possible methods for separation may be considered and the feasibility of each approach needs to be studied more extensively.

1. *Adherence*. A substantial proportion of macrophages adhere rapidly and firmly to plastic or glass, and this should allow such cells to be separated from most tumor cells, which tend to take longer to adhere well. However, this procedure would not be likely to deplete most of the macrophages from a tumor cell suspension, since some macrophages are only weakly adherent.

2. *Fc Receptors*. It is clear that most macrophages have receptors for the Fc portion of IgG (FcR). With the exception of some lymphomas, tumor cells either have no detectable Fc receptors or have low affinity receptors, detectable only by special techniques (see Tϕnder, this volume). The observations of some FcR on some freshly harvested tumor cells may in fact be attributable to binding to tumor cells of FcR shed from host lymphoid cells, since cultured tumor cells have been found to be consistently devoid of FcR. In any event, the Fc receptors on macrophages are clearly much more avid than those on tumor cells and this should provide a useful separation procedure.

C. Types of Lymphoid Cells in Human Tumors

Information in this area is scanty and there is a need for more careful enumeration of the various subpopulations of host lymphoid cells. It is becoming increasingly clear to investigators in this field that most of the available studies are inadequate, having relied on assessment of histologic sections of tumors. For reasons that are not entirely clear, some types of infiltrating cells, particularly macrophages, seem to be underestimated on conventionally prepared slides. Therefore, it will be important to perform more detailed studies on suspensions of cells isolated from human tumors after disaggregation and harvesting by procedures most likely to give optimal yields of cells (see Section I). Drs. G. Cannon and J. Gerson have noted that suspensions of cells from many carcinomas of the lung, breast, or colon contain 10-20% macrophages. There is also insufficient documentation of the proportions of T cells and B cells in carcinomas and other human tumors. It has been relatively straightforward to perform studies on malignant effusions since the cells are already in suspension. In one such study, high proportions of T cells were detected (Djeu *et al.*, 1976). The proportion of cells forming high-affinity rosettes with sheep erythrocytes was frequently higher than that in the peripheral blood of the same patients. Ioachim is one of the few investigators to note considerable numbers of B cells in lung cancers and some other tumors (see Ioachim, this volume).

D. Functional Activities of Immune Factors in Tumors

Overall, information in this important area is inadequate and fragmentary. Only some of the recent data on various types of functional activities and some of the major gaps in our knowledge will be identified and described.

In regard to lymphocytes, it is of particular interest to assess the possible antitumor reactivities of these cells. Several investigators (e.g., Klein, this volume) have noted that some *in situ* lymphocytes can form rosettes or conjugates with tumor cells, suggesting that they may have receptors for antigens or other surface structures on tumor cells. This is supported by a few observations of cytotoxic reactivity against tumor cells by tumor lymphocytes (e.g., Klein, this volume, reports on the infrequent occurrence of cytotoxicity against autologous sarcomas and lung cancers). It is unclear why it has been quite difficult to detect cytotoxic reactivity by lymphocytes in most human tumors. One possible explanation relates to the techniques usually employed for isolation of the lymphocytes and for measuring cytotoxic activity. Exposure of the cells to proteolytic enzymes may lead to their inactivation, which may not be readily reversible by *in vitro* incubation. Contamination of the lymphoid cell preparations by an appreciable number of tumor cells could easily obviate detection of cytotoxicity against radiolabeled tumor cells, since the unlabeled tumor cells could act as competitive inhibitors (Ortiz de Landazuri and Herberman, 1972). An additional major consideration is the target cells used for the cytotoxicity assays. It is unclear how much restriction of cytotoxic activity against human tumor cells by immune T cells is imposed by the major histocompatibility complex. If histocompatible target cells are required for optimal detection of immune T cell cytotoxicity, then assays should rely mainly on autologous tumor target cells rather than the more commonly employed and convenient allogeneic cell lines. In addition, any cytotoxicity by *in situ* lymphoid cells needs to be characterized in regard to the nature of the effector cells. Reactivity by NK cells within the tumor would present a particular problem since they do not have sufficiently characteristic cell surface properties to allow easy separation from immune T cells. Monitoring for NK cells by assays with K562 target cells, and attempts to deplete NK activity by removal of FcR-bearing cells, may not be adequate. There have been recent indications that some NK cells may react against other target cells but not K562 and these effector cells may be less likely to have detectable FcR (Bolhuis, 1977; Eremin *et al.*, 1978). To date, little or no NK activity has been detected in human tumors (see Klein *et al.* and Herberman *et al.*, this volume). However, only K562 has been used as target cells. It is also possible that immune T cells and/or NK cells are present within many human tumors but are not sufficiently activated or are inhibited by the presence of tumor cells or suppressor cells. Attempts to generate or augment cytotoxic reactivity of *in situ* lymphocytes seem warranted, as do efforts to eliminate potentially inhibitory or suppressive cells.

There is even less information available regarding other possible activities of *in situ* lymphocytes. Some preliminary studies of their proliferative responses to autologous tumor cells have been performed (see Klein *et al.*, this volume), but only infrequent and low levels of activity have been detected. There are virtually no data on lymphokine production (e.g., leukocyte inhibitory factor, macrophage migration inhibitory factor) by lymphocytes within human tumors.

In contrast to the many studies of the functions of macrophages within rodent tumors, comparable studies of human macrophages are virtually nonexistent. This can be attributed largely to the unavailability of assays for measuring cytotoxic or other activities of human macrophages. However, assays for cytostatic (Jerrels *et al.*, 1978) and cytolytic (Mantovani *et al.*, 1979) activities of human monocytes have recently been developed and these should be directly applicable to tumor-derived macrophages.

Recently increased attention has been directed toward immunoglobulins in human tumors or in effusions (see Iochim and von Kleist *et al.*, this volume). Of fundamental interest is whether some of the immunoglolubins attached to tumor cells or in fluids are antibodies directed against tumor-associated antigens. This is of particular concern in regard to IgG since much of this class of immunoglobulins could be brought in or trapped by infiltrating lymphoid cells bearing FcR.

E. Concluding Remarks

It should be apparent from the above discussion that there are many interesting and important questions regarding *in situ* immunity to human tumors which need to be adequately studied. We are just at the beginning of most of these studies and current knowledge is at best preliminary and inadequate. Since it is now technically and logistically possible to approach most of the major issues, and since attention has now been focused on this area, one would hope and anticipate that rapid progress will soon be made.

IV. REFERENCES

A. Problems (Technical and Interpretive) Associated with the Isolation of Immune Effector Cells from Tumors

Abraham, R., and Barbolt, T. A., 1978, Lysosomal enzymes in macrophages of colonic tumors induced in rats by 1,2-dimethylhydrazine dihydrochloride, *Cancer Res.* 38: 2763-2767.

Amsterdam, A., and Jamieson, J. D., 1974, Studies on dispersed pancreatic exocrine cells. I. Dissociation technique and morphologic characteristics of separated cells, *J. Cell Biol.* 63:1037-1056.

Boeryd, R., Eriksson, O., Knutson, F., Lundin, P. M., and Norrby, K., 1965, On the viability of tumour cells in artificially produced suspensions, *Acta Pathol. Microbiol. Scand.* **65**: 514-520.

Kerbel, R. S., Pross, H. F., and Elliott, E. V., 1975, Origin and partial characterization of Fc receptor-bearing cells found within experimental carcinomas and sarcomas, *Int. J. Cancer* **15**:918-932.

Lauder, I., Aherne, W., Stewart, J., and Sainsbury, R., 1977, Macrophage infiltration of breast tumours: A prospective study, *J. Clin. Pathol.* **30**:563-568.

Monis, B., and Weinberg, T., 1961, Cytochemical study of esterase activity of human neoplasms and stromal macrophages, *Cancer* **14**:369-377.

Moore, K., and Moore, M., 1977, Intra-tumour host cells of transplanted rat neoplasms of different immunogenicity, *Int. J. Cancer* **19**:803-813.

Normann, S. J., and Cornelius, J., 1978, Concurrent depression of tumor macrophage infiltration and systemic inflammation by progressive cancer growth, *Cancer Res.* **38**:3453-3459.

Pross, H. F., and Kerbel, R. S., 1976, An assessment of intratumor phagocytic and surface marker-bearing cells in a series of autochthonous and early passaged chemically induced murine sarcomas, *J. Natl. Cancer Inst.* **57**:1157-1167.

Rinaldini, L. M. J., 1958, The isolation of living cells from animal tissues, *Int. Rev. Cytol.* **7**:587-647.

Russell, S. W., and Gillespie, G. Y., 1977, Nature, function and distribution of inflammatory cells in regressing and progressing Moloney sarcomas, *J. Reticuloendothel. Soc.* **22**:159-168.

Russell, S. W., Doe, W. F., Hoskins, R. G., and Cochrane, C. G., 1976, Inflammatory cells in solid murine neoplasms. I. Tumor disaggregation and identification of constituent inflammatory cells, *Int. J. Cancer* **18**:322-330.

Tønder, O., Humphrey, L. J., and Morse, P. A., 1975, Further observations on Fc receptors in human malignant tissue and normal lymphoid tissue, *Cancer* **35**:580-587.

Wiepjes, F. G., and Prop, F. J. A., 1970, An improved method for preparation of single-cell suspensions from mammary glands of adult virgin mouse, *Exp. Cell Res.* **61**:451-454.

Witz, I. P., 1977, Tumor-bound immunoglobulins: *In situ* expressions of humoral immunity, *Adv. Cancer Res.* **25**:95-148.

Wood, G. W., and Gollahon, K. A., 1977, Detection and quantitation of macrophage infiltration into primary human tumors with the use of cell-surface markers, *J. Natl. Cancer Inst.* **59**:1081-1087.

Wood, G. W., and Gollahon, K. A., 1978, T-lymphocytes and macrophages in primary murine fibrosarcomas at different stages in their progression, *Cancer Res.* **38**:1857-1865.

Wood, G. W., Gillespie, G. Y., and Barth, R. F., 1975, Receptor sites for antigen-antibody complexes on cells derived from solid tumors: Detection by means of antibody sensitized sheep erythrocytes labeled with technetium-99m, *J. Immunol.* **114**:950-957.

Woods, A. E., and Papadimitriou, J. M., 1977, The effect of inflammatory stimuli on the stroma of neoplasms: The involvement of mononuclear phagocytes, *J. Pathol.* **123**:163-174.

B. The Biological Significance of Tumor-Associated Immune Components

Bansal, S. C., Hargreaves, R., and Sjögren, H. O., 1972, Facilitation of polyoma tumor growth in rats by blocking sera and tumor eluate, *Int. J. Cancer* **9**:97-108.

Becker, S., and Klein, E., 1977, Decreased natural killer effect in tumor-bearing mice and its relation to the immunity against oncorna virus determined cell surface antigens, *Eur. J. Immunol.* **6**:892-898.

Black, M. M., and Leis, H. P., 1971, Cellular responses to autologous breast cancer tissue. Correlation with stage and lymphoreticuloendothelial reactiveness, *Cancer* **28**:263-273.

Braslawsky, G. R., Yaakubowitcz, M., Frensdorff, A., and Witz, I. P., 1976, Receptors for immune complexes on cells within a non-lymphoid murine tumor, *J. Immunol.* **116**: 1571-1578.

Eccles, S., and Alexander, P., 1974, Macrophage content of tumors in relation to metastic spread and host immune reaction, *Nature (London)* **250**:667-669.

Evans, R., 1977, Macrophages in solid tumors, in: *The Macrophage and Cancer* (K. James, B. McBride, and A. Stuart, eds.), pp. 321-329, Econoprint, Edinburgh.

Haskill, J. S., Yamamura, Y., and Radov, L., 1975, Host responses within solid tumors: Non-thymus-derived specific cytotoxic cells within a murine mammary adenocarcinoma, *Int. J. Cancer* **16**:798-809.

Haskill, J. S., Häyry, P., and Radov, L. A., 1978, Systemic and local immunity in allograft and cancer rejection, in: *Contemporary Topics in Immunobiology*, Vol. 8 (N. L. Warner and M. D. Cooper, eds.), pp. 107-170, Plenum Press, New York.

Ioachim, H. L., Dorsett, B., and Paluch, E., 1976, The immune response at the tumor site in lung carcinoma, *Cancer* **38**:2296-2309.

Izsak, F. C., Brenner, H. J., Landes, E., Ran, M., and Witz, I. P., 1974, Correlation between clinico-pathological features of malignant tumors and cell surface immunoglobulins, *Isr. J. Med. Sci.* **10**:642-646.

Jacquemin, P. C., Saxinger, C., and Gallo, R. C., 1978, Surface antibodies of human my-elogenous leukemia leukocytes reactive with specific type-C viral reverse transcriptases, *Nature (London)* **276**:230-236.

Kerbel, R. S., and Pross, H. F., 1976, Fc receptor-bearing cells as a reliable marker for quantitation of host lymphoreticular infiltration of progressively growing solid tumors, *Int. J. Cancer* **18**:432-438.

Mantovani, A., 1978, Effects on *in vitro* tumor growth of murine macrophages isolated from sarcoma lines differing in immunogenicity and metastasizing capacity, *Int. J. Cancer* **22**: 741-746.

Moav, N., and Witz, I. P., 1978, Characterization of immunoglobulins eluted from murine tumor cells: Binding patterns of cytotoxic anti-tumor IgG, *J. Immunol. Meth.* **22**: 51-62.

Prehn, R. T., 1977, Immunostimulation of the lymphodependent phase of neoplastic growth, *J. Natl. Cancer Inst.* **59**:1043-1049.

Ran, M., and Witz, I. P., 1972, Tumor-associated immunoglobulins. Enhancement of syngeneic tumors by IgG$_2$-containing tumor eluates, *Int. J. Cancer* **9**:242-247.

Ran, M., Yaakubowicz, M., and Witz, I. P., 1978, Lymphocytotoxic auto antibodies eluted from *in vivo* propagating sarcoma cells of mice, *J. Natl. Cancer Inst.* **60**:1509-1513.

Ran, M., Yaakubowicz, M., and Witz, I. P., 1979, *In situ* expressions of humoral immunity within a polyoma-virus induced tumor, in: *Antiviral Mechanisms in the Control of Neoplasia* (P. Chandra, ed.), pp. 355-371, Plenum Press, New York.

Sjögren, H. O., Hellström, I., Bansal, S. C., Warner, G. A., and Hellström, K. E., 1972, Elution of "blocking factors" from human tumors, capable of abrogating tumor-cell destruction by specifically immune lymphocytes, *Int. J. Cancer* **9**:274-283.

Tracey, D. E., Pross, H. F., Jondal, M., and Witz, I. P., 1975, Antibody-dependent cell-mediated cytotoxic activity in syngeneic mouse ascites tumors, *Int. J. Cancer* **16**: 870-880.

Vánky, F., Trempe, G., Klein, E., and Stjernswärd, J., 1975, Human tumor-lymphocyte interaction *in vitro*: Blastogenesis correlated to detectable immunoglobulin in the biopsy, *Int. J. Cancer* **16**:113–124.

Vose, B. M., Vánky, F., Argov, S., and Klein, E., 1977, Natural cytotoxicity in man: Activity of lymph node and tumor infiltrating lymphocytes, *Eur. J. Immunol.* **7**:753–757.

Witz, I. P., 1977, Tumor-bound immunoglobulins: *In situ* expressions of humoral immunity, *Adv. Cancer Res.* **25**:95–148.

Wolosin, L. B., and Greenberg, A. H., 1979, Murine natural anti-tumor antibodies. I. Rapid *in vivo* binding of natural antibody by tumor cells in syngeneic mice, *Int. J. Cancer* **23**: 519–529.

Wood, G. W., and Gillespie, G. Y., 1975, Studies on the role of macrophages in regulation of growth and metastasis of murine chemically induced fibrosarcomas, *Int. J. Cancer* **16**: 1022–1029.

C. Difficulties and Significance of Clinical Studies on *in Situ* Tumor Immunity

Bolhuis, R. L. H., 1977, Cell-mediated immunity to carcinoma of the urinary bladder. Specificity of the reaction and the nature of the effector cells, Radiobiological Institute of the Organization for Health Research TNO, Fijawijk, The Netherlands, pp. 1–169.

Djeu, J. F., McCoy, J. L., Cannon, G. B., Reeves, W. J., West, W. H., and Herberman, R. B., 1976, Lymphocytes forming rosettes with sheep erythrocytes in metastatic pleural effusions, *J. Natl. Cancer Inst.* **56**:1051–1052.

Eremin, O., Coombs, R. R. A., Plumb, D., and Ashby, A., 1978, Characterization of the human natural killer (NK) cell in blood and lymphoid organs, *Int. J. Cancer* **21**:42–50.

Herberman, R. B., 1977, Existence of tumor immunity, in: *Mechanisms of Tumor Immunity* (S. Cohen and I. Green, eds), pp. 175–191, John Wiley & Sons, New York.

Jerrells, T. R., Dean, J. H., Richardson, G. L., McCoy, J. L., and Herberman, R. B., 1978, Role of suppressor cells in depression of in vitro lymphoproliferative responses of lung and breast cancer patients, *J. Natl. Cancer Inst.* **61**: 1001–1009.

Mantovani, A., Jerrells, T. R., Dean, J. H., and Herberman, R. B., 1979, Cytolytic and cytostatic activity of tumor cells of circulating human monocytes, *Int. J. Cancer* **23**:18–27.

Ortiz de Landazuri, M., and Herberman, R. B., 1972, Specificity of cellular immune reactivity to virus-induced tumors, *Nature (London) New Biol.* **238**:18–19.

Chapter 2

Separation of Individual Kinds of Cells from Tumors

Thomas G. Pretlow II and Theresa P. Pretlow

Department of Pathology
University of Alabama in Birmingham
Birmingham, Alabama 35294

I. INTRODUCTION

Cancers are composed of malignant cells and many different kinds of stromal and infiltrating host cells. In the past, the biochemical investigation of cancers has been based predominately upon the analysis of homogenates of whole tumors. The biochemical characterization of malignant cells from tumors would be facilitated if methods could be developed for the purification of malignant cells from tumors to be studied. Similarly, study of the host's infiltrating cells would be greatly facilitated by the development of methods for the purification of host cells from cancers. The culture of malignant cells from solid tumors has often been complicated by overgrowth of the malignant cells by host fibroblasts (Chaudhuri *et al.*, 1974; Feller *et al.*, 1972; Halpern *et al.*, 1975; Herberman and Oldham, 1975; Lasfargues *et al.*, 1972; Mavligit *et al.*, 1975); presumably, this difficulty could be circumvented by the culture of malignant cells purified from tumors. Since 1969 (T. G. Pretlow and Boone, 1969), our laboratory has been interested in the development of methods for the purification of single kinds of cells from cancers. While we have had some experience in the separation of individual kinds of cells from transplantable tumors of experimental animals (T. G. Pretlow and Boone, 1970; Stewart *et al.*, 1972; Zettergren *et al.*, 1973; T. P. Pretlow *et al.*, 1977a,b), there are several aspects of transplantable tumors which make their separation a much easier problem than the purification of cells from primary autochthonous tumors. In this review, we shall emphasize the purification of cells from autochthonous tumors. In addition, we shall emphasize work with human tumors. Rather than review the purification of cells from tumors in general, we shall focus on those techniques that are currently used in our laboratory, i.e., sedimentation and electrophoresis.

II. COMPOSITION OF TUMORS

While methods for the quantitative morphometric analysis of tissues have been available for many years (Chalkley, 1943; Weibel, 1963; Weibel et al., 1966), there have been surprisingly few quantitative morphometric studies of tumors. The absence of such quantitative studies is all the more surprising in view of the fact that pathologists have, for decades, expressed their subjective and semiquantitative opinions that specific kinds of lymphoid infiltrates influence the prognosis for some kinds of tumors (Black et al., 1955; Berg, 1959). Among human tumors, bronchogenic carcinoma is one of the few cancers which has been the object of quantitative morphometric studies (Gerstl et al., 1974, 1976). Ioachim has observed that the abundance of plasma cells in bronchogenic carcinomas is related both to the histologic type and to the degree of differentiation of these tumors (Ioachim et al., 1976). He has emphasized the potentially biologically different meanings associated with inflammatory infiltrates (1) surrounding tumors, (2) in bands of stroma separating cords of tumor cells, and (3) actually in the cords of tumor cells or in the malignant cells themselves. Ioachim (1976) has observed differences between primary human cancers and their metastases with respect to the quantity and quality of inflammatory infiltrates. These differences between primary and metastatic tumors have not often been emphasized and seem of particular importance since the therapy of cancer initially must depend upon the characterization of the primary tumor in most instances. Underwood (1974) reviewed 38 articles which attempted to correlate the prognoses of specific kinds of cancers with the quantity and quality of infiltrating inflammatory cells; in most instances, a relationship was reported to exist between prognosis and the nature of inflammatory infiltrates. Underwood (1972) was one of the first to attempt the morphometric analysis of human tumors.

Among the limited numbers of studies addressed to the morphometry of human tumors, some have been concerned with only limited aspects of the morphometry of tumors, i.e., the ratio of nucleus to cytoplasm, the proportion of fibrous tissue in the tumor, etc. It has been our impression in working with several human tumors that even tumors which lack prominent inflammatory infiltrates contain many inflammatory cells. One is often surprised by the large proportion of plasma cells, lymphocytes, macrophages, and granulocytes which are found in suspensions of cells from tumors which lack obvious inflammatory infiltrates when examined in 5-μm sections stained with hematoxylin and eosin.

This discrepancy, which we have noted to be especially prominent in human colonic carcinomas (Brattain *et al.*, 1977a,b), may result from the selective destruction of malignant cells during the disaggregation of human solid tumors. There may be an increased proportion of inflammatory cells in these suspensions because they survive the procedures which are used for obtaining cells in suspension. This possibility cannot be critically evaluated in the absence of morphometric data. Another possible explanation for this discrepancy lies in the fact that malignant cells are often larger than inflammatory cells. Large, darkly staining tumor cells may obscure smaller inflammatory cells.

We were interested to learn (H. R. MacDonald, personal communication) that tumor spheroids in syngeneic animals often yield large proportions of inflammatory cells after trypsinization even when histologic examination of these spheroids does not suggest a prominent infiltration by inflammatory cells. It seems unlikely that the malignant cells of transplantable spheroids which are trypsinized generation after generation are more susceptible to destruction by trypsin than the host inflammatory cells which have not been the object of selection by trypsinization. In our opinion, pathologists naturally underestimate the number of inflammatory cells in tumors probably in part because their training emphasizes the assessment and characterization of the malignant cells in cancers.

III. DISPERSAL OF TUMORS

Before one can attempt to purify individual kinds of cells, it is necesssary to evaluate the various available methods for obtaining cells in suspension. Shortman (1972) has emphasized the importance of obtaining suspensions of predominately single cells with minimal aggregates, red blood cells, debris, and other unwanted material. In selecting methods for the dispersal of a particular kind of tumor into suspensions of single cells, it is important to evaluate critically the consequences of the disaggregation process selected; the potential significance of investigations of suspensions of cells will be dependent upon the degree to which the cells which were obtained in suspension are truly representative of the intact tissue. Most of the available methods for obtaining suspensions of cells result in a less than quantitative yield of the cells available in tissues. The destruction and modification of cells secondary to the techniques utilized for obtaining them in suspension constitute an important variable in most such experiments. Too often, investigators focus on the functions of the cells that were obtained in suspension without giving serious consideration to the possibility that the functions of the suspended cells may not be representative of the functions of the corresponding types of cells in tissues. Suspended cells may fail to be representative of the corresponding types of cells in tissues either because of selective destruction of subpopulations of cells or because of modification of function consequent to the techniques employed for obtaining the cells in suspension.

It seems important to emphasize the common observation that different normal tissues and different tumors require different techniques. If tissues are to be obtained as suspensions of cells with high yields, age, species, and the type of tissue under study are all significant variables in the selection of techniques for obtaining cells in suspension. For example, we found that Pronase was more effective than collagenase or trypsin for obtaining *hamster* kidney cells in suspension (T. G. Pretlow *et al.*, 1974); on the other hand, trypsin was more effective than collagenase or Pronase for obtaining rat kidney cells in suspension (Kreisberg *et al.*, 1977*a*). In selecting a technique for obtaining cells in suspension from a particular tissue, one should consider the number of cells obtained per gram of tissue and the abilities of the cells obtained in suspension to exhibit specific functions. As a minimum, it seems important to report the number of cells obtained per gram of tissue and the proportion of cells which exclude trypan blue. On many occasions, we have found that additional data are required. For example, in work with the human tonsil (Willson *et al.*, 1976*b*), we found that trypsin and collagenase used in parallel gave us approximately equivalent yields of cells. In addition, whether trypsin or collagenase was used, similar proportions of cells excluded trypan blue. We obtained smaller numbers of cells when tonsils were obtained in suspension by purely mechanical techniques (mincing, teasing, etc.). If we had calculated only the number of cells obtained per gram of tissue and had observed only trypan blue as a measure of viability, we would have concluded (Willson *et al.*, 1976*b*) that trypsin and collagenase were approximately equally suited for work with human tonsil. Further study showed that cells obtained in suspension with collagenase incorporated only approximately one-half as much tritiated thymidine when stimulated with phytohemagglutinin, concanavalin A, or pokeweed mitogen as cells obtained in suspension with trypsin. Cells obtained in suspension mechanically exhibited an even lower response to mitogens than tonsillar cells obtained in suspension with collagenase. Despite the fact that we obtained approximately similar numbers of cells per gram of tonsil and an approximately similar proportion of cells that excluded trypan blue with trypsin or with collagenase, we obtained a very different frequency of different cell types in suspension with these two enzymes. Specifically, we obtained 394 ± 131 million cells per gram of tonsil with trypsin and 334 ± 131 million cells per gram of tonsil with collagenase. From the same three tonsils, $98 \pm 0.6\%$ of the cells obtained in suspension with trypsin excluded trypan blue and $96 \pm 1.5\%$ of the cells obtained in suspension with collagenase excluded trypan blue. As an example of the different frequencies of different cell types obtained in suspension with these two agents, we obtained $6.5 \pm 2.3\%$ plasma cells in our suspensions of trypsinized tonsils and less than 1% plasma cells in the suspensions obtained with collagenase.

In addition to the well known differences between different kinds of enzymes, it is important to emphasize the fact that different batches of particular enzymes may exhibit marked differences in their suitabilities for work with a particular tissue. In the case of trypsin, for example, it is widely acknowledged that batches of crude trypsin may be more effective than twice-crystallized trypsin for the dissociation of some tissues and that adulterating enzymes in the batches of trypsin may be responsible for the desired activity. Numerous investigators have noted marked differences among batches of trypsin (Heisto et al., 1971; Pine et al., 1969; Speicher and McCarl, 1974). In our own laboratory, we (Willson et al., 1976a) found that different batches of trypsin differed almost 10-fold with respect to the yield of cells that we could obtain per gram of human tonsil. The suitability of a particular batch of trypsin for work with the tonsil was not related to the assayed specific activity for trypsin. In addition to the marked differences in the number of cells that could be obtained per gram of tonsil, there were additional marked differences in the proportion of plasma cells obtained with different batches of trypsin. Differences in different batches of collagenase have been reported by other laboratories (Hilfer and B. Jwn, 1971; Kono, 1969; Kloppenborg et al., 1968), and we found marked differences among batches of collagenase with respect to their suitability for obtaining cells in suspension from myocardium (T. G. Pretlow et al., 1972). We have observed similar differences among batches of Pronase (T. G. Pretlow et al., unreported data). It might be helpful to note that we have found Pronase obtained from a particular supplier (EM Laboratories, Elmsford, NY) very consistent from batch to batch.

The various techniques which are available for obtaining cells in suspension have been reviewed comprehensively recently (T. G. Pretlow et al., 1975; Waymouth, 1974). Because of the extensive reviews which are available, we shall not treat these methods in detail here. The methods that are available may be broadly subsumed under three main categories: mechanical, enzymatic, and those which employ chelating agents. While mechanical methods for obtaining cells in suspension work well when the tissues are mouse lymphoid tissues and some other experimental rodent tissues, we are not aware of any published papers that report high yields of cells from human tumors obtained in suspension by purely mechanical methods. In our hands, human tumors have been consistently more effectively dissociated by treatment with enzymes than by mincing, teasing, sieving, the use of tissue presses, etc. Despite the paucity of work with human tumors in the literature, there are several published articles from different laboratories that confirm the general experience that human tumors are not obtained in suspension effectively by mechanical methods; these methods generally give suspensions with fewer than 50% viable cells (Mavligit et al., 1973, 1975; Wepsic, 1970; Nairn et al., 1971). Some investigators have had similar experience with tumors from experimental animals (Vaage, 1968). Similarly, in our purification of cells from Hodgkin's disease (T. G. Pretlow *et al.*, 1973; Willson *et al.*, 1977; McGuire *et al.*, 1979), prostatic carcinoma (Helms *et al.*, 1976), and colonic carcinoma (Brattain *et al.*, 1977*a,b*), we found in preliminary studies that mechanical methods were much less effective than the use of enzymes for the dissociation of these human tumors into suspensions of single cells.

Before leaving the discussion of methods for obtaining cells in suspension from human tumors, we should comment briefly on the use of DNase. DNase has been used alone or in combination with other enzymes to obtain cells in suspension from a variety of transplantable tumors in experimental animals (Carney and Malmgren, 1967; Knutson *et al.*, 1971; Norrby *et al.*, 1966; Oppenheimer and Humphreys, 1971). While DNase is undoubtedly useful for dispersing the gels that are often encountered in the dissociation of tissues, we should emphasize our experience that many of the gels obtained in the dissociation of human tumors are not dispersed by DNase. In our investigations of various methods to obtain cells in suspension from the tumor of Hodgkin's disease, prostatic carcinoma, and colonic carcinoma, we found that the addition of DNase to the digestion mixture did not result in either improved yield or improved viability. In the final analysis, it is necessary to compare the available enzymes with each new kind of tumor to be investigated.

Some have opposed the use of proteolytic enzymes to obtain cells in suspension because of possible alterations in the surfaces of cells treated with enzymes. Such changes undoubtedly occur. There have been many studies of altered antigenicity and/or electrophoretic mobilities of cells after treatment with proteolytic enzymes (Simon-Reuss *et al.*, 1964; Hayry *et al.*, 1965; Vaage, 1968; Fayet *et al.*, 1970; Hommes *et al.*, 1970; Maslow, 1970; Schlesinger and Gottesfeld, 1971; Gibofsky and Terasaki, 1972; Rosenberg and Rogentine, 1972; Wallach and Esandi, 1964; Bosmann *et al.*, 1973; Weiss and Horoszewicz, 1971; Vassar, 1963; Vassar *et al.*, 1973; Woo and Cater, 1972; Seaman and Uhlenbruck, 1963; Wiig, 1974; Weiss *et al.*, 1972). In deciding whether to use proteolytic enzymes or mechanical methods, one must balance the advantages to be obtained from a much larger yield of cells from human tumors with enzymatic methods against the alterations in cell surface which are often associated with the use of proteolytic enzymes. Many alterations of cell surfaces by proteolytic enzymes are reversible. Turner *et al.* (1972) observed that most of the HL-A2 removed by digestion with papain was regenerated within 6 h *in vitro*. Hughes *et al.* (1972) reported the regeneration of surface components digested from ascites tumor cells with neuraminidase. Several laboratories (Kono and Barham, 1971; Soderman *et al.*, 1973; Shafie *et al.*, 1977) have reported the regeneration of insulin receptors removed from cell membranes with trypsin after only 90 min *in vitro* in the presence of soybean trypsin inhibitor. McClay *et al.* (1977) reported the regeneration of "trypsin-sensitive cell-surface components" of embryonic neural retina cells after 4–5 h in culture. Thompson *et al.* (1976) found that antigens on most mammary epithelial cells were removed by trypsinization but regenerated in culture. In our own laboratory, we (Willson *et al.*, 1976b) observed the regeneration of sheep red blood cell receptors on human tonsillar lymphocytes after culture for 20 h following trypsinization. In summary, while treatment of cells with proteolytic enzymes is undoubtedly injurious in some instances, this injury is often able to be repaired after brief periods of culture.

IV. SEPARATION OF CELLS

In our discussion of the available methods for the purification of cells from tumors, we shall emphasize the methods with which we are most familiar, i.e., electrophoresis and sedimentation.

A. Electrophoresis of Cells

In 1902, Dr. Ralph S. Lillie (1902) described the movement of isolated nuclei, leukocytes, muscle cells, and red blood cells in an electric field in an isotonic solution of cane sugar as viewed through a microscope. Among his several observations, he noted that "The resistance of the sugar-solution is very high and only a slight current passes . . ." As discussed in Section IV.A.1, more than half a century later, the development of electrophoretic buffers of low conductivity that are made isosmolar with saccharides has become an important innovation in the modern electrophoresis of cells. Two years later, Girard-Mangin and Henri (1904) described somewhat similar experiments in the electrophoresis of cells in Europe.

The long history of the electrophoresis of cells is reviewed in the symposium edited by Ambrose (1965) and subsequently by us (T. G. Pretlow *et al.*, 1975). Despite its venerable antiquity, cell electrophoresis was not used extensively for the preparative purification of viable cells until the 1970s. During the first half-century of cell electrophoresis, investigators were preoccupied with such concerns as the design of apparatus, the construction of model systems, the electrophoresis of red blood cells, and alterations of electrophoretic mobility following the exposure of cells to lytic enzymes. In the 1970s, the techniques, apparatus, and buffers of Hannig and Zeiller (Hannig, 1972) were applied to a variety of problems in cell separation and demonstrated the utility of the electrophoresis of cells for the separation of large numbers (10^8–10^9 cells/h) of viable cells for biochemical and biological investigations. The theory and applications of cell electrophoresis have been reviewed elsewhere by us (T. G. Pretlow *et al.*, 1975), and we shall simply touch on the relevant aspects of cell electrophoresis here.

1. Medium for Electrophoresis

Much has been written about the effect of the medium selected for the electrophoresis of cells on the electrophoretic mobility of cells. The mobilities of cells are affected by many properties of the medium, including ionic strength, dielectric constant, temperature, viscosity, pH, and the ability of the medium to maintain cell viability (Weiss, 1966; Zeiller et al., 1975a; Mehrishi and Thomson, 1968). Several investigators have emphasized changes in the electrophoretic mobilities of cells associated with the death of cells (Leise and LeSane, 1974; Carstensen et al., 1968; Weiss, 1966). Hannig (1971) reviewed the properties that are desirable for media to be used for specific problems in electrophoresis and reviewed the several kinds of media that have been employed for specific problems. Hannig (1972) has pointed out that "In the electrophoretic separation of particle suspensions (cells and cell organelles), the ionic strength of the particles plays a minor role owing to their relatively small surface charge . . ." and that "A higher conductivity of the buffer solution is unfavorable, not only because of increased production of unwanted Joule heat but also because the absolute and relative electrophoretic mobility of the components to be separated drops." This decrease in electrophoretic mobility with increase in conductivity of the suspending medium was known much earlier from work with bacterial cells (Brown and Broom, 1935); however, practical advantage of this knowledge was not taken before Hannig and his associates emphasized this important point. In our laboratory, we have found that the buffers of Zeiller and Hannig have been most satisfactory in permitting us to separate rat proximal tubule cells (Kreisberg et al., 1977b) and human tonsillar cells (T. G. Pretlow et al., 1980).

2. Neoplastic, Dividing, and Immature Cells

Subject to the limitations and exceptions that are inherent in generalizations about cells, there is a large body of evidence that suggests that immature and proliferating cells have greater electrophoretic mobilities than mature and resting cells. In general, malignant, neoplastic cells have been found to have electrophoretic mobilities that are similar to or more rapid than dividing or immature, normal cells.

(a) Hepatoma Cells.   In 1956, Ambrose et al. (1956) measured the electrophoretic mobilities of rat cells from normal liver, normal kidney, and tumors from liver and kidney induced with butter yellow and stilbesterol, respectively. Cells were obtained in suspension from all tissues by perfusion of the tissues with culture medium containing various chelating agents. Under these conditions, kidney tumor cells showed higher electrophoretic mobilities than cells from normal kidneys; liver tumor cells showed higher electrophoretic mobilities than normal liver cells. Similar data were published with greater detail together with the characterization of cells from several ascites tumors (Lowick et al., 1961).

Normal, fetal, regenerating, and neoplastic liver have provided an interesting series of comparisons. Ben-Or et al. (1960) observed that regenerating liver cells have higher electrophoretic mobilities than normal liver cells. Eisenberg et al. (1962) demonstrated that the electrophoretic mobility of rat liver cells decreased from birth to 21 days of age. In the younger animals, these investigators observed ". . . numerous, small, round cells . . .", which they believed to be hemopoietic cells and excluded from their investigations. In addition, they expanded their earlier observations (Ben-Or et al., 1960) that cells from regenerating liver have a higher electrophoretic mobility than normal liver cells. The highest electrophoretic mobility was observed 48 h after partial hepatectomy.

Extending these studies of liver cells, Fuhrmann (1965) observed that the electrophoretic mobility of cells from the regenerating liver increased ". . . parallel to that of the mitotic index taken in the morning . . ."; however, they observed a diurnal variation in the mitotic rate, which made it necessary that this correlation be observed in the morning. They also observed that the electrophoretic mobilities of regenerating liver cells were little affected by treatment with neuraminidase, while the electrophoretic mobilities of malignant cells from an ascitic hepatoma were markedly decreased by treatment with neuraminidase. When these experiments were conducted in vivo by injection by neuraminidase intraperitoneally into animals with ascitic tumors, the mobilities of the ascites tumor cells decreased rapidly and returned to pretreatment levels over the following 1–3 days. Similar decreased electrophoretic mobility of HeLa cells was observed after treatment with neuraminidase. The transplantability of ascitic hepatoma cells and culturability of the HeLa cells were not altered by treatment with neuraminidase. Subsequently, Woo and Cater (1972) confirmed the observation that the mobilities of hepatoma cells are decreased by treatment with neuraminidase and noted that fetal liver cells were affected similarly.

(b) Ascites Tumors. In addition to the studies of ascites tumors mentioned above (Lowick et al., 1961), there have been several other studies of ascites tumors. Like blood cells, ascites tumor cells have the advantage that they already are obtained in suspension. Cook et al. (1962) used Ehrlich cells to study alterations of electrophoretic mobility according to altered pH and treatments with trypsin, neuraminidase, and aldehyde fixatives. Mayhew (1968) reported that the electrophoretic mobilities of Ehrlich cells varied with the age of the tumor; he observed that treatment of Ehrlich ascites tumor cells with neuraminidase and ribonuclease alone and in combination caused decreased electrophoretic mobility. Hartveit et al. noticed that the electrophoretic mobilities of Bf 8 and Ehrlich ascites tumor cells changed on successive days following transplantation (Hartveit et al., 1968).

(c) Lymphoma and Leukemia. There have been many studies of electrophoresis of cells from mouse and human lymphomas and leukemias. As in the several other organ systems described above, it would appear that electrophoretic mobility is at least crudely related to the maturity of the cells under study. In

both the rat and man, cells from bone marrow show a somewhat more rapid electrophoretic mobility than the more mature cells found in peripheral blood (Arnold, 1965; Ruhenstroth-Bauer, 1965). In human marrow (Ruhenstroth-Bauer, 1965), there is a small subpopulation of granulocytes with electrophoretic mobilities similar to those of granulocytes in the peripheral circulation; however, the majority of granulocytes from the marrow have a more rapid electrophoretic mobility. In both virally produced leukemia in rats (Arnold, 1965) and "naturally occurring" leukemia in man (Ruhenstroth-Bauer, 1965), the transformation to acute leukemia is associated with an increased electrophoretic mobility. Data obtained by Lichtman and Weed (1970) essentially confirmed Ruhenstroth-Bauer's characterization of mature peripheral blood cells, marrow cells, and leukemic cells; in addition, these authors found that the electrophoretic mobilities of all tested cell types was decreased by treatment with neuraminidase. Leukemia cells, like normal blood cells and ascites tumor cells, have been used extensively to study the surface properties of cells as a function of pH (Mehrishi and Thomson, 1968; Cook and Jacobson, 1968) and as altered by neuraminidase, aldehyde fixation, and other chemical alterations (Cook and Jacobson, 1968).

3. Electrophoresis of Cultured Benign and Malignant Cells

Heard et al. (1961) found that cultured fibroblasts from mouse embryos manifested greater electrophoretic mobility than cultured fibroblasts from adult animals. Fibroblasts from the 20-methylcholanthrene-treated strain L fibroblasts exhibited an electrophoretic mobility intermediate between fibroblasts from embryos and adult mice. In the same vein, Forrester et al. (1962) observed that polyoma-transformed hamster fibroblasts exhibited both more heterogeneous and higher electrophoretic mobilities than fibroblasts from the same population not transformed. Latner and Turner (1974) found smaller differences between virus-transformed and "normal" BHK_{21} cells than have been characteristic of transformed and "normal" cells in other systems.

Attempts have been made to correlate electrophoretic mobility with the aggressiveness of cells from different tumors. Purdom et al. (1958) studied several sublines of the same transplantable tumor and concluded that "... the selection for a biological characteristic, namely, the ease of producing the ascites form, which also leads to the appearance of early metastases, is correlated with the progressive increase in negative electrical charge . . . ." Bosmann et al. (1973) found that sublines of a melanoma developed by Fidler (1973) differed prior to confluency but became similar when the cultures reached confluency. The sublines differed with respect to their propensities to give rise to metastases in vivo; in sparse cultures, the line with the greatest propensity to metastasize exhibited the higher electrophoretic mobility.

In summary, electrophoretic characterization of cells has, with few exceptions, shown that mature, normal cells have lower electrophoretic mobilities than cells from embryos, regenerating cells, and neoplastic cells. Most of the studies of cells other than those from the lymphoid and hemopoietic systems have been carried out with equipment that does not permit the separation and recovery of a sufficient number of cells to permit biochemical, morphological, and other kinds of characterization. With the development of free-flow electrophoresis, it should be possible to separate a sufficient number of cells to permit much more detailed characterization than was formerly possible.

4. Viability and Function after Electrophoresis

There are few published data to suggest that electrophoresis is harmful to cells. Except for a study performed with microorganisms (Hamilton and Sale, 1967), there has been little investigation of the mechanisms by which cells may be injured by exposure to electrical fields. There are considerable data which support the working hypothesis that electrophoresis performed properly does little harm to viability or function. After electrophoresis, Boltz et al. (1973) found that electrophoresed cells exhibited 75% of the plating efficiency observed prior to electrophoresis. Zeiller (Zeiller et al., 1972c) observed little change in the number of mouse marrow cells with the capacity to form colonies in the spleens of irradiated mice after electrophoresis. Ganser et al. (1968) evaluated electrophoretically separated nucleated blood cells by observing their capacities to exclude dye and to exhibit phagocytosis; they estimated that 70–80% of the electrophoretically separated cells were viable. Zeiller and his associates as well as others (Zeiller et al., 1970, 1972a,b, 1976; Schlegel et al., 1975a,b) have shown that antibody-forming cells still have the capacity to form plaques after electrophoretic separation. After electrophoretic separation, lymphocytes are able to function in the graft-versus-host reaction (Zeiller et al., 1971, 1974; Andersson et al., 1973a); in cytotoxicity reactions (Hayry and Anderson, 1975; Hayry et al., 1973); in mixed lymphocyte cultures as stimulating cells (Hayry et al., 1975b; von Boehmer, 1974) and as responding cells (Andersson et al., 1973b; Hayry et al., 1973; von Boehmer, 1974); in cultures stimulated with various mitogens including phytohemagglutinin, bacterial lipopolysaccharide, concanavalin A, and pokeweed mitogen (Hayry et al., 1973, 1975a; Andersson et al., 1973b, 1975; Stein et al., 1973; Stein, 1975b; Seiler et al., 1974; Shortman et al., 1975); and as antibody progenitor cells detected by passive transfer into syngeneic recipients (Schlegel et al., 1975a,b).

5. Free-Flow Electrophoresis

As discussed in Section IV.A, the electrophoresis of cells had been useful for analytical purposes since 1902. The electrophoresis of cells in sufficient quantities (10^8–10^9/h) to permit detailed characterization and biochemical studies became a possibility when Hannig, Zeiller, and their associates at the

Max Planck Institute in Munich introduced two major deviations from the electrophoresis of cells as practiced during the preceding half century. First, they employed Hannig's (Hannig, 1964, 1967, 1969, 1971, 1972) continuous flow electrophoresis apparatus to conduct a type of electrophoretic experiment termed "free-flow" electrophoresis by Hannig. Second, they developed a new series of buffers for electrophoresis that differed from those buffers in common use previously in that the buffers of Hannig and Zeiller were of lower conductivity. These buffers were made isosmotic with solutes of low ionic strength, such as glucose, sorbitol, and sucrose. Media of low ionic strength permitted Hannig and Zeiller to use sufficient voltages to obtain good separations while avoiding the thermoconvective problems commonly observed with more commonly employed salt solutions of higher conductivity.

Hannig, Zeiller, and their associates have applied free-flow electrophoresis to a wide variety of problems in experimental immunology and hematology (Hannig, 1964; Hannig and Krusmann, 1968; Ganser et al., 1968; Hannig and Zeiller, 1969; Zeiller and Hannig, 1971; Zeiller et al., 1970, 1971, 1972a-c, 1974, 1975a,b, 1976; Schubert et al., 1973; Zeiller and Pascher, 1973; Seiler et al., 1974; Mehrishi and Zeiller, 1974; Droege et al., 1974a,b; Hannig et al., 1975). Probably because of the expense of the equipment for free-flow electrophoresis and because of the difficulty in keeping the equipment in good repair, other laboratories were slow to use the technique until after it had been proved several times by Hannig and Zeiller. In 1972, the first of a series of experiments from Nordling, Andersson, and Hayry (Nordling et al., 1972) in which cells of the immune system were separated by free-flow electrophoresis appeared; later articles in this series from their laboratory have appeared regularly (Hayry et al., 1973, 1975a,b; Hayry and Andersson, 1975; Andersson et al., 1973a,b, 1975).

At almost the same time as Nordling et al. (1972) published their first application of the technique of Hannig and Zeiller, Stein (Stein et al., 1973) published his first use of free-flow electrophoresis for the separation of human lymphocytes. Stein has continued to employ free-flow electrophoresis for the separation of lymphoid cells (Stein, 1975a,b). A little later, Shortman, von Boehmer, Schlegel, and their associates began to report their applications of free-flow electrophoresis to the separation of lymphoid and hemopoietic cells (von Boehmer, 1974; von Boehmer et al., 1974; Schlegel et al., 1975a,b; Melchers et al., 1975; Roelants et al., 1975; Osmond et al., 1975). Other laboratories have studied lymphoid, hemopoietic, and/or blood cells by free-flow electrophoresis (Herve et al., 1975; Just et al., 1975).

In 1977, free-flow electrophoresis was first applied to the separation of proximal tubule cells from rats in our laboratory (Kreisberg et al., 1977b) and from rabbits by Heidrich and Dew (1977). Initially, we were guarded in our estimation of the breadth of applicability of this technique because we were skeptical about (1) possible injurious effects of the electrophoretic procedure on the cells to be studied, (2) possible injurious effects of the rather unusual electrophoretic buffers on the cells, and (3) the effects of the proteolytic enzymes that we have usually found necessary for work with human tissues on the separability of the cells to be electrophoresed. In order to examine these potential problems, we studied the separation of human tonsillar cells by electrophoresis. These cells were selected because we have had considerable experience in the separation, characterization, and culture of human tonsillar cells (Willson *et al.*, 1975, 1976*a,b*). To our surprise, the human tonsillar cells obtained in suspension with trypsin or collagenase responded to mitogens and excluded trypan blue equally as well before and after electrophoresis (T. G. Pretlow *et al.*, 1980). Of equal interest, while the electrophoretic mobilities of all cells were somewhat decreased as compared with human tonsillar cells obtained in suspension mechanically (without trypsin or collagenase), all cells were as well purified after being obtained in suspension with trypsin as after being obtained in suspension mechanically. This group of cells in our laboratory has shown no evidence of injury or decreased viability after electrophoresis with the technique of Hannig and Zeiller and after exposure to their buffers for several minutes at 4.0°C.

6. Potential Applications of Free-Flow Electrophoresis to Cancer Cells

In light of the extensive evidence reviewed above that cancer cells have greater electrophoretic mobilities than normal cells, free-flow electrophoresis may provide a broadly applicable method for the separation of malignant cells from stromal cells. In contrast to the techniques which were available for the electrophoretic separation of tumor cells during the first half of this century, free-flow electrophoresis is a preparative technique. To our knowledge, there have been no reports of the purification of cells from solid tumors by free-flow electrophoresis. In recent months, experiments carried out in our laboratory with a limited variety of tumors have demonstrated that malignant cells migrate more rapidly than benign cells in the buffers and apparatus of Hannig and Zeiller, and we are hopeful that free-flow electrophoresis may be broadly applicable to problems in the purification of malignant cells from cancers.

B. Sedimentation

1. Techniques and Definitions

The theory of gradient sedimentation as applied to mammalian cells has been reviewed extensively previously (T. G. Pretlow *et al.*, 1975) and will not be reviewed here. Briefly, cells possess two physical properties that are useful to the investigator who wants to employ sedimentation for their purification: density and diameter. If cells are to be separated on the basis of differences in density, one centrifuges the cells with sufficient force and for a sufficient period of time to bring them to the location in the density gradient at which the density of the gradient is equal to the densities of the respective cells. This type of centrifugation, termed "isopycnic" sedimentation, has not been broadly applicable to the purification of individual kinds of cells from tumors.

If one wishes to separate cells that differ with respect to their diameters, one carries out "velocity" sedimentation. In velocity sedimentation, one allows the sedimentation of the cells to proceed for a much shorter period of time and/or with a lower centrifugal force than required for isopycnic sedimentation. Optimally, gradients for velocity sedimentation should be designed such that the cells remain at locations that are remote from their respective densities. Early in velocity sedimentation, the diameters of cells are more important than their densities in determining their *rates* of sedimentation. As the cells approach their densities in the gradients, density becomes a more important factor. The details of the theory have been reviewed previously (T. G. Pretlow *et al.*, 1975). The commonly employed methods for velocity sedimentation are sedimentation at unit gravity, isokinetic sedimentation, and elutriation.

In addition to the types of sedimentations described in the previous paragraph, sedimentation can be carried out in discontinuous gradients. When neutral density separations and discontinuous gradient separations were first employed in the 1940s, 1950s, and early 1960s (Vallee *et al.*, 1947; Fawcett *et al.*, 1950; Fawcett and Vallee, 1952; Alexander and Spriggs, 1960; Spriggs and Alexander, 1960), these rather crude instruments represented important new advances in cell separation. One would hope that these rather crude techniques would be of primarily historical interest; however, they continue to be used even in the 1970s. The artifacts which are associated with the use of discontinuous gradients have been reviewed often (T. G. Pretlow *et al.*, 1975; Shortman, 1972; Leif, 1970). An eminent authority on centrifugation has stated (de Duve, 1971): "The discontinuous gradient is essentially a device for generating artificial bands. This may be a convenient way of compressing together for preparative purposes certain segments of the distributions observed in continuous gradients. But it is also a dangerous procedure, in that it creates the illusion of clear-cut separation." The discontinuous gradient is never an optimal means for the separation of cells that differ in respect to density and/or diameter.

2. Medium

For both isopycnic and velocity cell sedimentation techniques, one would prefer media that are not toxic. In the case of isopycnic sedimentation, it seems desirable to us that the medium be a medium that will permit one to construct isosmotic density gradients easily. In 1975, we (T. G. Pretlow *et al.*, 1975) reviewed the densities of several dozen different kinds of cells as determined in the three most commonly employed media for isopycnic gradient sedimentation, i.e., Ficoll, albumin, and colloidal silica. We concluded from this review that the densities of cells are approximately equal in all three of these media. Contrary to this conclusion, Wolff (1977) has stated that in colloidal silica particles exhibit "... a different (lighter) specific gravity (density) than observed in sucrose or Ficoll gradients." Wolff does not present any data to support this conclusion, and there is ample data to refute this conclusion in the previously cited review (T. G. Pretlow *et al.*, 1975).

A number of other media have been advocated for isopycnic centrifugation. Without reviewing these, we should express the opinion that each new medium for isopycnic sedimentation generates much more excitement than is merited by isopycnic centrifugation as a technique for the purification of cells. Each new medium for isopycnic sedimentation is heralded as the final solution to the difficult problem of separating cells; however, to our knowledge, there are only two or three examples of mixtures of cells that can be as well separated by isopycnic sedimentation as by velocity sedimentation. In most cases, velocity sedimentation is far more effective for the purification of cells. If isopycnic sedimentation and velocity sedimentation are equally effective for a problem in cell separation, it appears to us that velocity sedimentation is vastly preferable because of the lower centrifugal forces to which cells are subjected during velocity sedimentation. In short, isopycnic sedimentation is not very useful for the purification of cells.

For velocity sedimentation, the choice of a medium has considerable importance since the separation that will be achieved will be dictated by properties of the gradient medium other than density. While the density of the gradient is an important consideration in velocity sedimentation, in well-designed experiments the density of the gradient medium is deliberately minimized. Because of the low densities of the solutions employed, viscosity becomes a very important consideration. If one is to repeat an experiment in velocity sedimentation, it will be important that one work with a gradient having a viscosity profile which is constant from experiment to experiment. For this reason, it seems desirable to us that a synthetic medium of defined molecular weight be employed. Ficoll has a defined average molecular weight of 400,000, and the viscosity of Ficoll is consistent from batch to batch. As reviewed in detail previously (T. G. Pretlow *et al.*, 1975), it is possible to alter the physical properties of Ficoll by using a suboptimal method to obtain Ficoll in solution. The methods which we recommend have been described in detail (T. G. Pretlow *et al.*, 1975). We should mention that Ficoll is stable in solution at neutral pH for only 3–4 days; however, it can be stored in solution at $-20°C$ at neutral pH for periods in excess of 3 months.

3. Isopycnic Sedimentation

One of the earliest isopycnic separations of cells from tumors was that of Pertoft (1970). Pertoft did not report a specific purity for his cells separated from the Furth transplantable mast cell tumor by isopycnic centrifugation; how-ever, he did observe that among those cells that ". . . were banded at densities 1.06 and 1.08; practically all contained metachromatic granules." Subsequently (Helting *et al.*, 1972), these cells were termed "mast cells" without additional evidence to support their identification. In work with this same transplantable tumor some years later, we (T. P. Pretlow *et al.*, 1977a) found that metachro-matic granules were often found in macrophages as well as in malignant cells in this mast cell tumor. The experimentally determined densities for the cells from the Furth mast cell tumor were very similar in our laboratory in Ficoll gradients and in Pertoft's laboratory in gradients of colloidal silica. Like Pertoft, we found that malignant mast cells could be purified from this tumor by isopycnic sedi-mentation in greater than 90% purity (T. P. Pretlow *et al.*, 1977a); however, cells from this tumor were more effectively purified by velocity sedimentation in the isokinetic gradient. We mention the comparison of velocity sedimentation and isopycnic sedimentation for the purification of cells from the Furth mast cell tumor because this comparison illustrates a principle which we have found to be *true for every tumor which we have examined to date:* cells have been more effectively purified by velocity sedimentation than by isopycnic sedimentation. While exceptions to this generalization may become apparent with further investigation, we have not encountered such exceptions up to the present time. In fact, malignant cells were more effectively purified from the Furth mast cell tumor than from any other tumor which we have examined. We believe that our success and Pertoft's success in purifying malignant mast cells from this tumor is related to the fact that these malignant cells contain very dense cytoplasmic granules similar to those found in mature mast cells. Mature mast cells are among the densest cells which we have ever encountered (T. G. Pretlow and Cassady, 1970; T. P. Pretlow *et al.*, 1977a).

Grdina (Grdina *et al.*, 1974, 1975, 1976, 1977, 1978) has had considerable, carefully documented experience in the separation of cells from mouse fibrosar-comas by isopycnic sedimentation in continuous gradients of Renografin. After labeling this cell with tritiated thymidine, they found that the distribution of the radioactivity in the density gradients closely paralleled the distribution of cells (Grdina *et al.*, 1974). Five broadly overlapping subpopulations of cells were identified after isopycnic sedimentation (Grdina *et al.*, 1975). These subpopula-tions differed with respect to their sensitivity to ionizing radiation. The sensitivity of the subpopulations of cells to ionizing radiation was affected by the presence or absence of hypoxia (Grdina *et al.*, 1976). After separating cells from these fibrosarcomas by isopycnic sedimentation in Renografin and by elutriation (Grdina *et al.*, 1977), it was shown that the abilities of the separated cells to form lung colonies was more related to density than to the sizes of the cells. The ability to form colonies in lungs was not closely related to cell-cycle parameters. Gamma radiation affected the cells differently from neutron radiation (Grdina *et al.*, 1978). Grdina pointed out that cell separation methods "reduce the heterogeneity found in the solid tumor by allowing for the isolation of subpopulations which can be studied either individually or in relation to the entire tumor." A similar, very careful study of conditions for the dissociation and isopycnic sedimentation of cells from a mouse fibrosarcoma in albumin gradients has been reported recently (Sheridan and Finlay-Jones, 1977).

Recently, Ng and Inch (1978) described the densities of EMT6 cells grown as monolayers, spheroids, and solid tumors. Interestingly, the densities of these malignant cells grown as speroids were similar to the densities observed in cells from solid tumors derived from EMT6 cells. The cells from monolayers were less dense than cells from spheriods and solid tumors. In many ways, this report is a model of our view of the appropriate manner for the description of isopycnic sedimentation. The investigators carefully tested band capacity. It would appear that many of those who separate cells by isopycnic centrifugation on continuous density gradients are unaware of the concept of band capacity. This is a very important aspect of all gradient centrifugation. These investigators reported that the recovery of cells from their isopycnic gradients ranged between 62 and 83%. They tested the statistical significance of the differences they observed between different kinds of EMT6 cells. They rebanded their cells to determine the repeatability of the measured densities.

We have had a considerable interest in the separation of cells from a variety of normal and malignant tissues over the past several years. The purification of malignant cells by isopycnic sedimentation has been unimpressive with the only exception being the purification of cells from the Furth mast cell tumor (see earlier this section). Our first effort in the purification of cells with solid tumors was a study of transplantable malignant melanomas (T. G. Pretlow and Boone, 1970). The velocity sedimentation described in that report was carried out in a gradient that was much cruder than those which we have used more recently; despite the fact that this gradient for velocity sedimentation was less than optimally designed, velocity sedimentation resulted in a greater purification than isopycnic sedimentation. Subsequent studies of cells from tumors in our laboratory have been carried out in the isokinetic gradient. Separation of lymphocytes, macrophages, and malignant cells from an ascites myeloma showed that all cell types were better purified by velocity sedimentation than by isopycnic sedimentation (Stewart *et al.*, 1972). Cells from the tumor of Hodgkin's disease were more effectively purified by velocity sedimentation in our isokinetic gradient than by isopycnic centrifugation (T. G. Pretlow *et al.*, 1973). While in some cases isopycnic sedimentation proved to be a useful third and final step in the purification of lymphocytes from a series of transplantable tumors (Zettergren *et al.*, 1973), velocity sedimentation in the isokinetic gradient was the most useful of the three steps in the purification of lymphocytes from these transplantable tumors. More recently, we have described work with two transplantable tumors from which we could separate lymphocytes in 89–90% purity by a one-step sedimentation in the isokinetic gradient (T. P. Pretlow *et al.*, 1977a,b). The malignant cells from both of these tumors were better purified by velocity sedimentation in the isokinetic gradient than by isopycnic sedimentation. Our work with human colonic carcinoma (Brattain *et al.*, 1977a,b) has resulted in a marked concentration of epithelial cells from human colonic carcinomas. These cells could be cultured in soft agar after purification. The purified epithelial cells showed an increased content of carcinoembryonic antigen and of hexosaminidase as compared with the cells prior to separation in the isokinetic gradient. Isopycnic sedimentation was not as effective for the purification of cells from these tumors. A variety of stromal cells were purified from human colonic carcinomas in these experiments. Epithelial cells were obtained from human prostatic carcinomas more effectively by velocity sedimentation than by isopycnic sedimentation (Helms *et al.*, 1976).

4. Velocity Sedimentation

(a) Unit Gravity. Despite the enormous volume of work that has been carried out with lymphoid cells with velocity sedimentation at unit gravity, there has been surprisingly little application of this technique to the separation of different kinds of cells from tumors. The largest and some of the best documented work is that of Haskill and his associates (Haskill *et al.*, 1975a,b, 1976; Haskill, 1977; Holden *et al.*, 1976). Working with a methylcholanthrene-induced, transplantable sarcoma, Haskill succeeded in separating fractions of cells at unit gravity which contained "over 90% macrophages." The "remaining cells were granulocytes and lymphocytes" (Haskill *et al.*, 1975a) in the "host" cell fractions. In work with another transplantable tumor, Haskill and his associates (Haskill *et al.*, 1975b) studied a tumor that would progress or regress depending on the conditions of transplantation. "Regressive tumors" contained only 9% malignant cells. Haskill found (Haskill *et al.*, 1975b) very different patterns of sedimentation at unit gravity for "progressor" and "regressor" tumors. Again, these investigators found that they could separate "host" cells from malignant cells; however, it is difficult to assess just how homogeneous the fractions of host cells were with respect to morphology and/or function. In a subsequent review of work with this same line of transplantable tumor cells (Haskill *et al.*, 1976), it is apparent that after velocity sedimentation theta-positive cells, cells having the capacity to form rosettes with sheep red blood cells coated with mouse antibodies, and eosinophils were broadly overlapping in the gradient (see Fig. 1 of Haskill *et al.*, 1976). Phagocytic cells were found throughout the portion of the gradient which contained malignant cells. From the data presented, it is not possible to determine whether or not phagocytic cells were present among the cells in fractions containing "theta-positive" cells.

In a similar study of cells from regressing murine sarcoma virus-induced tumors, Holden, Haskill, Kirchner, and Herberman (1976) studied the distributions of "host" cells in cell separations performed at unit gravity. Macrophages, T cells, and B cells were found in broadly overlapping areas of the gradient. Again with cells from transplantable tumors, Haskill (1977) demonstrated that cells demonstrating "antibody-dependent" cellular cytotoxicity sedimented at a modal location which was different from, but broadly overlapping with, "armed monocytes."

Aside from the work of Haskill, we are aware of only two other applications of sedimentation at unit gravity to the separation of cells from tumors. MacDonald (MacDonald *et al.*, 1978) demonstrated that cells infiltrating allografted spheroids had velocity sedimentation properties similar to small lymphocytes. These cells formed a different modal population of cells from the EMT6 cells capable of forming clones *in vitro*. Davis and Ralph (1975) employed sedimentation at unit gravity to "compare cell sizes" of cells from mastocytoma grown intraperitoneally. There are several features of this paper that make it uninterpretable for us. First, it is not possible to compare the sizes of cells by any method for velocity sedimentation without first knowing their densities (T. G. Pretlow and Pretlow, 1977; Catsimpoolas and Griffith, 1977). Second, it was assumed that changes in velocity of sedimentation after the administration of drugs resulted from changes in the sizes of malignant cells. Changes in patterns of velocity sedimentation may indeed have resulted from changes in size; however, changes in such patterns could have resulted from changes in density and/or the frequency distribution of cell types among the unseparated cells. There was no evidence presented that the observed changes did or did not result from changes in the frequency distribution of lymphocytes, macrophages, malignant cells, and other cell types present in the peritoneal cavities of the mice. Based on work in our laboratory with ascites tumors, it is highly likely that most of the cells in the peritoneal cavities studied under the conditions described by Davis and Ralph were not malignant cells at all, but macrophages. It is important to emphasize that these investigators left the cells in the peritoneal cavities for slightly more than 2 days. We have studied several ascites tumors (Stewart *et al.*, 1972; T. G. Pretlow and Pretlow, unpublished observations); after the injection of 1 million cells, we have not encountered an ascites tumor which contains a majority of malignant cells after growth for only 2 days. Tulp and Welagen (1976) obtained a degree of synchronization of some ascites tumor cells by sedimentation at unit gravity for 6 h and 40 min.

(b) Isokinetic Gradient. Since the original description of the isokinetic gradient that we employ (T. G. Pretlow, 1971), this technique has had several applications to the separation of cells from tumors. We shall first describe the work in other laboratories; later, we shall describe work in our own laboratory.

Russell, Gillespie, Hansen, and Cochrane (1976) were the first group other than our own to report the purification of cells from tumors by sedimentation in the isokinetic gradient (T. G. Pretlow, 1971). These investigators found that suspensions of cells from regressing Moloney sarcomas contained approximately 22% T lymphocytes. In the first step of their purification, they removed adherent cells and found that their enriched suspensions contained 38.9% lymphocytes. As a second step they employed isokinetic sedimentation, and their "pooled" gradient fractions that contained T lymphocytes consisted of 60% T lymphocytes.

In 1978, using a technique similar to one used in our laboratory for the separation of lymphocytes from tumors in a one-step procedure (T. P. Pretlow et al., 1977a,b), Blazar and Heppner published a very detailed account of their meticulous separation of lymphocytes from autochthonous mouse mammary tumors (Blazar and Heppner, 1978a,b; Blazar et al., 1978). In their very careful study of autochthonous mouse mammary tumors, Blazar and Heppner found that digestion of the tumors with trypsin, collagenase, and DNase gave them both a larger number of cells per gram of tumor and a higher viability than was possible using simply mechanical techniques for obtaining the cells in suspension (Blazar and Heppner, 1978a). In early experiments, they found that they could separate mouse thymus cells from cultured cells of a mouse mammary tumor cell line (Blazar and Heppner, 1978a).

In their first report, these investigators described the distribution of several kinds of cells from mammary tumors in the isokinetic gradient. We would like to emphasize that, in contrast to work with sedimentation of tumor cells at unit gravity as reviewed above, Blazar and Heppner's separation of tumor cells in the isokinetic gradient (their Fig. 8) gave fractions of lymphocytes which were almost totally devoid of macrophages and monocytes. Our experience in the separation of cells from tumors in the isokinetic gradient has also given almost complete separation of lymphocytes from monocytes (T. P. Pretlow et al., 1977a,b). This observation would suggest to us that the isokinetic gradient gives better resolution for the separation of lymphocytes and monocytes from tumors than has been achieved at unit gravity. Interestingly, they found that the separations of mammary tumor cell lines resulted in the purification of cells that were as readily cultured after cell separation as before cell separation, i.e., similarly to our reported observations they could find no toxic effect of Ficoll at the concentrations employed in the isokinetic gradient. Blazar and Heppner (1978b) separated cells with theta-positivity, cells reacting with antilymphocyte serum, cells with surface immunoglobulin, cells with Fc receptors, and cells that were phagocytic from a large number of autochthonous tumors in the isokinetic gradient. In a third report (Blazer et al., 1978), these investigators demonstrated that lymphoid cells purified from autochthonous mammary tumors actually stimulated the growth of epithelial cells from these tumors. To our knowledge, this is the first demonstration of the stimulation of malignant epithelial cells from tumors by lymphoid populations of cells in the tumors. These investigators noted that "even when lymph node cells of the tumor bearer were cytotoxic to the tumor cells, the separated tumor-associated lymphoid cells were markedly stimulatory." They found that the stimulatory activity of the lymphoid cells purified from the tumors was abrogated by treatment of the lymphoid cells with antilymphocyte serum and complement. In addition, they found that they could (Blazar *et al.*, 1978) "separate cytotoxicity and stimulation into different fractions" of cells from the lymph nodes of tumor-bearing animals. Yarlott and McKhann (1976) separated "specifically immune lymphocytes" which had adhered to a monolayer of cultured tumor cells; lymphocytes were separated from the tumor cells in the isokinetic gradient in greater than 99% purity.

Attempts in our laboratory to purify cells from transplantable tumors were begun with a relatively crude gradient which varied from 2.4 to 6.1% Ficoll. The slope of this gradient was somewhat steeper than optimal. Despite this we were able to purify cells from hamster "melanotic malanomas" in 89-91% purity (T. G. Pretlow and Boone, 1970). With the development of the isokinetic gradient (T. G. Pretlow, 1971), we had a more powerful instrument for the velocity sedimentation of cells from tumors. Our first application of the isokinetic gradient to the purification of cells from transplantable tumors was the separation of lymphocytes, macrophages, and malignant cells from an ascites myeloma (Stewart *et al.*, 1972). After these cell separations, lymphocytes were 98.9 ± 0.4%; macrophages, 79.3 ± 12.1%; and malignant cells, 52.1 ± 6.9% of nucleated cells in the purest fractions. Fractions that contained the most highly purified lymphocytes and macrophages, as well as the modal populations of these cells, contained less that 0.2% myeloma cells. Approximately 2000 cells from the purified malignant cells were found to be tumorigenic. Animals that received more than 1 million cells from "host" cell fractions failed to develop tumors. In the following year, we (Zettergren *et al.*, 1973) purified lymphocytes from a variety of transplantable tumors. The unseparated suspensions of cells contained 0.6-4.8% lymphocytes. A three-step procedure was used employing isokinetic sedimentation, isopycnic sedimentation, and filtration. The purified fractions from these transplantable tumors contained 58.4-96.8% lymphocytes. To our knowledge, this was the first description of a broadly applicable technique for the purification of lymphocytes from solid tumors.

More recently, we have observed two transplantable tumors from which lymphocytes can be purified as 89-90% of cells in a one-step sedimentation in the isokinetic gradient. The first of these tumors is the Furth mast cell tumor and has the advantage that the malignant cells uniformly contain metachromatic granules. Occasionally, one also observes metachromatic granules in macrophages which have phagocytized tumor cells. Depending upon the size of the tumors when the animals are sacrificed, the unseparated cells contain 2.4-32.9% lymphocytes (T. P. Pretlow *et al.*, 1977*a*). After separation, lymphocytes are 88.9 ± 10.1%

of nucleated cells in the purest fraction; granulocytes, $49.4 \pm 12.4\%$; macrophages, $17.3 \pm 14.0\%$; and malignant cells, $97.2 \pm 1.9\%$. Purified cells were injected into animals. Animals receiving as few as 16 malignant mast cells developed tumors. No animals that received purified lymphocytes (up to 57,000) developed tumors. Similar experiments were possible with the transplantable Ward adenocarcinoma of the colon in Fischer rats. Lymphocytes were obtained in $90.4 \pm 5.0\%$ purity. Most rats that received greater than 100,000 purified malignant cells intramuscularly developed tumors; rats that received more than 1 million cells from the modal population of lymphocytes failed to develop tumors (T. P. Pretlow *et al.*, 1977*b*).

In our first work with human tumors, we separated cells from the splenic tumor of Hodgkin's disease. Relatively mature-appearing lymphoid cells were purified from the tumor in 98.4% purity. Fractions which were enriched with respect to Hodgkin's cells and Reed–Sternberg cells were obtained. The Hodgkin's and Reed–Sternberg cells (T. G. Pretlow *et al.*, 1973) were able to be cultured from the purified fractions. In later studies (Willson *et al.*, 1977), we found that lymphocytes purified from the tumor of the mixed-cellularity type of Hodgkin's disease failed to respond to phytohemagglutinin, concanavalin A, and pokeweed mitogen. In contrast, lymphocytes purified from other lymphoid tissues including human spleens, tonsils, and blood responded to these mitogens. In the case of spleens and tonsils, the tissues were dissociated and treated in exactly the same fashion as the tumors of the patients with Hodgkin's disease. Failure of lymphocytes purified from the tumor of Hodgkin's disease to respond to phytohemagglutinin was not the result of an absence of T cells, since the purified "lymphocytes" contained more than 61% cells capable of forming non-immune rosettes with sheep red blood cells. Earlier, we had demonstrated (Willson *et al.*, 1976*b*) that lymphocytes purified from human tonsils responded slightly less vigorously than unseparated cells from human tonsils and that the addition of rapidly sedimenting cells (presumably macrophages) to the fractions of purified tonsillar lymphocytes enhanced the response of tonsillar lymphocytes to mitogens. In contrast, addition of more rapidly sedimenting cells (including macrophages) to the purified lymphocytes from Hodgkin's tumor did not result in a detectable response to mitogens. Similarly, in some experiments we added rapidly sedimenting cells (including macrophages) from adjacent, uninvolved spleen to the lymphocytes purified from splenic tumor of the same patient. Again, the addition of macrophages from this uninvolved spleen failed to facilitate the response of tumor lymphocytes to mitogens. Addition of macrophages from uninvolved spleen to purified splenic lymphocytes enhanced their response to mitogens in a fashion similar to that reported for human tonsillar cells (Willson *et al.*, 1976*b*).

The purification of Hodgkin's cells and Reed–Sternberg cells from the tumor of Hodgkin's disease facilitated our demonstration that the cells which contain the tumor-associated antigen described by Order and Hellman (Order *et al.*, 1971, 1972; Katz *et al.*, 1973) are the lymphocytes which are rosetted about the Hodgkin's cells and Reed–Sternberg cells (T. G. Pretlow *et al.*, 1976, 1978). These lymphocytes differ from most lymphocytes from the tumor of Hodgkin's disease in that they are very tenaciously attached to the Hodgkin's cells and Reed–Sternberg cells. Because of this attachment they are found at the gradient-cushion interface after the described cell separation (T. G. Pretlow *et al.*, 1973), while the majority of lymphocytes from Hodgkin's disease are found closer to the sample–gradient interface than to the gradient–cushion interface (Willson *et al.*, 1977; T. G. Pretlow *et al.*, 1973). The opportunity to observe fractions enriched with respect to Hodgkin's cells and Reed–Sternberg cells resulted in our chance observation that there appears to be a correlation between the prognosis of patients with Hodgkin's disease and the proportion of Hodgkin's cells and Reed–Sternberg cells with attached lymphocytes (McGuire *et al.*, 1979). Patients which have a high proportion of Hodgkin's cells and Reed–Sternberg cells with attached lymphocytes do not develop recurrent disease, while, based on the observation of a limited number of patients, those who have a low proportion of Hodgkin's cells and Reed–Sternberg cells with attached, antigenic lymphocytes develop recurrent disease.

Our more recent work with human solid tumors has been with colonic carcinoma and prostatic carcinoma. We have obtained highly purified stromal cells from colonic carcinomas; we have been impressed with the variability of the inflammatory infiltrates observed. Photomicrographs of fractions of stromal cells from human colonic carcinoma have been published (Brattain *et al.*, 1977*b*). The purification of malignant epithelial cells from human colonic carcinomas markedly facilitated the culture of malignant cells in soft agar (Brattain *et al.*, 1977*a,b*). The purification of malignant cells from human colonic carcinomas led to a study of hexosaminidase isoenzymes in normal human colons, human colonic carcinomas, and purified cells from human colonic carcinomas (Brattain *et al.*, 1977*c*). We found that the beta isoenzyme of hexosaminidase is markedly elevated in the malignant cells from human colonic carcinomas as compared with epithelial cells from normal colon. This led to our observation of beta-hexosaminidase in the urine of patients with colonic carcinoma. This isoenzyme promises to be a useful marker in the follow-up of patients with this disease (Brattain *et al.*, 1979).

We have also succeeded in purifying epithelial cells from carcinoma of the prostate (Helms *et al.*, 1976) and from hyperplastic prostates (Helms *et al.*, 1975). The purification of epithelial cells from these tissues has facilitated the biochemical characterization of acid phosphatases from prostatic epithelial cells (Helms *et al.*, 1977).

It would appear to us that the purification of cells from human tumors will facilitate studies of "host" cells and of the malignant cells. In our experience, most human cancers contain approximately one-half "host" cells. Any studies of isoenzymes from autochthonous human tumors must therefore be biased by the presence of these benign cells in homogenates of whole tumor. The precise quantitation of biochemical alterations associated with specific kinds of human malignancies will be dependent upon the availability of purified malignant cells which are representative of the malignant cells in the tumors. Obviously, if the purified malignant cells are to be truly representative of the cells from the tumor, a large proportion of the cells available in tumors must be obtained in suspension. The problem of obtaining representative suspensions of cells from human tumors has received very little study, and the costs and time involved in the study of human tumors when they become available are much greater than the costs and time required for the study of rodent tumors.

(c) Elutriation. In 1948, Lindahl reported the development of a special centrifuge for the separation of cells (Lindahl, 1948). The history of this instrument was reviewed by us in 1975 (T. G. Pretlow *et al.*, 1975). In the late 1960s, the Beckman Instrument Company made one of these instruments and has made it commercially available in the 1970s. They have termed their instrument an "Elutriator," and Lindahl's counterstreaming centrifugation has become Beckman's elutriation. One of the early applications of counterstreaming centrifugation or elutriation was the purification of small, probably inflammatory cells from malignant cells of an ascites tumor (Lindahl and Klein, 1955). Other separations of cells from ascites tumors were reported from Lindahl's group (Lindahl, 1962; Sorenby and Lindahl, 1964). In collaboration with Meistrich, Suzuki *et al.* (1977) separated cells from a cell line derived from a methlcholanthrene-induced fibrosarcoma. Despite an extreme degree of variability among different experiments, they demonstrated that they could achieve some degree of concentration of cells having the capacity to form lung colonies. In one experiment, cells having the capacity to form lung colonies were concentrated 17.6-fold; however, in two other experiments the concentration was 2- to 3-fold. Cells forming colonies in soft agar did not appear to be concentrated by elutriation in these experiments. Since we are never told what proportion of the cells introduced into the elutriator was recovered, it is not possible to know what proportion of this highly variable purification of cells is caused by separation in the elutriator and what proportion is caused by the selective destruction of cells unable to form colonies in lungs. Meistrich (Meistrich *et al.*, 1977) has also reported the purification of cells from hypotetraploid transplantable mouse tumors by elutriation. Cells that had been labeled with tritiated thymidine were concentrated more than twofold in some fractions as compared with other fractions. Meistrich (Meistrich *et al.*, 1977) emphasizes a general problem which we believe has been emphasized too little in the literature: "One limitation appears to be the ability to obtain cells in a good single-cell suspension." This problem is particularly important when autochthonous tumors are the objects of study.

Recently, we have reviewed 43 published articles which have applied elutriation to the separation of cells. It would appear to us that, as suggested by Lindahl (reviewed by T. G. Pretlow et al., 1975), elutriation offers the principal advantage that one can separate as many as 10^8-10^9 cells per centrifugation. Depending upon the kinds of cells studied, the capacity of each elutriation experiment may vary between these limits. As suggested by Lindahl (reviewed by T. G. Pretlow et al., 1975), the principal limitations of elutriation result from the fact that sedimentation by elutriation is not ideal, i.e., there are many artifacts.

(d) Advantages of Various Methods for Velocity Sedimentation. It is our opinion that each of the above described methods for velocity sedimentation has advantages and disadvantages. In our opinion, isokinetic sedimentation and cell separation at unit gravity have approximately the same capacity for resolving cells having different velocities of sedimentation if one assumes that the cells under study will not aggregate in the several hours required for sedimentation at unit gravity. Both techniques lend themselves to work under sterile conditions and show relatively few evidences of toxicity for most cells. Both isokinetic sedimentation and sedimentation at unit gravity can be carried out in most laboratories with very little expense. Both techniques lend themselves to problems that require the separation of 10^7-10^8 cells. The principal disadvantages of sedimentation at unit gravity stem from the fact that the actual sedimentation process requires 3 h or more in most laboratories. While most lymphoid cells and transplantable tumors tolerate the conditions used for sedimentation at unit gravity for 3 h, we prefer to use the shorter period (i.e., 10–20 min) required for cell separation in our isokinetic gradients for work with most kinds of autochthonous tumors or epithelial cells freshly prepared from organs. For many kinds of epithelial cells aggregation is a major problem; it seems preferable for that reason to complete their separation without the necessity that they sit together and aggregate for several hours as required in the technique for cell separation at unit gravity.

Elutriation probably has a lesser capacity for separating cells having different diameters than isokinetic sedimentation or sedimentation at unit gravity; however, the capacity of each experiment with centrifugal elutriation is greater than the capacities of the other two techniques. Meistrich has had extensive experience with both sedimentation at unit gravity and elutriation, and it is his opinion that sedimentation at unit gravity (M. L. Meistrich, personal communication) has a greater capacity for resolving cells with small differences in velocity of sedimentation. Currently, the elutriation rotor costs approximately as much as a large refrigerated centrifuge and, in order to use the elutriator, one needs both an elutriation rotor and a particular kind of refrigerated centrifuge. Recently, Wells and his associates (Wells et al., 1977) have reported the purification of CFU-C, cells which respond to phytohemagglutinin, and cells which respond to concanavalin A in a shallow gradient of Ficoll in tissue culture medium in the Sorvall

SZ-14 reorienting gradient zonal rotor. This rotor separates approximately the same number of cells as can be separated by elutriation. It appears that the SZ-14 rotor is both much cheaper than the elutriator and free of some of the artifacts which are inherent in the design of the elutriator. Much more experience with the SZ-14 rotor and with the elutriator will be required before they can be compared rigorously.

V. CRITERIA FOR THE DOCUMENTATION OF CELL SEPARATION

Probably the most critical deficiency in the literature on the separation of cells is the absence of well-established and generally accepted criteria for the documentation of cell separations. Sophisticated techniques for the separation of cells have been developed during the past decade, and the literature in the multiple areas of cell separation is expanding exponentially. Despite the fact that there appears to be wide recognition of the usefulness of cell separation procedures for a variety of purposes, many of the reports of cell separation currently in excellent journals lack sufficient data to permit us to evaluate them critically. Investigators have been purifying enzymes for many decades, and the criteria by which one evaluates the degree of enzyme purification are well established. One would not consider reporting the purification of an enzyme or even attempting the purification of an enzyme in the absence of a suitable assay for the determination of specific activity. Unfortunately, not all investigators have recognized the need for similar specific methods for the quantitative evaluation of cell separations. In an excellent review on methods for purification, de Duve (1971) wrote ". . . in the early days of centrifugal fractionation, adequate purification of a subcellular organelle was quite unattainable technically, and there were practically no means of evaluating the purity of a preparation. This is how, for instance, nuclei came to be credited with such a wealth of cytoplasmic enzyme activities . . . . Even today, with all of our technical improvements, and with the vast advances in our knowledge, preparative fractionation remains a hazardous undertaking." In an area such as cell separation in which the criteria for purification are both diverse and not well established, the critical assessment of purification is at least as difficult. In the case of separation of cells from tumors, often the concentrations of malignant cells have been judged purely on the basis of morphology, without specific markers for the cells; yet the reader has not been shown photomicrographs to substantiate even this criterion for purity. Not infrequently, investigators have avoided the use of numbers totally and simply reported that the "enriched" cells or the fractions which consisted "primarily of tumor cells" were tested with a biochemical or immunological technique. The most sophisticated biochemical and immunological techniques are of little value when they are used for the analysis of uncharacterized cells.

The first question that must be asked in approaching any purification is: How well does the suspension of cells represent the cells which were present *in situ* in the tissue? One must determine how many cells per gram of tissue were obtained, and one would like to know what proportion of the cells available in the tissue were obtained in suspension. When the number of cells obtained in suspension per gram of tissue is not reported, it is impossible for an investigator in another laboratory to compare work in his laboratory with that carried out in the first laboratory. It is important to know, not just the proportions of lymphocytes, neutrophils, macrophages, tumor cells, etc., in the suspensions obtained from tumors, but the *absolute number* of cells which were obtained in suspension. These data are important (1) for making an estimate of the degree to which the cells in suspension represent the cells in the tissue, and (2) for determining what proportion of the unseparated cells are recovered after cell separation procedures. Numerous reports have omitted these critical data. Without such data, one cannot know if fractions that are "enriched" contain higher concentrations of specific components than the cells prior to separation. It is quite possible that "enriched" or "depleted" fractions from cell separation procedures both contain higher or lower concentrations of a particular component than the starting material, i.e., the separation procedures may be selectively destructive for a particular kind of cell. In the absence of data which give the absolute recovery of each component, we cannot assess whether components are "purified" because of the resolution of the technique or because of selective destruction of other components in the unseparated material. If only a minute proportion of the cells in the starting sample suspension is recovered it is impossible to know just how selective the attrition may have been.

In addition to a numerical expression of the composition of the starting sample suspension of cells and of the fractions of purified cells, it is important for investigators to give some indication of the degree of variability that was encountered among experiments. In surveying the literature in the area of cell separation by a wide variety of techniques, one is tempted to believe that many investigators are not convinced that standard deviations and confidence intervals are of practical importance. Cells are fragile. In our experience, lymphoid cells are less fragile than malignant cells from primary tumors, and it is absolutely essential to give quantitative data that will allow other investigators to evaluate the degree of variability encountered among different experiments.

Ideally, one would like an objective marker that would allow one to quantitate the proportions of cells in suspension before and after purification. Such markers are available in the cells from some kinds of tumors, e.g., uniformly melanotic melanomas; mast cell tumors that make metachromatic, heparin-containing granules; and myeloma cells that make specific immunoglobulins. Unfortunately, reliable markers are not available for most kinds of cancer cells. In the absence of such markers, investigators who want to work with important human tumors are frequently left with only conventional cytology. While conventional cytology is often very helpful, we believe that it is critical that investigators who use conventional cytology as a major criterion for the purification of cells supply readers with photomicrographs that allow the readers to critically evaluate the cytological criteria employed. Such photomicrographs should have sufficient magnification to allow one to appraise the cytology of individual cells accurately. The number of cells photographed should be sufficient to be representative of purified fractions. We believe that photomicrographs are an important kind of data that ought to be supplied with most reports of cell separation. Photomicrographs are inexpensive and communicate both qualitative and quantitative data that readers can interpret and evaluate critically for themselves. In our experience, permanent, stained preparations are much more valuable than "wet preparations." Stained preparations are both permanent records of the experiments that can be critically evaluated by others and much more instructive than wet preparations even in very experienced hands.

In addition to evaluating the degree of purification by morphological markers or other markers that allow one to determine the precise proportion of cells in purified preparations, it is important to determine whether or not the functions of cells have been compromised by the technique for purification. Assays of function have been reviewed by us previously (T. G. Pretlow *et al.*, 1975) and are very familiar to the readers of this series. We shall therefore not dwell on techniques for assessing functions of cells.

VI. CONCLUDING REMARKS

In concluding, we wish to reemphasize the importance of methods for cell separation in the characterization of malignant cells from solid tumors. In view of the common experience that often more than half of cells obtained in suspensions from tumors are "stromal" and "host" cells, the biochemical characterization of alterations associated with neoplastic transformation *in vivo* are dependent upon obtaining pure fractions of malignant cells which are representative of the cells *in situ* in the tumors. Additionally, if the specific functions of "host" cells in tumors are to be investigated, it will be necessary to develop methods that allow investigators to purify specific types of "host" cells in a sufficient yield to be representative of these cells in tumors. Interest in this area of investigation has developed only in recent years, and most of the techniques for purifying "host" cells from tumors have been reported without quantitative estimations of the yields that were achieved. If we are to evaluate accurately the degree to which the functions of purified cells reflect the functions of these cells in tumors, it will be essential that all investigators begin to report the number of cells they obtain per gram of tumor and the proportions of each type of cell in the starting sample suspensions that are recovered after purification. The application of quantitative morphometric techniques to the characterization of autochthonous tumors is in its infancy and is another important requirement if the significance of "host" cells in primary tumors is to be appreciated quantitatively.

ACKNOWLEDGMENTS

This work was supported by Grants CA 13148 and CA 23922 from the National Cancer Institute, and Grant PDT-9B from the American Cancer Society. Dr. Thomas Pretlow was supported by NIH Research Career Development Award K4-CA 70584.

VII. REFERENCES

Alexander, R. F., and Spriggs, A. I., 1960, The differential diagnosis of tumour cells in circulating blood, *J. Clin. Pathol.* 13:414.

Ambrose, E. J. (ed.), 1965, *Cell Electrophoresis*, Little, Brown, and Company, Boston.

Ambrose, E. J., James, A. M., and Lowick, J. H. B., 1956, Differences between the electrical charge carried by normal and homologous tumour cells, *Nature (London)* 177:576.

Andersson, L. C., Nordling, S., and Hayry, P., 1973a, Fractionation of mouse T and B lymphocytes by preparative cell electrophoresis. Efficiency of the method, *Cell Immunol.* 8:235.

Andersson, L. C., Nordling, S., and Hayry, P., 1973b, Proliferation of B and T cells in mixed lymphocyte cultures, *J. Exp. Med.* 138:324.

Andersson, L. C., Nordling, S., and Hayry, P., 1975, Electrophoretic fractionation of guinea pig lymphocytes: Evidence for different subsets of T and B cells in spleen and lymph node, *J. Immunol.* 114:1226.

Arnold, R., 1965, Pathological haemocytopherograms of rats and mice, in: *Cell Electrophoresis*, (E. J. Ambrose, ed.), p. 36, Little, Brown and Company, Boston.

Ben-Or, S., Eisenberg, S., and Doljanski, F., 1960, Electrophoretic mobilities of normal and regenerating liver cells, *Nature (London)* 188:1200.

Berg, J. W., 1959, Inflammation and prognosis in breast cancer. A search for host resistance, *Cancer* 12:714.

Black, M. M., Opler, S. R., and Speer, F. D., 1955, Survival in breast cancer cases in relation to the structure of the primary tumor and regional lymph nodes, *Surg. Gynecol. Obstet.* 100:543.

Blazar, B. A., and Heppner, G. H., 1978a, *In situ* lymphoid cells of mouse mammary tumors. I. Development and evaluation of a method for the separation of lymphoid cells from mouse mammary tumors, *J. Immunol.* 120:1876.

Blazar, B. A., and Heppner, G. H., 1978b, *In situ* lymphoid cells of mouse mammary tumors. II. The characterization of lymphoid cells separated from mouse mammary tumors, *J. Immunol.* 120:1881.

Blazar, B. A., Miller, F. R., and Heppner, G. H., 1978, *In situ* lymphoid cells of mouse mammary tumors. III. *In vitro* stimulation of tumor cell survival by lymphoid cells separated from mammary tumors, *J. Immunol.* 120:1887.

Boltz, R. C. Jr., Todd, P., Streibel, M. G., and Louie, M. K., 1973, Preparative electrophoresis of living mammalian cells in a stationary ficoll gradient, *Prep. Biochem.* 3:383.

Bosmann, H. B., Bieber, G. F., Brown, A. E., Case, K. R., Gersten, D. M., Kimmerer, T. W., and Lione, A., 1973, Biochemical parameters correlated with tumour cell implantation, *Nature (London)* **246**:487.

Brattain, M. G., Kimball, P. M., Pretlow, T. G., II, and Pitts, A. M., 1977a, Partial purification of human colonic carcinoma cells by sedimentation, *Br. J. Cancer* **35**:850.

Brattain, M. G., Pretlow, T. P., and Pretlow, T. G., II, 1977b, Cell fractionation of large bowel cancer, *Cancer* **40**:2479.

Brattain, M. G., Kimball, P. M., and Pretlow, T. G., II, 1977c, β-Hexosaminidase isozymes in human colonic carcinoma, *Cancer Res.* **37**:731.

Brattain, M. G., Kimball, P. M., Durant, J. R., Pretlow, T. G., II, Smith, D., Carpenter, J., and Marks, M., 1979, Urinary hexosaminidase in patients with lung carcinoma, *Cancer* **44**:2267.

Brown, H. C., and Broom, J. C., 1935, The importance of electric charge in certain aspects of immunity, *Trans. R. Soc. Trop. Med. Hyg.* **28**:357.

Carney, P. G., and Malmgren, R. A., 1967, Comparison of techniques for obtaining single cell suspensions from tumors, *Transplantation* **5**:455.

Carstensen, E. L., Fuhrmann, G. F., Smearing, R. W., and Klein, L. A., 1968, The influence of conductivity on the electrophoretic mobility of red blood cells, *Biochim. Biophys. Acta* **156**:394.

Catsimpoolas, N., and Griffith, A. L., 1977, Preparative density gradient electrophoresis and velocity sedimentation at unit gravity of mammalian cells, in: *Methods of Cell Separation*, Vol. I (N. Catsimpoolas, ed.), p. 1, Plenum Press, New York.

Chalkley, H. W., 1943, Method for the quantitative morphologic analysis of tissues, *J. Natl. Cancer Inst.* **4**:47.

Chaudhuri, S., Koprowska, I., Putong, P. B., and Townsend, D. E. R., 1974, Human *in vitro* system for the detection of uterine cervical preinvasive carcinoma, *Cancer Res.* **34**:1335.

Cook, G. M. W., and Jacobson, W., 1968, The electrophoretic mobility of normal and leukaemic cells of mice, *Biochem. J.* **107**:549.

Cook, G. M. W., Heard, D. H., and Seaman, G. V. F., 1962, The electrokinetic characterization of Ehrlich ascites carcinoma cell, *Exp. Cell Res.* **28**:27.

Davis, J., and Ralph, R. K., 1975, Regulation of growth of mouse mastocytoma cells, *Cancer Res.* **35**:1495.

de Duve, C., 1971, Tissue fractionation. Past and present, *J. Cell Biol.* **50**:20D.

Droege, W., Zucker, R., and Jauker, U., 1974a, Cellular composition of the mouse thymus: Developmental changes and the effect of hydrocortisone, *Cell. Immunol.* **12**:173.

Droege, W., Zucker, R., and Hannig, K., 1974b, Developmental changes in the cellular composition of the chicken thymus, *Cell. Immunol.* **12**:186.

Eisenberg, S., Ben-Or, S., and Doljanski, F., 1962, Electro-kinetic properties of cells in growth processes. I. The electrophoretic behavior of liver cells during regeneration and post-natal growth, *Exp. Cell Res.* **26**:451.

Fawcett, D. W., and Vallee, B. L., 1952, Studies on the separation of cell types in sero-sanguinous fluids, blood, and vaginal fluids by flotation on bovine plasma albumin, *J. Lab. Clin. Med.* **39**:354.

Fawcett, D. W., Vallee, B. L., and Soule, M. H., 1950, A method for concentration and segregation of malignant cells from bloody, pleural, and peritoneal fluids, *Science* **111**:34.

Fayet, G., Pacheco, H., and Tixier, R., 1970, Sur la reassociation *in vitro* des cellules isolees de thyroide de porc et la thyrogloubline. I. Conditions pour l'induction des reassociations cellulaires par la thyreostimuline, *Bull. Soc. Chim. Biol.* **52**:299.

Feller, W. F., Stewart, S. E., and Kantor, J., 1972, Primary tissue culture explants of human breast cancer, *J. Natl. Cancer Inst.* **48**:1117.

Fidler, I. J., 1973, Selection of successive tumour lines for metastasis, *Nature (London) New Biol.* **242**:148.

Forrester, J. A., Ambrose, E. J., and Macpherson, J. A., 1962, Electrophoretic investigations of a clone of hamster fibroblasts and polyoma-transformed cells from the same population, *Nature (London)* **196**:1068.

Fuhrmann, G. F., 1965, Cytopherograms of normal, proliferating and malignant rat liver cells, in: *Cell Electrophoresis* (E. J. Ambrose, ed.), p. 92, Little Brown and Company, Boston.

Ganser, M., Hannig, K., Krusmann, W. F., Pascher, G., and Ruhenstroth-Bauer, G., 1968, The separation of blood cells using continuous carrier-free flow electrophoresis, *Klin. Wochenschr.* **46**:809.

Gerstl, B., Switzer, P., and Yesner, R., 1974, A morphometric study of pulmonary cancer, *Cancer Res.* **34**:248.

Gerstl, B., Wong, S., and Yesner, R., 1976, Quantitative microscopy of epidermoid lung carcinoma: Correlation with survival time, *J. Natl. Cancer Inst.* **56**:463.

Gibofsky, A., and Terasaki, P. I., 1972, Trypsinization of lymphocytes for HL-A typing, *Transplantation* **13**:192.

Girard-Mangin, M., and Henri, M. V., 1904, Etude du phenomene d'agglutination. I. Agglutination des globules rouges par l'hydrate ferrique colloidal, *C. R. Soc. Biol.* **56**:866.

Grdina, D. J., Milas, L., Mason, K. A., and Withers, H. R., 1974, Separation of cells from a fibrosarcoma in Renografin density gradients, *J. Natl. Cancer Inst.* **52**:253.

Grdina, D. J., Basic, I., Mason, K. A., and Withers, H. R., 1975, Radiation response of clonogenic cell populations separated from a fibrosarcoma, *Radiat. Res.* **63**:483.

Grdina, D. J., Basic, I., Guzzino, S., and Mason, K. A., 1976, Radiation response of cell populations irradiated *in situ* and separated from a fibrosarcoma, *Radiat. Res.* **66**:634.

Grdina, D. J., Hittelman, W. N., White, R. A., and Meistrich, M. L., 1977, Relevance of density, size, and DNA content of tumour cells to the lung colony assay, *Br. J. Cancer* **36**:659.

Grdina, D. J., Linde, S., and Mason, K., 1978, Response of selected tumour cell populations separated from a fibrosarcoma following irradiation *in situ* with fast neutrons, *Br. J. Radiol.* **51**:291.

Halpern, B. C., Ezzell, R., Hardy, D. N., Clark, B. R., Ashe, H., Halpern, R. M., and Smith, R. A., 1975, Effect of methionine replacement by homocystine in cultures containing both malignant rat breast carcinosarcoma (Walker-256) cells and normal adult rat liver fibroblasts, *In Vitro* **11**:14.

Hamilton, W. A., and Sale, A. J. H., 1967, Effects of high electric fields on microorganisms. II. Mechanism of action of the lethal effect, *Biochim. Biophys. Acta.* **148**:789.

Hannig, K., 1964, Eine neuentwicklung der tragerfreien kontinuierlichen elektrophorese, *Hoppe-Seyler's Z. Physiol. Chem.* **338**:211.

Hannig, K., 1967, Preparative electrophoresis, in: *Electrophoresis: Theory, Methods, and Applications*, Vol. 2 (M. Bier, ed.), p. 423, Academic Press, New York.

Hannig, K., 1969, The application of free-flow electrophoresis to the separation of macromolecules and particles of biological importance, in: *Modern Separation Methods of Macromolecules and Particles*, Vol. 2 (T. Gerritson, ed.), p. 45, Wiley-Interscience, New York.

Hannig, K., 1971, Free-flow electrophoresis. A technique for continuous preparative and analytical separation, in: *Methods in Microbiology*, Vol. 5B (J. R. Norris and D. W. Ribbons, eds.), p. 513, Academic Press, New York.

Hannig, K., 1972, Separation of cells and particles by continuous free-flow electrophoresis, in: *Techniques of Biochemical and Biophysical Morphology*, Vol. 1 (D. Glick and R. M. Rosenbaum, eds.), p. 191, Wiley-Interscience, New York.

Hannig, K., and Krusmann, W-F., 1968, Die anwendung der tragerfreien kontinuierlichen elektrophorese zur auftrennung der weiben blutzellen aus humanblut, *Hoppe-Seyler's Z. Physiol. Chem.* **349**:161.

Hannig, K., and Zeiller, K., 1969, Separation and characterization of immunocompetent cells with the aid of the free-flow continuous electrophoresis, *Hoppe-Seyler's Z. Physiol. Chem.* **350**:467.

Hannig, K., Wirth, H., Meyer, B-H., and Zeiller, K., 1975, Free-flow electrophoresis. I. Theoretical and experimental investigations of the influence of mechanical and electrokinetic variables on the efficiency of the method, *Hoppe-Seyler's Z. Physiol. Chem.* **356**:1209.

Hartveit, F., Cater, D. B., and Mehrishi, J. N., 1968, Changes in the electrophoretic mobility of mouse lymphocytes, thymocytes, macrophages, and tumour cells following immunisation, *Br. J. Exp. Pathol.* **49**:634.

Haskill, J. S., 1977, ADCC effector cells in a murine adenocarcinoma. I. Evidence for bloodborne bone-marrow-derived monocytes, *Int. J. Cancer* **20**:432.

Haskill, J. S., Proctor, J. W., and Yamamura, Y., 1975a, Host responses within solid tumors. I. Monocytic effector cells within rat sarcomas, *J. Natl. Cancer Inst.* **54**:387.

Haskill, J. S., Yamamura, Y., and Radov, L., 1975b, Host responses within solid tumors: Non-thymus-derived specific cytotoxic cells within a murine mammary adenocarcinoma, *Int. J. Cancer* **16**:798.

Haskill, J. S., Yamamura, Y., Radov, L., and Parthenais, E., 1976, Discussion paper: Are peripheral and *in situ* tumor immunity related?, *Ann. N.Y. Acad. Sci.* **276**:373.

Hayry, P., and Andersson, L. C., 1975, Generation of T memory cells in one-way mixed lymphocyte culture. III. Homing and lifetime of "secondary" lymphocytes, *Cell. Immunol.* **17**:165.

Hayry, P., Penttinen, K., and Saxen, E., 1965, The different effects of some methods of disaggregation on the electrophoretic mobility of the HeLa-cell, *Ann. Med. Exp. Fenn.* **43**:91.

Hayry, P., Andersson, L. C., and Nordling, S., 1973, Electrophoretic fractionation of mouse T and B lymphocytes. Efficiency of the method and purity of separated cells, *Transpl. Proc.* **5**:87.

Hayry, P., Andersson, L. C., Gahmberg, C., Roberts, P., Ranki, A., and Nordling, S., 1975a, Fractionation of immunocompentent cells by free-flow cell electrophoresis, *Isr. J. Med. Sci.* **11**:1299.

Hayry, P., Kontiainen, S., Nordling, S., and Andersson, L. C., 1975b, Comparison between thymus-dependent and thymus-independent lymphocytes as stimulator cells in allogeneic mixed lymphocyte culture, *Acta Pathol. Microbiol. Scand. Sect. C* **83**:249.

Heard, D. H., Seaman, G. V. F., and Simon-Reuss, I., 1961, Electrophoretic mobility of cultured mesodermal tissue cells, *Nature (London)* **190**:1009.

Heidrich, H.-G., and Dew, M. E., 1977, Homogeneous cell populations from rabbit kidney cortex. Proximal, distal tubule, and renin-active cell isolated by free-flow electrophoresis, *J. Cell Biol.* **74**:780.

Heisto, H., Jensen, L., and Knuds, F., 1971, Studies on trypsin treatment of red cells with special reference to differences between trypsin preparations, *Vox Sang.* **21**:115.

Helms, S. R., Brazeal, F. I., Bueschen, A. J., and Pretlow, T. G., II, 1975, Separation of cells with histochemically demonstrable acid phosphatase activity from suspensions of human prostatic cells in an isokinetic gradient of Ficoll in tissue culture medium, *Am. J. Pathol.* **80**:79.

Helms, S. R., Pretlow, T. G., II, Bueschen, A. J., Lloyd, K. L., and Murad, T. M., 1976, Separation of cells with histochemically demonstrable acid phosphatase activity from suspensions of cells from human prostatic carcinomas in an isokinetic gradient of Ficoll in tissue culture medium, *Cancer Res.* 36:481.

Helms, S. R., Brattain, M. G., Pretlow, T. G., II, and Kreisberg, J. I., 1977, "Prostatic acid phosphatase?" A comparison of acid phosphatase activities in epithelial cells, granulocytes, monocytes, lymphocytes, and platelets purified by velocity sedimentation in isokinetic gradients of Ficoll in tissue culture medium, *Am. J. Pathol.* 88:529.

Helting, T., Ogren, S., Lindahl, U., Pertoft, H., and Laurent, T., 1972, Glycosaminoglycan synthesis in mouse mastocytoma, *Biochem. J.* 126:587.

Herberman, R. B., and Oldham, R. K., 1975, Problems associated with study of cell-mediated immunity to human tumors by microcytotoxicity assays. *J. Natl. Cancer Inst.* 55:749.

Herve, P., Masse, M., Lenys, R., and Peters, A., 1975, Application des methodes preparatives en veine liquide a la separation des cellules sanguines, *Rev. Fr. Transfus. Immunohematol.* 18:439.

Hilfer, S. R., and Brown, J. M., 1971, Collagenase. Its effectiveness as a dispersing agent for embryonic chick thyroid and heart, *Exp. Cell Res.* 65:246.

Holden, H. T., Haskill, J. S., Kirchner, H., and Herberman, R. B., 1976, Two functionally distinct anti-tumor effector cells isolated from primary murine sarcoma virus-induced tumors, *J. Immunol.* 117:440.

Hommes, F. A., Draisma, M. I., and Molenaar, I., 1970, Preparation and some properties of isolated rat liver cells, *Biochim. Biophys. Acta* 222:361.

Hughes, R. C., Sanford, B., and Jeanloz, R. W., 1972, Regeneration of the surface glycoproteins of a transplantable mouse tumor cell after treatment with neuraminidase, *Proc. Natl. Acad. Sci. USA* 69:942.

Ioachim, H. L., 1976, The stromal reaction of tumors: An expression of immune surveillance, *J. Natl. Cancer Inst.* 57:465.

Ioachim, H. L., Dorsett, B. H., and Paluch, E., 1976, The immune response at the tumor site in lung carcinoma, *Cancer* 38:2296.

Just, W. W., León-V., J. O., and Werner, G., 1975, Isoelectric focusing in continuous-flow electrophoresis. I. Separation of mixed red blood cells of different species, *Anal. Biochem.* 67:590.

Katz, D. H., Order, S. E., Graves, M., and Benacerraf, B., 1973, Purification of Hodgkin's disease tumor-associated antigens, *Proc. Natl. Acad. Sci. USA* 70:396.

Kloppenborg, P. W. C., Island, D. P., Liddle, G. W., Michelakis, A. M., and Nicholson, W. E., 1968, A method of preparing adrenal cell suspensions and its applicability to the *in vitro* study of adrenal metabolism, *Endocrinology* 82:1053.

Knutson, F., Lundin, P. M., and Norrby, K., 1971, Syngeneic serum and ascitic fluid in enzymatically produced tumour cell suspensions, *Pathol. Eur.* 6:34.

Kono, T., 1969, Roles of collagenases and other proteolytic enzymes in the dispersal of animal tissues, *Biochim. Biophys. Acta* 178:397.

Kono, T., and Barham, F. W., 1971, The relationship between the insulin-binding capacity of fat cells and the cellular response to insulin. Studies with intact and trypsin-treated fat cells, *J. Biol. Chem.* 246:6210.

Kreisberg, J. I., Pitts, A. M., and Pretlow, T. G., II, 1977a, Separation of proximal tubule cells from suspensions of rat kidney cells in density gradients of Ficoll in tissue culture medium, *Am. J. Pathol.* 86:591.

Kreisberg, J. I., Sachs, G., Pretlow, T. G., II, and McGuire, R. A., 1977b, Separation of proximal tubule cells from suspensions of rat kidney cells by free-flow electrophoresis, *J. Cell. Physiol.* 93:169.

Lasfargues, E. Y., Coutinho, W. G., and Moore, D. H., 1972, Pitfalls in the isolation of a human breast carcinoma virus in tissue culture, *J. Natl. Cancer Inst.* 48:1101.

Latner, A. L., and Turner, G. A., 1974, Surface modification and electrophoresis of normal and transformed BHK_{21} cells, *J. Cell Sci.* **14**:203.

Leif, R. C., 1970, Buoyant density separation of cells, in: *Automated Cell Identification and Cell Sorting* (G. L. Wied and G. F. Bahr, eds.), p. 21, Academic Press, New York.

Leise, E. M., and LeSane, F., 1974, Isoelectric focusing of peripheral lymphocytes, *Prep. Biochem.* **4**:395.

Lichtman, M. A., and Weed, R. I., 1970, Electrophoretic mobility and N-acetyl neuraminic acid content of human normal and leukemic lymphocytes and granulocytes, *Blood* **35**:12.

Lillie, R. S., 1902, On differences in the direction of the electrical convection of certain free cells and nuclei, *Am. J. Physiol.* **8**:273.

Lindahl, P. E., 1948, Principle of a counter-streaming centrifuge for the separation of particles of different sizes, *Nature (London)* **161**:648.

Lindahl, P. E., 1962, Lipid content in hyperdiploid and hypertetraploid cells isolated from the hyperdiploid Ehrlich ascites tumour, *Nature (London)* **194**:589.

Lindahl, P. E., and Klein, G., 1955, Separation of Ehrlich ascites tumour cells from other cellular elements, *Nature (London)* **176**:401.

Lowick, J. H. B., Purdom, L., James, A. M., and Ambrose, E. J., 1961, Some microelectrophoretic studies of normal and tumour cells, *J. R. Microsc. Soc.* **80**:47.

MacDonald, H. R., Howell, R. L., and McFarlane, D. L., 1978, The multicellular spheroid as a model tumor allograft, *Transplantation* **25**:141.

Maslow, D. E., 1970, Electrokinetic surfaces of trypsin-dissociated embryonic chick liver cells, *Exp. Cell Res.* **61**:266.

Mavligit, G. M., Gutterman, J. U., and Hersh, E. M., 1973, Separation of viable from nonviable tumor cells using Ficoll–Hypaque density solution, *Immunol. Commun.* **2**:463.

Mavligit, G. M., Barsales, P. B., Gutterman, J. U., Mackay, B., and Hersh, E. M., 1975, A rapid method for establishing short-term primary cultures of human tumor cells from fresh tumor biopsies, *Proc. Soc. Exp. Biol. Med.* **150**:597.

Mayhew, E., 1968, Electrophoretic mobility of Ehrlich ascites carcinoma cells grown *in vitro* or *in vivo*, *Cancer Res.* **28**:1590.

McClay, D. R., Gooding, L. R., and Fransen, M. E., 1977, A requirement for trypsin-sensitive cell-surface components for cell–cell interactions of embryonic neural retina cells. *J. Cell Biol.* **75**:56.

McGuire, R. A., Jr., Pretlow, T. G., II, Wareing, T. H., and Bradley, E. L., 1979, Hodgkin's cells and attached lymphocytes: A possible prognostic indicator in splenic tumor, *Cancer* **44**:183.

Mehrishi, J. N., and Thomson, A. E. R., 1968, Relationship between pH and electrophoretic mobility for lymphocytes circulating in chornic lymphocytic leukaemia, *Nature (London)* **219**:1080.

Mehrishi, J. N., and Zeiller, K., 1974, T and B lymphocytes: Striking differences in surface membranes, *Br. Med. J.* **1**:360.

Meistrich, M. L., Grdina, D. J., Meyn, R. E., and Barlogie, B., 1977, Separation of cells from mouse solid tumors by centrifugal elutriation, *Cancer Res.* **37**:4291.

Melchers, F., Cone, R. E., von Boehmer, H., and Sprent, J., 1975, Immunoglobulin turnover in B lymphocyte subpopulations, *Eur. J. Immunol.* **5**:382.

Nairn, R. C., Nind, A. P. P., Guli, E. P. G., Muller, H. K., Rolland, J. M., and Minty, C. C. J., 1971, Specific immune response in human skin carcinoma, *Br. Med. J.* **4**:701.

Ng, C. E., and Inch, W. R., 1978, Comparison of the densities of clonogenic cells from EMT6 fibrosarcoma monolayer cultures, multicell spheroids, and solid tumors in Ficoll density gradients, *J. Natl. Cancer Inst.* **60**:1017.

Nordling, S., Andersson, L. C., and Hayry, P., 1972, Thymus-dependent and thymus-independent lymphocyte separation: Relation to exposed sialic acid on cell surface, *Science* **178**:1001.

Norrby, K., Knutson, F., and Lundin, P. M., 1966, On the single cell state in enzymatically produced tumor cell suspensions, *Exp. Cell Res.* **44**:421.

Oppenheimer, S. B., and Humphreys, T., 1971, Isolation of specific macromolecules required for adhesion of mouse tumour cells, *Nature (London)* **232**:125.

Order, S. E., Porter, M., and Hellman, S., 1971, Hodgkin's disease: Evidence for a tumor-associated antigen, *N. Engl. J. Med.* **285**:471.

Order, S., Chism, S. E., and Hellman, S., 1972, Studies of antigens associated with Hodgkin's disease, *Blood* **40**:621.

Osmond, D. G., Miller, R. G., and von Boehmer, H., 1975, Characterization of immuno-globulin-bearing and other small lymphocytes in mouse bone marrow by sedimentation and electrophoresis, *J. Immunol.* **114**:1230.

Pertoft, H., 1970, Separation of cells from a mast cell tumor on density gradients of colloidal silica, *J. Natl. Cancer Inst.* **44**:1251.

Pine, L., Taylor, G. C., Miller, D. M., Bradley, G., and Wetmore, H. R., 1969, Comparison of good and bad lots of trypsin used in the production of primary monkey kidney cells. A definition of the problem and comparison of certain enzymatic characteristics, *Cytobios* **2**:197.

Pretlow, T. G., 1971, Estimation of experimental conditions that permit cell separations by velocity sedimentation on isokinetic gradients of Ficoll in tissue culture medium, *Anal. Biochem.* **41**:248.

Pretlow, T. G., II, 1978, Isolation of lymphocyte populations, *Natl. Cancer Inst. Monogr.* **49**:79.

Pretlow, T. G., and Boone, C. W., 1969, Separation of mammalian cells using programmed gradient sedimentation, *Exp. Mol. Pathol.* **11**:139.

Pretlow, T. G., and Boone, C. W., 1970, Separation of malignant cells from transplantable rodent tumors, *Exp. Mol. Pathol.* **12**:249.

Pretlow, T. G., II, and Cassady, I. M., 1970, Separation of mast cells in successive stages of differentiation using programmed gradient sedimentation, *Am. J. Pathol.* **61**:323.

Pretlow, T. G., II, and Pretlow, T. P., 1977, Separation of viable cells by velocity sedimentation in an isokinetic gradient of Ficoll in tissue culture medium, in: *Biological Separations. Methods of Cell Separation*, Vol. I (N. Catsimpoolas, ed.), p. 171, Plenum Press, New York.

Pretlow, T. G., Glick, M. R., and Reddy, W. J., 1972, Separation of beating cardiac myocytes from suspensions of heart cells, *Am. J. Pathol.* **67**:215.

Pretlow, T. G., Luberoff, D. E., Hamilton, L. J., Weinberger, P. C., Maddox, W. A., and Durant, J. R., 1973, Pathogenesis of Hodgkin's disease: Separation and culture of different kinds of cells from Hodgkin's disease in a sterile isokinetic gradient of Ficoll in tissue culture medium, *Cancer* **31**:1120.

Pretlow, T. G., II, Jones, J., and Dow, S., 1974, Separation of cells having histochemically demonstrable glucose-6-phosphatase from suspensions of hamster kidney cells in an isokinetic density gradient of Ficoll in tissue culture medium, *Am. J. Pathol.* **74**:275.

Pretlow, T. G., II, Weir, E. E., and Zettergren, J. G., 1975, Problems connected with the separation of different kinds of cells, *Int. Rev. Exp. Pathol.* **14**:91.

Pretlow, T. G., II, Jones, C. M., and Pretlow, T. P., 1976, Separation of tumor cells by density gradient centrifugation: Recent work with human tumors and a discussion of the kind of quantitation needed in cell separation experiments, *Biophys. Chem.* **5**:99.

Pretlow, T. P., Glover, G. L., and Pretlow, T. G., II, 1977*a*, Separation of lymphocytes and mast cells from the Furth transplantable mast cell tumor in an isokinetic gradient of Ficoll in tissue culture medium, *Cancer Res.* **37**:578.

Pretlow, T. P., Glover, G. L., and Pretlow, T. G., II, 1977b, Purification of malignant cells and lymphocytes from a rat transplantable mucinous adenocarcinoma of the colon by isokinetic sedimentation in gradients of Ficoll, *J. Natl. Cancer Inst.* **59**:981.

Pretlow, T. G., II, Pretlow, T. P., and Crockett, F., 1980, Electrophoretic separation of tonsillar cells, manuscript in preparation.

Purdom, L., Ambrose, E. J., and Klein, G., 1958, A correlation between electrical surface charge and some biological characteristics during the stepwise progression of a mouse sarcoma, *Nature (London)* **181**:1586.

Roelants, G. E., Loor, F., von Boehmer, H., Sprent, J., Haag, L.-B., Mayor, K. S., and Ryden, A., 1975, Five types of lymphocytes Ig$^-\Theta^-$, Ig$^-\Theta^{+\text{weak}}$, Ig$^-\Theta^{+\text{strong}}$, Ig$^+\Theta^-$ and Ig$^+\Theta^+$) characterized by double immunofluorescence and electrophoretic mobility. Organ distribution in normal and nude mice, *Eur. J. Immunol.* **5**:127.

Rosenberg, S. A., and Rogentine, G. N., Jr., 1972, Natural human antibodies to "hidden" membrane components, *Nature (London) New Biol.* **239**:203.

Ruhenstroth-Bauer, G., 1965, The normal and pathological haemocytopherogram of man, in: *Cell Electrophoresis* (E. J. Ambrose, ed.), p. 66, Little, Brown and Company, Boston.

Russell, S. W., Gillespie, G. Y., Hansen, C. B., and Cochrane, C. G., 1976, Inflammatory cells in solid murine neoplasms. II. Cell types found throughout the course of Moloney sarcoma regression or progression, *Int. J. Cancer* **18**:331.

Schlegel, R. A., Shortman, K., Stocker, J. W., and Odgers, M., 1975a, Antigen-dependent B lymphocyte differentiation. A comparison of the electrophoretic mobilities of AFC-progenitors, induced AFC and background AFC specific for several antigens, *Aust. J. Exp. Biol. Med. Sci.* **53**:117.

Schlegel, R. A., von Boehmer, H., and Shortman, K., 1975b, Antigen-initiated B lymphocyte differentiation. V. Electrophoretic separation of different subpopulations of AFC progenitors for unprimed IgM and memory IgG responses to the NIP determinant, *Cell. Immunol.* **16**:203.

Schlesinger, M., and Gottesfeld, S., 1971, The effect of neuraminidase on expression of cellular antigens, *Transpl. Proc.* **3**:1151.

Schubert, J. C. F., Walther, F., Holzberg, E., Pascher, G., and Zeiller, K., 1973, Preparative electrophoretic separation of normal and neoplastic human bone marrow cells, *Klin. Wochenschr.* **51**:327.

Seaman, G. V. F., and Uhlenbruck, G., 1963, The surface structure of erythrocytes from some animal sources, *Arch. Biochem. Biophys.* **100**:493.

Seiler, F. R., Johannsen, R., Sedlacek, H. H., and Zeiller, K., 1974, Characterization of lymphocyte subpopulations of nonhuman primates separated by free-flow electrophoresis, *Transpl. Proc.* **6**:173.

Shafie, S. M., Gibson, S. L., and Hilf, R., 1977, Effect of insulin and estrogen on hormone binding in the R3230AC mammary adenocarcinoma, *Cancer Res.* **37**:4641.

Sheridan, J. W., and Finlay-Jones, J. J., 1977, Studies on a fractionated murine fibrosarcoma. A reproducible method for the cautious and a caution for the unwary, *J. Cell. Physiol.* **90**:535.

Shortman, K., 1972, Physical Procedures for the separation of animal cells, *Ann. Rev. Biophys. Bioeng.* **1**:93.

Shortman, K., von Boehmer, H., Lipp, J., and Hopper, K., 1975, Subpopulations of T lymphocytes, *Transpl. Rev.* **25**:163.

Simon-Reuss, I., Cook, G. M. W., Seaman, G. V. F., and Heard, D. H., 1964, Electrophoretic studies on some types of mammalian tissue cell, *Cancer Res.* **24**:2038.

Soderman, D. D., Germershausen, J., Katzen, H. M., 1973, Affinity binding of intact fat cells and their ghosts to immobilized insulin, *Proc. Natl. Acad. Sci. USA* **70**:792.

Sorenby, L., and Lindahl, P. E., 1964, On the concentrating of ascites tumour cells in stages of pre-mitosis and mitosis by counter-streaming centrifugation, *Exp. Cell Res.* 35:214.

Speicher, D. W., and McCarl, R. L., 1974, Pancreatic enzyme requirements for the dissociation of rat hearts for culture, *In Vitro* 10:30.

Spriggs, A. I., and Alexander, R. F., 1960, An albumin gradient method for separating the different white cells of blood, applied to the concentration of circulating tumour cells, *Nature (London)* 188:863.

Stein, G., 1975a, Separation of human lymphoid cells by preparative cell electrophoresis. II. Free-flow electrophoretic separation of human blood cells, *Biomedicine* 23:5.

Stein, G., 1975b, Separation of human lymphoid cells by preparative cell electrophoresis, *Z. Immunol. Forsch.* 150:68.

Stein, G., Flad, H. D., Pabst, R., and Trepel, F., 1973, Separation of human lymphocytes by free-flow electrophoresis, *Biomedicine* 19:388.

Stewart, M. J., Pretlow, T. G., II, and Hiramoto, R., 1972, Separation of ascites myeloma cells, lymphocytes and macrophages by zonal centrifugation on an isokinetic gradient, *Am. J. Pathol.* 68:163.

Suzuki, N., Frapart, M., Grdina, D. J., Meistrich, M. L., and Withers, H. R., 1977, Cell cycle dependency of metastatic lung colony formation, *Cancer Res.* 37:3690.

Thompson, K., Ceriani, R. L., Wong, D., and Abraham, S., 1976, Immunologic methods for the identification of cell types. I. Specific antibodies that distinguish between mammary gland epithelial cells and fibroblasts, *J. Natl. Cancer Inst.* 57:167.

Tulp, A., and Welagen, J. J. M. N., 1976, Fractionation of ascites tumour cells at 1g: Separation of cells in specific stages of the life cycle, *Eur. J. Cancer* 12:519.

Turner, M. J., Stroominger, J. L., and Sanderson, A. R., 1972, Enzymic removal and re-expression of a histocompatibility antigen, HL-A 2, at the surface of human peripheral lymphocytes, *Proc. Natl. Acad. Sci. USA* 69:200.

Underwood, J. C. E., 1972, A morphometric analysis of human breast carcinoma, *Br. J. Cancer* 26:234.

Underwood, J. C. E., 1974, Lymphoreticular infiltration in human tumours: Prognostic and biological implications: A review, *Br. J. Cancer* 30:538.

Vaage, J., 1968, A mechanical technique for obtaining high yields of viable, dispersed tumor cells, *Transplantation* 6:137.

Vallee, B. L., Hughes, W. L., Jr., and Gibson, J. G., II, 1947, A method for the separation of leukocytes from whole blood by flotation on serum albumin, *Blood (Special Issue)* 1:82.

Vassar, P. S., 1963, The electric charge density of human tumor cell surfaces, *Lab. Invest.* 12:1072.

Vassar, P. S., Hards, J. M., and Seaman, G. V. F., 1973, Surface properties of human lymphocytes, *Biochem. Biophys. Acta* 291:107.

von Boehmer, H., 1974, Separation of T and B lymphocytes and their role in the mixed lymphocyte reaction, *J. Immunol.* 112:70.

von Boehmer, H., Shortman, K., and Nossal, G. J. V., 1974, The separation of different cell classes from lymphoid organs. X. Preparative electrophoretic separation of lymphocyte subpopulations from mouse spleen and thoracic duct lymph, *J. Cell. Physiol.* 83:231.

Wallach, D. F. H., and Esandi, M. V. D. P., 1964, Sialic acid and the electrophoretic mobility of three tumor cell types, *Biochim. Biophys. Acta* 83:363.

Waymouth, C., 1974, To disaggregate or not to disaggregate. Injury and cell disaggregation, transient or permanent? *In Vitro* 10:97.

Weibel, E. R., 1963, Principles and methods for the morphometric study of the lung and other organs, *Lab. Invest.* 12:131.

Weibel, E. R., Kistler, G. S., and Scherle, W. F., 1966, Practical stereological methods for morphometric cytology, *J. Cell Biol.* 30:23.

Weiss, L., 1966, Effect of temperature on cellular electrophoretic mobility phenomena, *J. Natl. Cancer Inst.* 36:837.

Weiss, L., and Horoszewicz, J. S., 1971, Some biophysical aspects of E-B virus adsorption to the surfaces of three types of mammalian cells, *Int. J. Cancer* 7:149.

Weiss, L., Zeigel, R., Jung, O. S., and Bross, I. D. J., 1972, Binding of positively charged particles to glutaraldehyde-fixed human erythrocytes, *Exp. Cell Res.* 70:57.

Wells, J. R., Opelz, G., and Cline, M. J., 1977, Characterization of functionally distinct lymphoid and myeloid cells from human blood and bone marrow. II. Separation by velocity sedimentation, *J. Immunol. Meth.* 18:79.

Wepsic, H. T., 1970, Separation of viable tumor cells from non-viable tumor cells by flotation on bovine serum albumin. A short communication, *J. Natl. Cancer Inst.* 45:1031.

Wiig, J. N., 1974, Effect of neuraminidase on lymphoid cells, *Scand J. Immunol.* 3:357.

Willson, J. K. V., Luberoff, D. E., Pitts, A., and Pretlow, T. G., 1975, A method for the separation of lymphocytes and plasma cells from the human palatine tonsil using sedimentation in an isokinetic gradient of Ficoll in tissue culture medium, *Immunology* 28:161.

Willson, J. K. V., Pretlow, T. G., II, Zaremba, J. L., and Brattain, M. G., 1976a, Heterogeneity among preparations of crude trypsin used to disaggregate the human tonsil, *Immunology* 30:157.

Willson, J. K. V., Jr., Zaremba, J. L., Pitts, A. M., and Pretlow, T. G., II, 1976b, A characterization of human tonsillar lymphocytes after separation from other tonsillar cells in an isokinetic gradient of Ficoll in tissue culture medium, *Am. J. Pathol.* 83:341.

Willson, J. K. V., Jr., Zaremba, J. L., and Pretlow, T. G., II, 1977, Functional characterization of cells separated from suspensions of Hodgkin disease tumor cells in an isokinetic gradient, *Blood* 50:783.

Wolff, D. A., 1977, Rapid separation of living cells by colloidal silica density gradient centrifugation, *Tissue Cult. Assoc. Man.* 3:717.

Woo, J., and Cater, D. B., 1972, A study of the cell surface of tumour, foetal and lymph-node cells by cell electrophoresis after antibody and enzymic treatment, *Biochem. J.* 128:1273.

Yarlott, M. A., Jr., and McKhann, C. F., 1976, Discussion paper: *In vitro* augmentation of tumor immunity in a murine methylcholanthrene sarcoma system, *Ann. N.Y. Acad. Sci.* 277:533.

Zeiller, K., and Hannig, K., 1971, Free-flow electrophoretic separation of lymphocytes. Evidence for specific organ distributions of lymphoid cells, *Hoppe-Seyler's Z. Physiol. Chem.* 352:1162.

Zeiller, K., and Pascher, G., 1973, Detection of T and B cell-specific heteroantigens on electrophoretically separated lymphocytes of the mouse, *Eur. J. Immunol.* 3:614.

Zeiller, K., Pascher, G., and Hannig, K., 1970, The formation of 19S hemolysin-producing cells in intestinal lymph nodes of the rat, *Hoppe-Seyler's Z. Physiol. Chem.* 351:435.

Zeiller, K., Hannig, K., and Pascher, G., 1971, Free-flow electrophoretic separation of lymphocytes. Separation of graft versus host reactive lymphocytes of rat spleens, *Hoppe-Seyler's Z. Physiol. Chem.* 352:1168.

Zeiller, K., Holzberg, E., Pascher, G., and Hannig, K., 1972a, Free-flow electrophoretic separation of T and B lymphocytes. Evidence for various subpopulations of B cells, *Hoppe-Seyler's Z. Physiol. Chem.* 353:105.

Zeiller, K., Pascher, G., and Hannig, K., 1972b, Preparative electrophoretic separation of antibody forming cells, *Prep. Biochem.* 2:21.

Zeiller, K., Schubert, J. C. F., Walther, F., and Hannig, K., 1972c, Free-flow electrophoretic separation of bone marrow cells. Electrophoretic distribution analysis of *in vivo* colony forming cells in mouse bone marrow, *Hoppe-Seyler's Z. Physiol. Chem.* **353**:95.

Zeiller, K., Pascher, G., Wagner, G., Liebich, H. G., Holzberg, E., and Hannig, K., 1974, Distinct subpopulations of thymus-dependent lymphocytes. Tracing of the differentiation pathway of T cells by use of preparatively electrophoretically separated mouse lymphocytes, *Immunology* **26**:995.

Zeiller, K., Loser, R., Pascher, G., and Hannig, K., 1975a, Free-flow electrophoresis. II. Analysis of the method with respect to preparative cell separation, *Hoppe-Seyler's Z. Physiol. Chem.* **356**:1225.

Zeiller, K., Schindler, R. K., and Liebich, H.-G., 1975b, The T lymphocyte surface in development. A study of the electrokinetic, antigenic and ultrastructural properties of T lymphocytes in mouse thymus and lymph nodes, *Isr. J. Med. Sci.* **11**:1242.

Zeiller, K., Pascher, G., and Hannig, K., 1976, B lymphocyte subpopulations in the mouse spleen. A study of the differentiation pathway using free flow electrophoretically separated subpopulations of direct PFC progenitor cells, *Immunology* **31**:863.

Zettergren, J. G., Luberoff, D. E., and Pretlow, T. G., 1973, Separation of lymphocytes from disaggregated mouse malignant neoplasms by sedimentation in gradients in Ficoll in tissue culture medium, *J. Immunol.* **111**:836.

Chapter 3

Immunologic Reactivity of Lymphoid Cells in Tumors

Ronald B. Herberman, Howard T. Holden, Luigi Varesio,
Tadayoshi Taniyama, Paolo Puccetti, Holger Kirchner,
James Gerson, Sandra White, and Yona Keisari

Laboratories of Immunodiagnosis and Immunobiology
National Cancer Institute
Bethesda, Maryland 20205

and

J. Stephen Haskill

Medical University of South Carolina
Charleston, South Carolina 29401

I. INTRODUCTION

There have been many studies of immune responses against tumors and almost all of these have focused on the reactivity in the blood or spleen. From such studies, it has become clear that a wide variety of effector cells and types of immune functions may be involved in antitumor responses. Particular attention has been directed toward T cells that may be directly cytotoxic against tumor cells or may proliferate or produce lymphokines upon stimulation with tumor antigens. However, other effector mechanisms may be involved and need to be considered. These include B cells, which can produce antibodies that affect tumor cells directly or that interact with K cells or macrophages and thereby mediate antibody-dependent cell-mediated cytotoxicity; macrophages and monocytes, which are spontaneously cytotoxic or can be activated to become cytotoxic against tumor cells; and natural killer (NK) cells, a subpopulation of lymphocytes with spontaneous cytotoxic reactivity against tumor cells.

It is unclear which of these effector mechanisms are represented within tumors. Immune factors that are found *in situ* would be more likely to have a role in resistance against tumor growth. Conversely, failure to find in tumors some immune activities that are well represented in central lymphoid organs might provide clues to the usual inability of the immune response to success-fully limit tumor progression. Therefore, recent attention has been directed toward studies of *in situ* immunologic reactivity. It has been possible to isolate lymphoid cells from tumors, to separate subpopulations of these cells according to their functional or physical characteristics, and to evaluate their functional activity in a number of *in vitro* assays. Such studies have revealed a considerable variety of lymphoid cell functions, with subpopulations of cells exerting anti-tumor activity and with some cells actually suppressing immune responses, such as lymphocyte proliferation and lymphokine production.

Most of our studies in experimental animals have been performed on C57BL/6 or other strains of mice, in which primary tumors were induced by intramuscular inoculation of murine sarcoma virus (MSV). This has provided a good model system for analyzing the various facets of the systemic and *in situ* immune re-ponse, since techniques have been developed to consistently detect specific and nonspecific effector mechanisms in tumor-bearing mice. In addition, it has been possible to compare immune responses in mice which can completely regress their tumors to those in mice which eventually die from progressively growing tumors. After inoculation of the usual stock of Moloney MSV into adult, immuno-competent mice, tumors appear rapidly, reach peak size at about 14 days, and then usually regress completely by 21–28 days. In contrast, progressively growing tumors can be induced by inoculating the same stock of virus into immunologi-cally deficient mice, e.g., nude mice or very young mice, or by inoculating adult mice with a variant stock of MSV (Lavrin *et al.*, 1973; Takeichi *et al.*, 1978).

Based on some of the techniques developed in the experimental tumor systems, and on the results of those studies, we have also performed some pre-liminary studies on effector cells in human tumors. Most of our attention thus far has been focused on whether natural killer cell activity can be detected at the tumor site.

II. REACTIVITY OF IMMUNE T CELLS

A. Reactivity of Cells in Spleen and Other Lymphoid Organs

In mice bearing regressing MSV tumors, high levels of specific T-cell-mediated cytotoxicity have been detected in 4-h ^{51}Cr release assays against Rauscher or Moloney leukemia virus-induced lymphomas (Lavrin *et al.*, 1973) and in longer term visual or isotopic microcytotoxicity assays (Fossati *et al.*, 1975). Cytotoxic reactivity in the spleen, blood, most lymph nodes, and peritoneal cavity reached a peak at about 14 days after MSV inoculation and then rapidly declined. Reactivity was widely distributed among the various lymphoid organs. The lymph nodes draining the site of virus inoculation became reactive very early and this reactivity persisted for a longer period of time (Herberman et al., 1976). Mice injected with variant stocks of virus that produced progressive tumor growth had low levels of cytotoxic reactivity, but the kinetics of response were very similar to those seen with regressors.

T cells in the spleens of regressor mice also produce the lymphokine, migration inhibitory factor (MIF), upon incubation with intact tumor cells or 3 M KCl extracts of tumors (Landolfo et al., 1977a). Different mechanisms appeared to be involved in the responses to the different types of antigens (Landolfo et al., 1977b, 1978).

By 1g velocity sedimentation, it has been possible to determine the subpopulations of T cells responsible for each type of reactivity. The cytotoxic T cells in the spleen were relatively large, sedimenting with a velocity of about 5.0 mm/h (Holden et al., 1976). The lymphocytes producing MIF in response to intact tumor cells had the same sedimentation profile, but the T cells producing MIF in response to soluble tumor extracts appeared to be smaller cells, sedimenting at about 3.5 mm/h (Landolfo et al., 1980).

B. Reactivity of T Cells Isolated from MSV-Induced Tumors

Tumors at 14 days after inoculation of the regressor strain of MSV have been studied (Holden et al., 1976). Host cells were isolated by enzymatic disaggregation of the tumors and fractionated by 1g velocity sedimentation. T cells within the tumors were found to have high and specific cytotoxic reactivity, with the levels considerably higher than observed in spleens of the same mice (Table I). In contrast to the large size of the cytotoxic T cells in the spleen, the reactive cells from the tumor were small, sedimenting at 3.5-4.0 mm/h (Fig. 1). However, the effector cells were shown to be T cells, being nonadherent and sensitive to treatment with anti-Thy-1.2 plus complement (Holden et al., 1976). A similar pattern of results was obtained with T cells isolated from MSB, an MSV-

Table I. Cytotoxic Reactivity of Cells from MSV Tumors
and of Cells from the Spleens of the Same Mice

	Cytotoxicity (%)	
Responder cells	200:1[a]	50:1
Unfractionated cells from tumors	33	24
Spleen cells	22	15

[a]Attacker:target cell ratio.

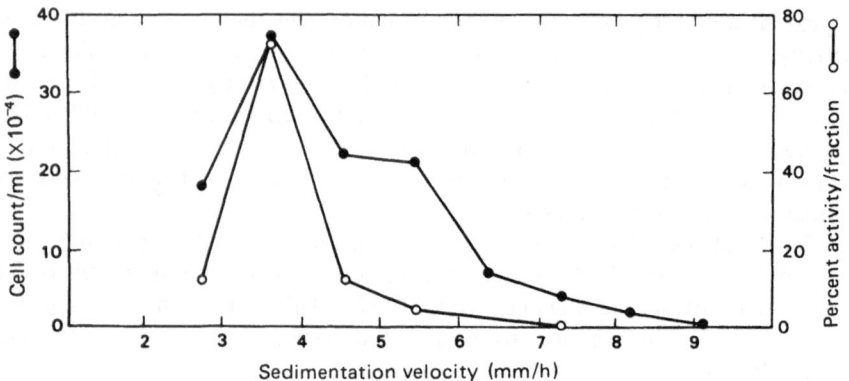

Figure 1. Velocity sedimentation (1*g*) of cytotoxic T lymphocytes from MSV-induced tumors. MSV-induced tumors were enzymatically dissociated and separated by 1*g* velocity sedimentation. Fractions were tested for their cytotoxic activity against RBL-5 tumor targets in a 4-h ^{51}Cr release assay. The results from that testing were normalized to account for the number of cells per fraction and the percent activity per fraction was calculated. •——•, Cell count/ml ($\times 10^{-4}$) in each fraction; ○——○, percent activity/fraction.

induced transplantable tumor line. It seems likely that the cytotoxic cells were generated in the spleen and other lymphoid organs, and only the small, more mature lymphocytes could migrate into the tumor. Alternatively, at the time of testing, the cytotoxic cells within the tumor may have already differentiated and become smaller.

In contrast to the high levels of cytotoxic reactivity by T cells isolated from MSV tumors, to date we have been unable to detect any MIF production by lymphocytes isolated from these tumors when cultured with intact tumor cells (Holden *et al.*, 1980; Varesio *et al.*, 1979). As shown in Table II, unfractionated cells from the tumors did not produce MIF upon culture with RBL-5 tumor cells. Even after removal of the adherent suppressor cells described below, no reactivity was observed. The combined treatment with the carbonyl iron/magnet technique and passage over a rayon column was shown to be quite effective in depleting macrophages, with the concentration of remaining phagocytic cells being less than 0.5%. In contrast, similarly treated spleen cells from the same mice produced more migration inhibition.

III. REACTIVITY OF MACROPHAGES

A. Reactivity of Macrophages in Spleen and Peritoneal Cavity

Macrophages in the spleens and peritoneal cavity of MSV tumor-bearers have been shown to have strong cytostatic reactivity, as measured by inhibition of

Table II. Effect of Macrophage Depletion on MIF Production in Response to RBL-5 Tumor Cells by Cells from Tumors and by Spleen Cells from the Same Mice

Responder cells	Treatment	RBL-5 added (%)	
		10	1
Cells from tumors	None	9^a	10
	Iron/magnet	-6	-5
	Rayon column	12	-2
	Iron/magnet + rayon column	-5	10
Spleen cells	None	25	20
	Iron/magnet	50	28
	Rayon column	32	30
	Iron/magnet + rayon column	37	40

[a]Percent migration inhibition.

incorporation of [^{3}H] thymidine into a lymphoma cell line (Kirchner et al., 1975a,b). Peak activity was seen at 14 days after MSV inoculation and the effects were nonspecific, with some antigenically unrelated cell lines strongly inhibited. The activity measured in this assay was actually due to inhibition of proliferation of the target cells, since similar results were obtained by visual counting of the target cells (Puccetti and Holden, 1979). By 1g velocity sedimentation, the cytostatic macrophages were found to be a heterogeneous population of cells, sedimenting with velocities between 3, 5, and 6 mm/h (Holden et al., 1976).

Peritoneal macrophages from MSV tumor-bearers also have been shown to have cytolytic activity, detectable in an 18-h ^{51}Cr release assay (Puccetti and Holden, 1979). Such a long-term assay was necessary to detect the macrophage-mediated activity, with little or no lysis seen after incubation for only 4 h. As with the cytostatic activity, the peak of macrophage-mediated cytolytic activity was also at 14 days after MSV inoculation and the effects were not antigenically specific. However, all of the activity seen in the cytostasis assay could not be attributed entirely to lysis of the target cells. At low ratios of effector cells to target cells, between 1:1 and 10:1, marked cytostasis occurred without significant lysis (Puccetti and Holden, 1979). Lysis usually was only seen at ratios greater than 10:1. These results indicate either that lysis requires more effector cells or that the subpopulations of macrophages or the levels of macrophage activation are different for each effect.

B. Reactivity of Macrophages in Tumors

Nonspecifically cytostatic macrophages also have been isolated from MSV-induced tumors (Holden et al., 1976). The effector cells had characteristics similar to those in the spleen, being adherent to rayon and resistant to treatment with anti-Thy-1.2 plus complement. As in the spleen, the effector cells were heterogeneous in size, with two peaks in 1g velocity sedimentation gradients, at velocities of 4 and 6 mm/h (Fig. 2). In addition, most of the cytostatic effector cells were shown to have receptors for the Fc portion of IgG, forming rosettes with antibody-coated erythrocytes and thus sedimenting more rapidly.

Adherent cells isolated from the tumors induced by the regressor strain of MSV were also found to be cytolytic, with considerably higher activity than peritoneal macrophages (Table III) (Puccetti and Holden, 1979). The effector cells were phagocytic, being inactivated by silica and carrageenan and removed by the carbonyl iron/magnet technique, and were not affected by treatment with anti-Thy-1.2 plus complement. By 1g velocity sedimentation, as in the growth inhibition assay, the cytolytic macrophages were heterogeneous in size, with peaks at 4-5 and 6-7 mm/h, and sometimes a third, small peak at about 7-8 mm/h (Fig. 3). More recently, we have performed a comparative study of cytolytic activity within regressing tumors and within progressing tumors in

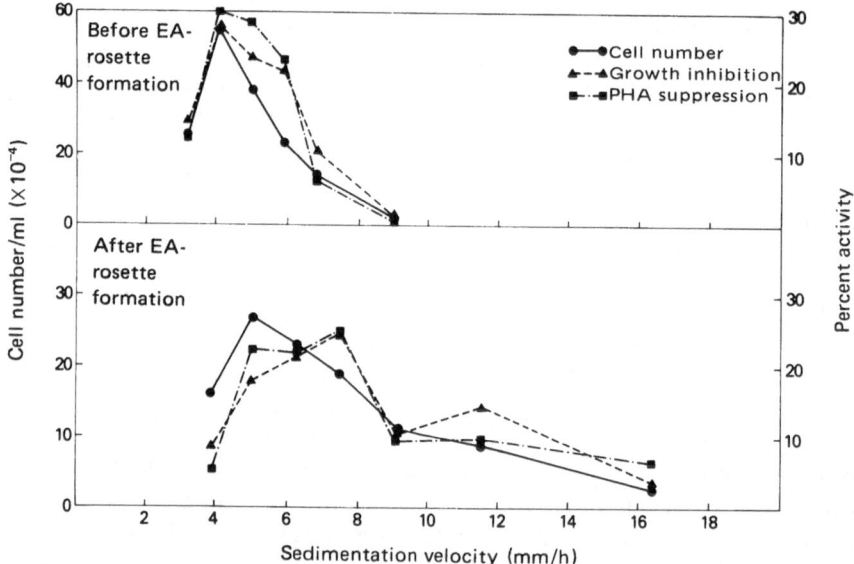

Figure 2. Velocity sedimentation (1g) of growth inhibitory and suppressor cell activity before and after erythrocyte rosette formation. Day 14 MSV-induced tumors were enzymatically dissociated. The resulting single cell suspension was divided into two pools; one was separated immediately by 1g velocity sedimentation while the other was first mixed with sheep erythrocytes coated with IgG antibodies to sheep erythrocytes (EA) to form rosettes via the Fc receptor and then separated by 1g velocity sedimentation. The fractions from both sedimentations were then tested for their growth inhibitory or suppressor activity. The results were normalized to account for the number of cells per fraction.

**Table III. Cytolytic Activity against RBL-5 Tumor
Cells by Adherent Cells from Different Sources**

Source of macrophages	^{51}Cr release (%)		
	200:1[a]	100:1	50:1
MSV tumor bearer			
Tumor	58	51	46
Peritoneum	43	34	24
Normal peritoneal cells	2	1	1

[a]Attacker: target cell ratio.

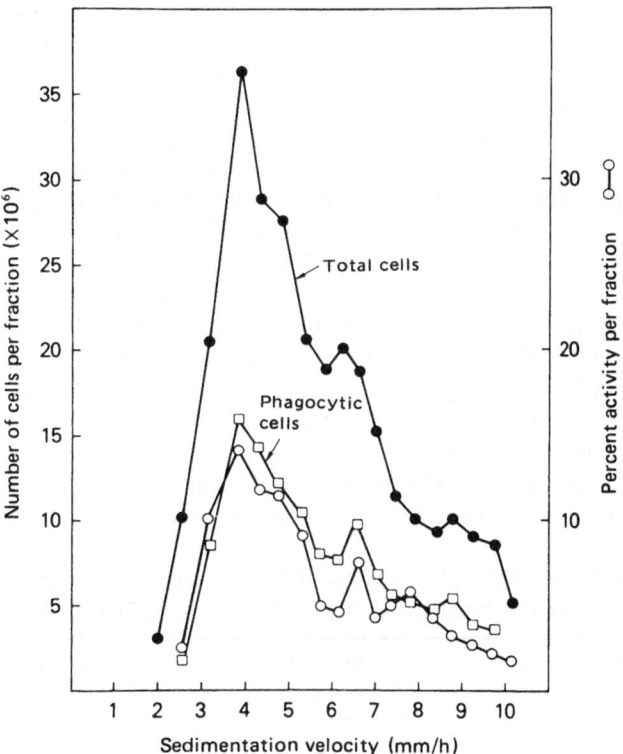

Figure 3. Velocity sedimentation (1g) of macrophage-mediated cytotoxicity of cells isolated from tumors induced by regressor MSV. Tumors from animals inoculated 14 days earlier with the regressor strain of MSV were removed and enzymatically dissociated into single cell suspensions. The cells were treated with anti-Thy-1.2 plus complement and then fractionated by 1g velocity sedimentation. Each fraction was assessed for phagocytic activity by latex ingestion and for macrophage-mediated cytotoxicity by an 18-h ^{51}Cr release assay.

conventional mice and in nude mice (Holden *et al.*, 1980; Taniyama and Holden, 1979). Furthermore, the cells isolated from the tumors were separated by 1*g* velocity sedimentation to see if the cytotoxic macrophages in the different types of MSV tumors had divergent characteristics. At 14 days after inoculation, cells from tumors in conventional mice that were induced by either the regressor or the progressor stock of MSV had similar levels of cytolytic activity (Table IV) (Taniyama and Holden, 1979). Later in the course of tumor progression, around 60 days after virus inoculation, the cytolytic activity of the macrophages in the tumors was substantially lower (Table IV). When cells from such progressing tumors were separated by velocity sedimentation, the distribution pattern of cytolytic activity was also different from that seen with regressing tumors (Fig. 4). There was only one peak of activity, with a velocity of 4 mm/h, even though the distribution profile of macrophages, as measured by latex ingestion, was the same as for macrophages from regressing tumors. No cytolytic activity was detected with the macrophages from progressor tumors in nude mice, even after separation of the cells by velocity sedimentation (Fig. 5). In some nude mice, adherent peritoneal exudate cells were cytotoxic but even in such animals the cells from the tumor were negative. Apparently the migration of cytolytically active macrophages into tumors, and to some extent the activation process itself, is dependent on the presence of thymus-dependent lymphocytes. This is analogous to a previous study of Grant *et al.* (1973) which also described a requirement for T cells in the activation of macrophages.

Recently, Russell *et al.* (1977, and this volume) also found that macrophages from progressing MSV-induced tumors had low or undetectable cytolytic activity. However, when assays were performed in the presence of bacterial lipopolysaccharide (LPS), strong cytolytic activity was induced. They suggested that the macrophages in progressor tumors were at an intermediate level of activation, with LPS further activating them to become cytolytic. In view of those findings, it was of considerable interest for us to determine whether macrophages from progressor tumors in nude mice, or the larger noncytolytic macrophages from

Table IV. Cytolytic Activity of Macrophages from Regressing or Progressing MSV-Induced Tumors in C57BL/6 Mice

MSV stock used to induce tumors	Days after MSV inoculation	Cytotoxicity against RBL-5 cells (%)[a]
Regressor	14	72
Progressor	14	65
Regressor	14	71
Progressor	50	30

[a]Attacker : target cell ratio, 50 : 1.

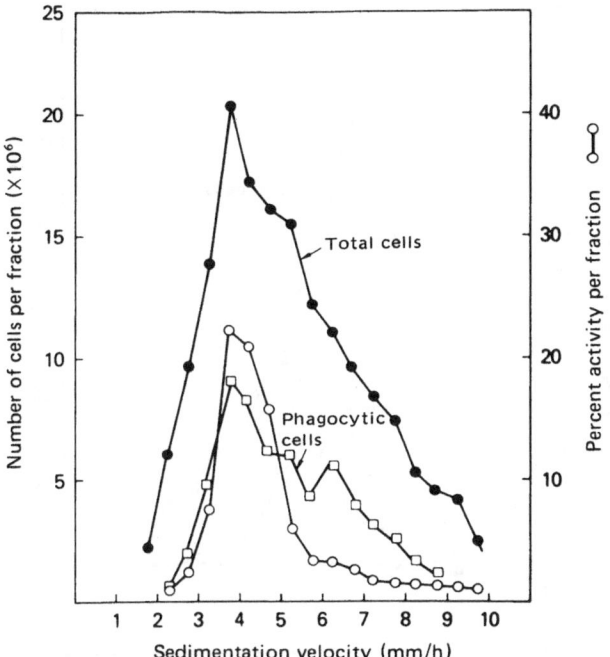

Figure 4. Velocity sedimentation (1g) of cells from tumors induced by progressor MSV: analysis of macrophage-mediated cytotoxicity. Tumors from mice inoculated 60 days earlier with the progressor strain of MSV were removed and enzymatically dissociated into single cell suspensions. The cells were treated with anti-Thy-1.2 plus complement and then fractionated by 1g velocity sedimentation. Each fraction was assessed for phagocytic activity by latex ingestion and for macrophage-mediated cytotoxicity in an 18-h ^{51}Cr release assay using RBL-5 target cells.

progressor tumors in conventional mice, could be similarly rendered cytolytic (Taniyama and Holden, 1979). Macrophages in populations with preexisting cytolytic activity developed higher levels of activity in the presence of LPS. However, the inactive macrophages from tumors of nude mice or conventional mice did not develop detectable cytolytic activity. Therefore, as yet we have not been able to obtain evidence in support of the hypothesis that some non-cytolytic populations of macrophages within tumors are partially activated and can be converted to cytolytic effector cells by stimulation with LPS. The reasons for the apparent discrepancies between out data and those of Russell and his colleagues (1977) are not entirely clear. However, there are a number of differences in the experimental system and the techniques used for measuring cytolysis. Our laboratories have recently performed some comparative experiments to resolve this issue and the main differences appear to be in the sensitivity of the

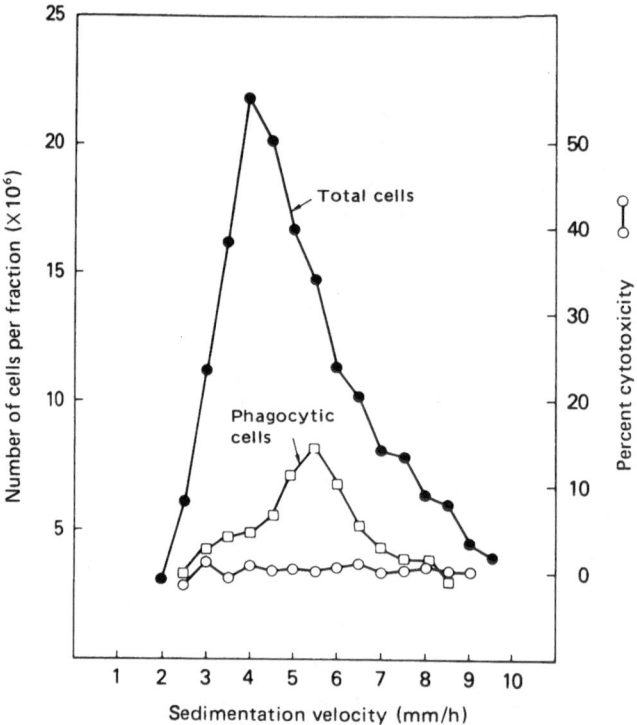

Figure 5. Velocity sedimentation (1*g*) cells from MSV-induced tumors in nude mice. Progressively growing tumors induced 14 days earlier by the inoculation of MSV were removed from the animals, enzymatically dissociated into single cell suspensions, and fractionated by 1*g* velocity sedimentation. Each fraction was assessed for phagocytic activity for latex ingestion and for macrophage-mediated cytotoxicity in an 18-h ^{51}Cr release assay.

assay systems. Our assay system appears to be somewhat more sensitive, so that macrophages from progressor mice might be more likely to display some activity even without stimulation by LPS.

IV. REACTIVITY OF NK CELLS

A. Reactivity of NK Cells in Spleen and Blood of Tumor Bearers

Considerable levels of cytolytic activity of NK cells against a variety of tumor target cells have been observed in the spleens and blood of young normal mice, between the ages of 4 and 10 weeks, and in the blood of most normal adult human donors (Herberman and Holden, 1978). In tumor-bearing mice (Herberman *et al.*,

1975; Becker and Klein, 1977) and patients that have large tumor burdens (McCoy et al., 1973; Pross and Baines, 1976; Takasugi et al., 1977), NK activity has been found to be depressed. Recent studies in our laboratory suggest that some of the depression of NK activity in MSV-tumor-bearing mice may be due to suppression mediated by prostaglandins, since treatment with indomethacin, an inhibitor of prostaglandin synthetase, has partially reversed the depression (M. Brunda, H. Holden, and R. B. Herberman, unpublished observations).

B. Reactivity of NK Cells in Tumors

There is little available information on the presence of NK cells in tumors. Becker and Klein (1977) reported on suggestive evidence for NK cells in MSV tumors induced in CBA mice, although NK cells have been undetectable in most human tumors studied (Vose et al., 1977). In recent studies we have detected NK cells in MSC-induced tumors in CBA and C57BL/6 mice (Gerson et al., 1979). The levels of NK activity in the tumors have appeared to parallel the levels in the spleen (Table V). The highest NK activity has been observed in tumors of 5- to 8-week-old CBA mice, which have high splenic NK activity, and in older mice (>10 weeks) with low systemic activity; only low levels have been detected in the tumors. Removal of adherent cells and incubation with interferon, a procedure known to augment NK activity of spleen cells (Djeu et al., 1979), caused a modest increase in the cytotoxicity by cells from the tumors.

In contrast to the consistent finding of similar levels of NK activity in the tumors and spleens of MSV-tumor-bearing mice, no NK activity was detected in any of the 29 human tumors (a variety of carcinomas and neuroblastomas) that

Table V. Natural Killer Cell Activity in Mice Bearing
MSV-Induced Tumors

Strain	Source of effector cells	Cytotoxicity (%)[a]	
		5–8 weeks[b]	>10 weeks
CBA	Normal spleen	74	6
	Tumor bearer		
	Spleen	64	5
	Tumor	62	2
C57BL/6	Normal spleen	45	1
	Tumor bearer		
	Spleen	16	1
	Tumor	14	2

[a] YAC-1 target cells, attacker : target cell ratio, 100 : 1.
[b] Age of mice at time of testing.

we have examined thus far. Some of the patients had depressed NK activity in the blood, but with others blood NK levels were in the normal range. It is as yet unclear whether NK cells usually fail to enter and persist in human tumors or whether the negative results were due to inhibitory factors or technical problems in preparing the cells. One possible explanation for some of our initial negative results was that the lot of collagenase used for disaggregation of the tumor could inactivate NK cells. A subsequent batch of collagenase has not had inhibitory effects on NK cells prepared from peripheral blood, but the cells from tumors disaggregated with this enzyme also had no detectable NK activity. Incubation of the cells from some tumors with interferon, under conditions that usually augment NK activity of cells in the blood normal donors (Herberman *et al.*, 1979) or cancer patients, did not induce appreciable levels of activity. In some preliminary experiments we have found that, when mixed together, cells from tumors inhibited the NK activity of blood lymphocytes. It remains to be determined whether this inhibitory activity was due to cold target inhibition by tumor cells or to suppressor cells.

Since MSV-induced tumors and human tumors gave divergent results, it seemed possible that the virus-induced regressing tumors with a short latent period were not an appropriate model for spontaneous human carcinomas and other tumors, which undoubtedly had been present for long periods of time and had already grown to rather large size. We have therefore examined some spontaneous mammary adenocarcinomas in C3H mice that are congenitally infected with mouse mammary tumor virus. Our preliminary results are interesting in that NK activity was more readily detected in small primary tumors than in more advanced lesions (Table VI). Larger tumors in this system may more closely resemble human tumors and further studies with this model may provide better insights into the role of NK cells in human tumors.

Table VI. Natural Killer Cell Activity in C3H Spontaneous Mammary Tumors

Effector cells	Cytotoxicity (%)[a]	
	Exp. 1	Exp. 2
Normal spleen	26	6
Tumor bearer (10–20-mm diameter)		
Spleen	5	8
Tumor	16	20
Tumor bearer (>30-mm diameter)		
Spleen	10	10
Tumor	5	5

[a]YAC-1 target cells, attacker: target cell ratio, 100:1.

V. FACTORS INHIBITING IMMUNE REACTIVITY

A. Suppressor Cells in Spleen or Peripheral Blood

There has been increasing interest in the possible role of suppressor cells in interfering with effective immune responses against tumors. In mice with MSV-induced tumors, spleen cells have been shown to have macrophages that can suppress lymphoproliferative responses to mitogens (Kirchner et al., 1974a,b), alloantigens (Fernbach et al., 1976), and tumor antigens (Kirchner et al., 1975b). Suppressor macrophages in the spleens of MSV-tumor-bearing mice could also inhibit the generation of cytotoxic T cells in response to tumor antigens (Glaser et al., 1976).

Recently, it has been shown that the depressed lymphoproliferative responses to mitogens or in mixed-leukocyte cultures of many patients with cancer, and depressed production of polyclonal immunoglobulins in patients with multiple myeloma, were due to suppression by monocytes (Broder et al., 1975; Berlinger et al., 1976; Goodwin et al., 1977; Zembala et al., 1977; Jerrells et al., 1978). We have recently performed a study of patients with carcinoma of the breast or lung who had depressed lymphoproliferative responses (Jerrells et al., 1978). Approximately one-half of the lung cancer patients with depressed reactivity had demonstrable suppressor cell activity which at least partially accounted for the low responses. The suppressor cells in two-thirds of these patients were adherent to Sephadex G-10 and in some instances were also shown to be phagocytic. With a few other lung cancer patients, the suppressor cells were nonadherent and their nature (suppressor T cells?) remains to be determined. With the breast cancer patients with depressed responses, a lower proportion had evidence of suppressor cells and more of these were not monocytic in nature. We have also found that the lack of lymphoproliferative responses of some lung or breast cancer patients to autologous tumor extracts (Dean et al., 1977, 1978) could be attributed to the presence of suppressor monocytes in the peripheral blood (Herberman et al., 1980).

B. Suppressor Cells and Inhibitory Factors in Tumors

We have also examined MSV tumors for the presence of lymphoid cells that might suppress immune responses. Macrophages from the the tumors, with the same velocity sedimentation characteristics as those active in cytostasis assays (Holden et al., 1976), have been found to inhibit lymphoproliferative responses to mitogens (Fig. 2). Even after rosetting with antibody-coated erythrocytes, the two activities could not be dissociated.

As discussed in Section II.B, T cells isolated from MSV tumors have not been found to produce MIF in response to tumor antigens. Since spleen cells from the same mice were reactive, and suppressor cells have been found in the tumors, it was of interest to determine whether suppressor cells could also account for the failure to observe MIF production. Indeed, macrophages from the tumors could abrogate MIF production by immune spleen cells in response to tumor antigens and alloantigens and by normal spleen cells in response to mitogens (Holden *et al.*, 1980; Herberman *et al.*, 1980) (Table VII). The production of MIF by lymphocytes has been shown to be independent of proliferation, with mitomycin-C-blocked cells fully capable of response. These results indicate that the primary effect of suppressor macrophages is on an early phase of the metabolic activity of stimulated lymphocytes and that at least some suppressive effects are independent of lymphoproliferation. It is as yet unclear why T cells isolated from MSV tumors and separated from macrophages were still unable to produce MIF. Immune T cells in MSV tumors may have had their activity blocked *in vivo* by their close contact with suppressor macrophages and this might not be readily reversible during the usual *in vitro* conditions.

Another possible explanation for low or undetectable immune reactivity within tumors is that tumors contain or release inhibitory substances. One category of potentially important inhibitory factors are proteases. Proteases derived from tumors have been shown to degrade immunoglobulins and may thereby interfere with humoral reactions against tumors cells (Keisari and Witz, 1975). To determine whether tumor-derived proteases might also inhibit cellular immune responses, MSV immune spleen cells were pretreated at 37°C for 6–12 h with lysosomal extracts (LE) from MSV-induced tumors. When these cells were tested in a 4-h ^{51}Cr release assay against RBL-5, their cytotoxicity was inhibited 30–57%. Lysosomal extracts from normal liver were equally or more inhibitory than tumor lysosomal extracts. In two representative experiments where tumor

Table VII. Suppressive Effect of Macrophages from MSV-Induced Tumors on MIF Production by Macrophage-Depleted C57BL/6 Spleen Cells

Immunization of responder	Stimulus	Suppressor cells[a]	Migration inhibition (%)
MSV	RBL-5 tumor cells	−	41
		+	−1
K36 (H-2^k)	K36 tumor cells	−	57
		+	−4
None	Concanavalin A	−	36
		+	−2

[a]Adherent cells (10%) from MSV tumors added to incubation mixture.

Table VIII. Inhibition of Cytotoxicity by MSV Immune T Cells by
Tumor and Normal Liver Lysosomal Extracts

Spleen cell treatment[a]	E:T ratio	Cytotoxicity (%)	Inhibition (%)
Exp. 1	200:1		
Media control		50	–
Tumor LE		35	30
Liver LE		27	46
Exp. 2	200:1		
Media control		38	–
Tumor LE		17	57
Liver LE		21	46
Exp. 3	25:1		
Media control		37	–
Tumor LE		20	46

[a]MSV immune spleen cells were pretreated 12 h at 37°C with lysosomal extracts (LE). After pretreatment, washed spleen cells were tested for their cytotoxicity in a 4-h ^{51}Cr release assay against RBL-5.

and liver LE were compared, the liver LE in both cases inhibited 46% of the cytotoxicity whereas the tumor LE inhibited 30 and 57% (Table VIII). This demonstration of a substance in normal tissue and within the tumor which can decrease cytotoxic reactivity by immune T cells points to another mechanism by which immune response to tumors might be subverted.

VI. CONCLUSIONS

From the above studies, it has become clear that tumors may contain a heterogeneous assortment of functional lymphoid cells and that these include both anti-tumor effector cells and immunosuppressive cells. It will be important to determine how the balance among these effects influences the pattern of tumor growth.

The findings with the MSV-induced tumors or spontaneous mammary tumors in mice may provide a useful model for performing analogous studies with human tumors. Considerably more extensive studies on lymphoid cells in human tumors are needed. Such studies of various human tumors should include determination of the subpopulations of cells and their functions. Cells from tumors and peripheral blood mononuclear cells can be compared in regard to the various functional properties discussed above for the experimental tumors. In addition, tumor cells separated from lymphoid cells should provide good sources of tumor antigens, and such tumor cells will be particularly important as target cells for autologous antitumor cytotoxicity.

VII. REFERENCES

Becker, S., and Klein, E., 1977, Decreased "natural killer"–NK–effect in tumor bearing mice and its relation to the immunity against oncorna virus determined cell surface antigens, *Eur. J. Immunol.* 6:892–898.

Berlinger, N. T., Lopez, C., and Good, R. A, 1976, Facilitation or attenuation of mixed leukocyte culture responsiveness by adherent cells, *Nature (London)* 260:145–146.

Broder, S., Humphrey, R., Durm, M., Blackman, M., Meade, B., Goldman, C., Strober, W., and Waldmann, T., 1975, Impaired synthesis of polyclonal (non-paraprotein) immunoglobulins by circulating lymphocytes from patients with multiple myeloma, *N. Engl. J. Med.* 293:887–892.

Dean, J. H., McCoy, J. L., Cannon, G. B., Leonard, C. M., Perlin, E., Kreutner, A., Oldham, R. K., and Herberman, R. B., 1977, Cell-mediated immune responses of breast cancer patients to autologous tumor-associated antigens, *J. Natl. Cancer Inst.* 58:549–555.

Dean, J. H., Jerrells, T. R., Cannon, G. B., Kibrite, A., Baumgardner, B., Weese, J. L., Silva, J., and Herberman, R. B., 1978, Demonstration of specific cell-mediated antitumor immunity in lung cancer to autologous tissue extracts, *Int. J. Cancer* 22:367–377.

Djeu, J. Y., Heinbaugh, J. A., Holden, H. T., and Herberman, R. B., 1979, Augmentation of mouse natural killer cell activity by interferon and interferon inducers. *J. Immunol.* 122:175–181.

Fernbach, B. R., Kirchner, H., Bonnard, G. D., and Herberman, R. B., 1976, Suppression of mixed lymphocyte responses in mice bearing primary tumors induced by murine sarcoma virus, *Transplantation* 21:381–386.

Fossati, G., Holden, H., and Herberman, R. B., 1975, Evaluation of the cell-mediated immune response to murine sarcoma virus by ^{125}iododeoxyuridine assay and comparison with ^{51}chromium and microcytotoxicity assays, *Cancer Res.* 35:2600–2608.

Gerson, J. M., Holden, H. T., Bonnard, G. D., and Herberman, R. B., 1979, Natural killer cell (NK) activity in murine and human tumors. *Proc. Am. Assoc. Cancer Res.* 20:238 (abstract).

Glaser, M., Kirchner, H., Holden, H. T., and Herberman, R. B., 1976, Inhibition of cell-mediated cytotoxicity against tumor-associated antigens by suppressor cells from tumor-bearing mice, *J. Natl. Cancer Inst.* 56:865–867.

Goodwin, J. S., Messner, R. P., Bankhurst, A. D., Peake, G. T., Saiki, J. H., and Williams, R. C., Jr., 1977, Prostaglandin-producing suppressor cells in Hodgkin's disease, *N. Engl. J. Med.* 297:963–968.

Grant, C. K., Evans, R., and Alexander, P., 1973, Multiple effector roles of lymphocytes in allograft immunity, *Cell. Immunol.* 8:136–146.

Herberman, R. B., and Holden, H. T., 1978, Natural cell-mediated immunity, in: *Advances in Cancer Research*, Vol. 27 (G. Klein and S. Weinhouse, eds.), pp. 305–377, Academic Press, New York.

Herberman, R. B., Nunn, M. E., and Lavrin, D. H., 1975, Natural cytotoxic reactivity of mouse lymphoid cells against syngeneic and allogeneic tumors. I. Distribution of reactivity and specificity, *Int. J. Cancer* 16:216–229.

Herberman, R. B., Kirchner, H., Holden, H. T., Glaser, M., Haskill, S., and Bonnard, G. D., 1976, Cell-mediated immunity in murine virus tumor systems, in: *Tumor Virus Infections and Immunity* (R. L. Crowell, H. Friedman, and J. E. Prier, eds.), pp. 147–164, University Park Press, Baltimore.

Herberman, R. B., Ortaldo, J. R., and Bonnard, G. D., 1979, Augmentation by interferon of human natural and antibody-dependent cell-mediated cytoxicity, *Nature (London)* 277:221–223.

Herberman, R. B., Holden, H. T., Djeu, J. Y., Jerrells, T. R., Varesio, L., Tagliabue, A., White, S. L., Oehler, J. R., and Dean, J. H., 1980, Macrophages as regulators of immune responses against tumors, in: *Macrophages and Lymphocytes: Nature, Functions, and Interaction* (M. R. Escobar and H. Friedman, eds.), Part B, pp. 361–379, Plenum Press, New York.

Holden, H. T., Haskill, J. S., Kirchner, H., and Herberman, R. B., 1976, Two functionally distinct anti-tumor effector cells isolated from primary murine sarcoma virus-induced tumors, *J. Immunol.* 117:440–446.

Holden, H. T., Varesio, L., Taniyama, T., and Puccetti, P., 1980, Functional heterogeneity and T cell-dependent activation of macrophages from murine sarcoma virus (MSV)-induced tumors, in: *Macrophages and Lymphocytes: Nature, Functions, and Interactions* (M. R. Escobar and H. Friedman, eds.), Part B, pp. 509–520, Plenum Press, New York.

Jerrells, T. R., Dean, J. H., Richardson, G. L., McCoy, J. L., and Herberman, R. B., 1978, Role of suppressor cells in depression of *in vitro* lymphoproliferative responses of lung and breast cancer patients, *J. Natl. Cancer Inst.* 61:1001–1009.

Keisari, Y., and Witz, I. P., 1975, The specific blocking of humoral immune cytolysis by anti-tumor antibodies degraded by lysosomal enzymes of tumor origin, *Eur. J. Immunol.* 5:790–795.

Kirchner, H., Chused, T. M., Herberman, R. B., Holden, H. T., and Lavrin, D. H., 1974a, Evidence of suppressor cell activity in spleens of mice bearing primary tumors induced by Moloney sarcoma virus, *J. Exp. Med.* 139:1473–1487.

Kirchner, H., Herberman, R. B., Glaser, M., and Lavrin, D. H., 1974b, Suppression of *in vitro* lymphocyte stimulation in mice bearing primary Moloney sarcoma virus-induced tumors, *Cell. Immunol.* 13:32–40.

Kirchner, H., Holden, H. T., and Herberman, R. B., 1975a, Inhibition of in vitro growth of lymphoma cells by macrophages from tumor-bearing mice, *J. Natl. Cancer Inst.* 55:971–975.

Kirchner, H., Muchmore, A. V., Chused, T. M., Holden, H. T., and Herberman, R. B., 1975a, Inhibition of proliferation of lymphoma cells and T lymphocytes by suppressor cell from spleens of tumor-bearing mice, *J. Immunol.* 114:206–210.

Landolfo, S., Herberman, R. B., and Holden, H. T., 1977a, Cellular immunity to murine sarcoma virus-induced tumors as measured by macrophage migration inhibition assays, *J. Natl. Cancer Inst.* 59:1675–1683.

Landolfo, S., Herberman, R. B., and Holden, H. T., 1977b, Two different mechanisms of stimulating migration inhibition factor (MIF) production in response to soluble tumor-associated antigens or intact tumor cells. *Nature (London)* 270:62–64.

Landolfo, S., Herberman, R. B., and Holden, H. T., 1978, Macrophage–lymphocyte interaction in migration inhibition factor (MIF) production against soluble or cellular tumor-associated antigens. I. Characteristics and genetic control of different mechanisms of stimulating MIF production, *J. Immunol.* 121:695–701.

Landolfo, S., Herberman, R. B., and Holden, H. T., 1980, Macrophage–lymphocyte interaction in migration inhibition factor (MIF) production. II. Identification of two subclasses of T lymphocytes producing MIF against soluble tumor-associated antigens, *J. Immunol.*, submitted.

Lavrin, D. H., Herberman, R. B., Nunn, M., and Soares, N., 1973, *In vitro* cytotoxicity studies of immune sarcoma virus (MSV)-induced immunity in mice, *J. Natl. Cancer Inst.* 51:1497–1508.

McCoy, J., Herberman, R., Perlin, E., Levine, P., and Alford, C., 1973, ^{51}Cr release cellular lymphocyte cytotoxicity as a possible measure of immunological competence of cancer patients, *Proc. Am. Assoc. Cancer Res.* 14:107 (abstract).

Pross, H. F., and Baines, M. G., 1976, Spontaneous human lymphocyte-mediated cytotoxicity against tumour target cells. I. The effect of malignant disease, *Int. J. Cancer* **18**:593–604.

Puccetti, P., and Holden, H. T., 1979 Cytolytic and cytostatic anti-tumor activities of macrophages from mice injected with murine sarcoma virus, *Int. J. Cancer* **23**:123–133.

Russell, S. W., Doe, W. F., and McIntosh, A. T., 1977, Functional characterization of a stable, noncytolytic stage of macrophage activation in tumors, *J. Exp. Med.* **146**:1511–1520.

Takasugi, M., Ramseyer, A., and Takasugi, J., 1977, Decline of natural non-selective cell-mediated cytotoxicity in patients with tumor progression. *Cancer Res.* **37**:413–418.

Takeichi, N., Boone, C. W., Holden, H. T., and Herberman, R. B., 1978, Immunological study of two stocks of Moloney sarcoma virus producing regressor and progressor tumors in C57BL/6 mice, *Int. J. Cancer* **21**:78–84.

Taniyama, T., and Holden, H. T., 1979, Cytolytic activity of macrophages isolated from primary murine sarcoma virus (MSV)-induced tumors, *Int. J. Cancer* **24**:151–160.

Varesio, L., Herberman, R. B., Gerson, J. M., and Holden, H. T., 1979, Suppression of lymphokine production by macrophages infiltrating murine virus-induced tumors, *Int. J. Cancer* **24**:97–102.

Vose, B. M., Vánky, F., and Klein, E., 1977, Human tumour-lymphocyte interaction *in vitro*. V. Comparison of the reactivity of tumour infiltrating, blood and lymph node lymphocytes with autologous tumour cells, *Int. J. Cancer* **20**:895–902.

Zembala, M., Mytar, B., Popiela, T., and Asherson, G. L., 1977, Depressed *in vitro* peripheral blood lymphocyte response to mitogens in cancer patients: The role of suppressor cells, *Int. J. Cancer* **19**:605–613.

Chapter 4

Separation and Characteristics of Tumor-Infiltrating Lymphocytes in Man

E. Klein, F. Vánky, U. Galili, B. M. Vose,* and M. Fopp†

Department of Tumor Biology
Karolinska Institute
Radiumhemmet, Karolinska Sjukhuset
S-104 01 Stockholm 60, Sweden

I. INTRODUCTION

During the initial phase of tumor immunology, when experiments were conducted with syngeneic systems, without the involvement of reactivities against histocompatibility antigens, the accumulation of important information was explosive. As usual with accumulating knowledge, the number of unanswered questions increased. It may seem disappointing that in spite of intense activity, progress has been relatively slow in two important areas that deal with the following questions: (1) Are there any immune parameters in man which can be

Abbreviations used in this chapter: (ATS) autologous tumor stimulation, (ALC) autologous lymphocyte cytotoxicity, (TIL) tumor-infiltrating lymphocytes, (PBL) peripheral blood lymphocytes, (T) thymus-dependent, (B) bursa-equivalent, (NK) natural killer, (NA) natural attachment, (BSS) balanced salt solution, (PBS) phosphate-buffered saline, (NHS) normal human serum, (HSA) human serum albumin, (FCS) fetal calf serum, (BSA) bovine serum albumin, (FI) Ficoll–Isopaque, (SRBC) sheep red blood cells, (E) cells with rosettes of SRBC, (SIg) surface immunoglobulin, (DNA) deoxyribonucleic acid, (DNase) deoxyribonuclease, (MLC) mixed lymphocyte culture, (MMC) mitomycin C, (cpm) counts per minute, (RI) reactivity index, (PHA) phytohemagglutinin, (EBV) Epstein–Barr virus, (MCA) methylcholanthrene, (NPC) nasopharyngeal carcinoma, (FITC) fluorescein isothiocyanate, (DCH) delayed cutaneous hypersensitivity.

*Present address: Department of Immunology, Paterson Laboratories, Christie Hospital and Holt Radium Institute, Manchester M20 9BX, England.
†Present address: Department of Oncology and Hematology, Clinic of Medicine, Kanton Spital, CH-9007 St. Gallen, Switzerland.

exploited for diagnosis or antitumor response? (2) What is the relevance of any *in vitro*-detected tumor-related reactivity for the events associated with tumor development *in vivo?*

In an effort to eliminate at least some of the factors which hamper interpretation of *in vitro* results when tumor cell lines are used as the antigen source, two tests have been designed in our laboratory for measuring cell-mediated antitumor recognition in man: autologous tumor stimulation (ATS) and autologous lymphocyte cytotoxicity (ALC). In both tests, tumor cells separated from biopsy specimens are allowed to react with autologous lymphocytes. We considered it advantageous to use biopsy cells because the modification and selective conditions imposed by tissue culture are avoided. In addition, due to the histocompatibility restriction of T-cell-mediated cytotoxicity, it is questionable whether established cell lines can be used as prototype targets. It is likely that in search for tumor-specific reactivities, experiments have to be performed in autologous systems. In fact, experiments with breast cancer patients performed with well-defined lymphocyte subsets devoid of natural killer (NK) cell activity failed to reveal selective cytotoxicity toward breast cancer-derived lines (Bakács *et al.*, 1978).

It is likely that lymphoid infiltration of tumor tissue is a manifestation of immunologic recognition. If so, it can be expected that the infiltrating lymphocytes bear the characteristics of immunologically active cells and even express specific functions directed against tumor cells. In most experiments in which tumor-derived lymphocytes were shown to be cytotoxic, the target cells carrying relevant antigens were selected for high sensitivity to cellular attack (e.g., Holden *et al.*, 1976). In fact there is no compelling evidence for the growth inhibitory function of tumor-infiltrating lymphocytes. If a host response occurs, the growing tumor may be composed of cells that were selected for immunoresistance or lymphoid infiltration may even cause stimulation of the tumor growth (Prehn, 1976). It is also likely that suppressor mechanisms or factors blocking the cellular or humoral attack counteract the host response (Witz, 1977; Ting *et al.*, 1977; Quan and Burtin, 1978; Bansal *et al.*, 1972).

We describe here our procedure for isolating the lymphocytes resident in human tumors, furnish evidence that some of them are in an activated state, and present our attempts to reveal specific reactivity with the tumor cells from the same biopsy. Finally, we relate the reactivity of blood lymphocytes in the ATS and ALC assays to the presence of lymphocytes within the tumor.

II. PROCEDURES FOR THE ISOLATION OF TUMOR-INFILTRATING LYMPHOCYTES

A. Tumors

Studies were performed on biopsy specimens from 82 human tumors, including lung, kidney, and colon carcinomas and various types of sarcomas. The specimens were obtained soon after the tumor removal, transported to the laboratory in sterile medium, and processing started within 30 min.

B. Dispersion of Tumor Specimens

Cell suspensions were prepared either mechanically and/or with the help of enzymes. Soft tumor specimens were dispersed by shaking the finely minced material in serum-free medium (RPMI 1640). The released cells of several harvests were collected. From tumors which were rich in stromal tissue, pieces free of macroscopic necrosis or hemorrhage were finely minced, mixed with serum-free medium containing collagenase (3 mg/ml) and DNase (0.2 mg/ml), and stirred with a magnet for 30-60 min until most of the tumor tissue was dispersed. Small clumps were removed by sedimentation for 3-4 min. The primary cell suspensions were washed twice with balanced salt solution (BSS) + 5% normal human serum (NHS).

C. Fractionation of the Tumor Suspension

The objectives of the procedure are to obtain suspensions enriched in viable tumor cells, to remove the stromal elements, and to separate the tumor-infiltrating lymphocytes. The latter was attempted in all cases in which the primary suspension contained at least 1% recognizable lymphoid cells.

Cell separation was performed by a combination of $1g$ velocity and density gradient sedimentation coupled with the exploitation of selective adherence properties of different cell types. The products of each step were inspected and checked for viability after addition of trypan blue, and their composition was determined first in unstained preparations and in parallel preparations of Türk solution mixed suspensions. A more thorough characterization of the cell morphologies were carried out on May–Grünwald–Giemsa-stained smears.

The discontinuous gradient for velocity sedimentation was made up from 10-ml layers of fetal calf serum, 100, 75, and 50% diluted with BSS, or of 0.5, 1.0, 1.5, or 2.0% human serum albumin (HSA) in phosphate-buffered saline.

Cell suspensions of the biopsies (about 5×10^7 cells in 10 ml of medium) were loaded on the velocity gradients (FCS or HSA) in the presence of 0.2 mg/ml of DNase and sedimented for 1-2 h at room temperature. Six fractions of 8 ml were collected from each gradient. The fastest sedimenting fractions usually contained the tumor cells, macrophages, and obvious nontumor stromal cells. The slowly sedimenting fractions contained lymphocytes, erythrocytes, and monocytes. The intermediate fractions were composed of mixtures of all these cells. These intermediate fractions were again sedimented on velocity gradients.

Further fractionation was carried out on density gradient of Ficoll–Isopaque (FI) solution made up from 75% of the stock solution (diluted with BSS) underlayered with the stock solution (density 1.077). The velocity gradient fractions were layered on FI. Depending on the number of cells, gradients of 6 or 20 ml were used. These were loaded with a maximum of 20×10^6 cells in 2 ml or 50×10^6 cells in 5 ml, respectively. The tubes were centrifuged at $800g$ for 10 min in a cold centrifuge. The FI density gradient separated the lymphocytes and the tumor cells from the erythrocytes and macrophages and the viable from the nonviable cells. The cells were recovered from the interphases.

In the intermediate fractions of the velocity sedimentation and in cases when clear separation of tumor cells and lymphocytes was not achieved, the discontinuous density gradient made up of 2 ml of 35, 31, 26, 23, or 21% BSA diluted in PBS. Cells ($10-20 \times 10^6$) in 2 ml were loaded on each gradient.

The tumor-cell-enriched fractions were purified from macrophages and stromal cells by incubation in plastic flasks (Falcon plastic 3024) at 37°C for 30 min in RPMI medium + 10% NHS. The majority of macrophages and small monocytes adhered to the plastic surface. The obvious contamination of tumor cells with stromal cells and lymphoid cells with macrophages after this stage was often under 3%. In some cases thereafter the supernatant cells were put on a FI gradient. Obviously the final tumor-cell-enriched preparations also contained a proportion of nonmalignant cells with separation characteristics similar to the tumor cells and without discriminative features in the stained smears.

The purity of cell suspensions was often checked by cell culture. In the majority of cultures after the first three to four passages the proportion of fibroblasts increased and overgrew the tumor cells.

The yield of viable tumor cells varied between 10^6 and 10^7 cells/g of tumor tissue, depending primarily on the type of tumor and the quality of the initial suspension. Approximately 60% of tumors were considered suitable for separation and in 70% of these the procedure gave success, i.e., the yield of cells was sufficient to set up *in vitro* tests.

Lymphocyte-containing fractions were further purified on FI density gradients. The lymphocytes were recovered from the interphase between the stock solution and its 75% dilution. Monocytes were eliminated by incubation of the washed suspensions on plastic surfaces at 37°C for 30 min in RPMI medium + 10% NHS.

Lymphocytes separated from the biopsies were used in functional tests only when the obvious contamination with tumor cells was less than 1% and with other cell types (stromal cells, monocytes) was less than 3%. The tumor-infiltrating lymphocytes (TIL) comprised 51% E-rosette-forming cells (range 37-81) and 22% cells with EA rosettes (range 10-28).

D. Lymphocyte Markers

T cells were detected by sheep red blood cell (SRBC) rosetting. SRBC were washed three times in BSS, adjusted to 1% in fetal calf serum (FCS), and mixed with an equal volume of the test cell suspension (5×10^6/ml in FCS). Following centrifugation, the tubes were incubated at 37°C for 15 min and thereafter for 2 h at 4°C. After resuspension the proportion of lymphocytes having more than three attached erythrocytes was counted. "Stable" E rosettes were detected similarly. In this case the cells were suspended in saline, and after centrifugation the pellet was incubated at 37°C for 30 min before being scored for rosettes.

Surface immunoglobulin (SIg) was detected by immunofluorescence. FITC-labeled goat anti-human Ig (Hyland Laboratories, Los Angeles, California, USA) was used at 1:30 dilution. The cells were stained for 45 min at 4°C. Three hundred cells were scored.

E. Attachment of Tumor- and Blood-Derived T Lymphocytes to a Variety of Cells

1. Attachment of Lymphocytes to Cells in Suspension

Lymphocytes and target cells were adjusted to 10^6 cells/ml. Lymphocyte aliquots (0.25 ml) were added to 0.05 ml of target cell suspensions in Falcon 2058 tubes. The tubes were centrifuged for 4 min at 200g, and the pellets were incubated at 37°C for 20 min. The pellets were gently resuspended, and SRBC were added for identification of the target-attached T lymphocytes. The number of lymphocytes with SRBC (E rosettes) attached to 100 target cells was determined.

2. Attachment of T Cells to Cells in Monolayers, Fibroblasts, Macrophages, CAMA-1, SKMES-1, and SW982

Three hundred target cells were seeded to the wells of Falcon 3034 microplates. The medium was removed and 20-μl aliquots of 10^6/ml lymphocyte suspensions were added. The plates were incubated for 4–20 h at 37°C in humidified atmosphere containing 5% CO_2. Thereafter, the plates were washed with saline to remove the nonadherent lymphocytes. Subsequently, 20 μl of SRBC suspension (in saline) were added to the wells and the plates were centrifuged for 3 min at 200g, and incubated for 30 min at room temperature (22-24°C). At the end of incubation, the plates were carefully washed three times with saline to remove excess SRBC. The T cells attached to the monolayer cells were identified by their SRBC binding. No T cells were seen attached to the plastic surface. The proportion of SRBC-rosetted lymphocytes attached to 100 target cells was scored.

F. Cell Lines

K562 cells (Lozzio and Lozzio, 1975) and Daudi cells (Klein *et al.*, 1968) were grown as stationary suspension cultures in RPMI 1640 medium supplemented with 10% FCS. The mammary carcinoma line CAMA-1, lung carcinoma line SKMES-1, and the fibrosarcoma line SW982 (received from Dr. J. Fogh, Sloan-Kettering, New York, USA) were kept as monolayers in Earle's medium with 10% FCS. Macrophages were obtained by culturing blood monocytes for 6-8 days. Human fibroblasts were used after 10-20 *in vitro* passages.

G. Peripheral Blood Lymphocytes (PBL)

Heparinized blood samples (50 ml) were taken on the morning of operation before premedication and allowed to stand in the syringe for 1 h at room temperature. The separation of lymphocytes was performed according to a modification (Vose *et al.*, 1977*a*) of the original methods (Bøyum, 1974). The adherent cells were removed by incubation in RPMI medium + 10% NHS in a Falcon culture flask for 30 min at 37°C. The floating cells were collected. They were either used or subjected to further separation on nylon fiber columns (Julius *et al.*, 1973). The fraction obtained by this procedure consisted of 85-95% SRBC-rosette-forming cells (T cells), 1-4% EA-rosette-forming cells (Fc-receptor-positive cells), and 1-2% cells with surface immunoglobulin (B cells).

H. Medium

RPMI 1640 medium with *L*-glutamine (200 mM solution, 1% by volume) benzylpenicillin (100 i.u./ml), streptomycin sulfate (100 μg/ml), Hepes buffer (0.1 mM/ml), and heat-inactivated serum from healthy male donors (added in 10% concentration) was used in all experiments (RPMI + NHS).

I. Estimation of DNA Synthesis and Autologous Tumor Stimulation (ATS) Test

The methods have been described in detail previously (Vánky and Stjernswärd, 1976). The ATS results were evaluated by calculating a reactivity index (RI) which is the ratio between the ^{3}[H]-TdR uptake (cpm) in the test sample and in the control where mitomycin C (MMC)-treated identical lymphocytes were added instead of tumor cells. RI exceeding 4.0 was considered positive when the difference between the values was statistically significant.

J. Autologous Lymphocyte Cytotoxicity (ALC) Test

A short-term ^{51}Cr-release microtest was used to register the lysis of biopsy cells. The procedure has been described in detail previously (Vose *et al.*, 1977*a*).

Lymphocytes were tested directly for killing effect, or after cocultivation with autologous tumor cells, secondary ALC (Vose *et al.*, 1978).

The ALC was evaluated by calculating the proportion of ^{51}Cr release for each tube from the formula:

$$\% \,^{51}\text{Cr release} = \frac{\text{supernatant counts} \times 100}{\text{supernatant} + \text{pellet counts}}$$

Percentage of cytotoxicity was then derived:

$$\% \text{ specific cytotoxicity} = \frac{\% \,^{51}\text{Cr release test} - \text{spontaneous release}}{\% \text{ maximum release} - \text{spontaneous release}} \times 100$$

Significance was calculated by Student's t-test and in all cases it was considered positive if the cytotoxicity was higher than 20%.

III. FUNCTIONS OF TUMOR-INFILTRATING LYMPHOCYTES

The two types of biopsy suspensions, mechanically- or enzyme-dispersed, were compared in 12 cases (Table I). The viability of the enzyme-dispersed suspensions was invariably superior. In some cases the difference was considerable (e.g., Nos. 1120 and 1246). These preparations had an often higher proportion of lymphoid cells. The poorer quality of the mechanically-dispersed suspension may reflect the damage caused by the procedure or simply the poor viability of the tumor cells.

Cells with obvious lymphoid character (small size, round shape, high nuclear : cytoplasm ratio) were seen in 29/77 biopsy preparations (38%) in variable proportions. Seminomas (2/2) and kidney carcinomas (3/3) always contained such cells; among lung tumors squamous cell carcinomas often contained more (8/14) than adenocarcinomas (5/12) and oat cell tumors (1/5). In 4/7 osteosarcoma suspensions, lymphocytes were present while they were absent in the 10 chondrosarcomas, 4 of the 5 fibrosarcomas, and in 7 of the 10 astrocytomas.

In some suspensions lymphoblastlike cells could be seen. However, since it was not possible to differentiate with certainty between lymphoblasts and tumor cells, this was never attempted.

The proportion of macrophages varied between 1 and 13%, estimated by stained smears.

A. Presence of SRBC-Rosetting Lymphocytes in the Biopsy Suspension

In 15 biopsies the suspensions obtained with enzyme treatment were studied for the presence of lymphocytes with T and B markers (Table II). In 7/15 cases

Table I. Composition of the Primary Cell Suspensions

Cell category	Liposarcoma 1119[a] e	m[b]	1120 e	m	Osteosarcoma 1010 e	m	1021 e	m	Squamous cell cancer 2204 e	m	2249 e	m	Adenocarcinoma 1246 e	m	1292 e	m	1295 e	m	Oat cell cancer 2205 e	m	Kidney cancer 505 e	m	Melanoma 800 e	m
Viable tumor cell[c]	99	45	81	18	88	42	95	54	83	23	97	33	93	11	89	29	95	55	98	49	86	30	84	63
Lymphoid cell[d]	8	3	0	0	15	8	3	2	46	15	39	14	45	6	1	1	18	10	39	21	54	18	16	11
Macrophage[d]	3	1	0	0	7	3	0	0	29	12	8	3	37	5	23	7	20	11	5	3	3	1	18	13
Erythrocyte[d]	7	3	129	41	22	13	9	5	77	25	24	9	271	67	27	12	15	7	14	9	5	2	33	22
Other (probably not tumor cell)[d]	8	2	3	4	27	19	50	27	9	3	6	2	17	3	1	1	7	3	0	0	0	0	12	9

Column groups: *Lung tumors* spans Squamous cell cancer, Adenocarcinoma, and Oat cell cancer. *Metastasis in lung* spans Kidney cancer and Melanoma.

[a] Patient number.
[b] e, The collagenase–DNase dispersed suspension; m, the mechanically dispersed suspension.
[c] Percentage of viable/all tumor cells.
[d] Number/100 tumor cells.

Table II. Proportion of E-Rosetting and SIg-Positive Lymphocytes in the Biopsy Suspension

| Patient No. | Diagnosis | Positive cells (%) | |
		E	SIg
	Sarcomas		
1119	Liposarcoma	39 (0)[a]	NT[b]
1021	Osteosarcoma	27 (0)	1
1003	Osteosarcoma	55 (2)	NT
	Lung carcinomas		
1295	Adenocarcinoma	80 (10)	3
2213	Adenocarcinoma	38 (11)	NT
1298	Squamous cell	18 (0)	1
2249	Squamous cell	54 (3)	NT
1281	Squamous cell	65 (6)	NT
1286	Squamous cell	54 (0)	1
2224	Squamous cell	60 (1)	NT
2203	Squamous cell	66 (0)	1
	Metastasis in lung		
2211	Kidney carcinoma	65 (7)	NT
2214	Kidney carcinoma	87 (14)	1
800	Melanoma	53 (3)	1
505	Seminoma	75 (20)	1

[a]The number of E-rosetting cells seen attached to 100 tumor cells, is in parentheses.
[b]NT, not tested.

the majority of lymphocytes bound SRBC. Only in 1/8 tumors were more than 1% SIg-positive cells detected.

B. Separation of Tumor Cells and Lymphocytes

Using the procedure delineated in the Section II, examples are given with six tumor specimens comprising four tumor types (Tables III–VII).

The use of fractions was decided on the basis of inspection. Some were discarded, some judged of sufficient purity for use in the experiments, some were subjected for further fractionation steps. The criteria for these decisions are obvious from the composition of the populations.

The major difficulty in the fractionation was the uncertainties involved in distinguishing between the cell types. It is also uncertain to what degree the enriched fractions represent the tumor cell and lymphocyte compartments of the tumor. At this stage of our experimentation the aim was to obtain fractions of sufficient purity and no attempt was made to recover the total population.

Table III. Protocol of Cell Separation—Myxoid Liposarcoma No. 1120[a]

| | | Fractions | | | | | | | | | | | |
| | | Step 1: HSA velocity gradient[c] | | | | Step 2: BSA density gradient[c] | | | | | Step 3: FI density gradient[c] | | |
Cell category	Composition of the suspension[b]	Bottom 1	2% 2	1% 3	0.5% 4	Bottom 5	35% 6	31% 7	26% 8	21% 9	Bottom 10	100% 11	75% 12
Viable tumor cell[d]	81	87	61	44	0	0	0	83	86	82	3	93	0
Lymphoid cell[e]	<1	<1	<1	<1	<1	<1	1	<1	0	0	0	<1	0
Macrophage[e]	<1	<1	<1	1	1	<1	0	0	0	0	0	0	0
Erythrocyte[e]	129	3	317	736	M	M	M	327	8	0	M	0	0
Other (probably not tumor cell)[e]	3	1	6	2	1	15	19	0	0	0	0	0	0
Use of fraction[f]:		Pooled to step 2			Disc.	Disc.	Pooled to step 3			Exp.[g]	Disc.	Exp.	

[a]Weight, 15 g; yield, 3.8×10^6 tumor cells/g.
[b]Suspension dispersed with collagenase–DNase mixture.
[c]HSA, human serum albumin; BSA, bovine serum albumin; FI, Ficoll–Isopaque.
[d]Percent of all tumor cells.
[e]Number/100 tumor cells (all, viable, and nonviable); M, majority of cells.
[f]Fractions 9 and 11 pooled for experiment, tumor-cell-enriched suspension.
[g]Fractions judged of sufficient purity for experiment.

Table IV. Protocol of Cell Separation—Myxoid Liposarcoma No. 1119[a]

Cell category	Composition of the suspension	Step 1: HSA velocity gradient				Step 2: Fl density gradient			Step 3: HSA velocity gradient				Step 4: BSA density gradient				
		Bottom	2%	1%	0.5%	Bottom	100%	75%	Bottom	2%	1%	0.5%	Bottom	35%	31%	26%	21%
		1	2	3	4	5	6	7	8	9	10	11	12	13	14	15	16
Viable tumor cell	99	96	94	68	69	21	85	99	71	87	<1	<1	<1	<1	<1	<1	<1
Lymphoid cell	8	2	6	50	50	6	14	0	<1	<1	M	M	17	M	310	5	<1
Macrophage	3	<1	2	<1	1	6	<1	<1	0	0	0	0	0	0	0	0	0
Erythrocyte	7	<1	<1	6	56	163	<1	0	0	0	<1	<1	<1	<1	0	0	0
Other (probably not tumor cell)	8	3	1	0	0	7	<1	<1	<1	0	0	0	0	0	0	0	0
Use of fractions[b]:		Exp.	To step3	Pooled to step 2		Disc.	To step 3	Pooled for exp.	Pooled for exp.	Pooled to step 4			Disc.	Pooled for exp.		Disc.	

[a]Weight, 22 g; yield, 7.2×10^6 tumor cells/g.
[b]Fractions 1, 7, 8, and 9 were pooled, tumor-cell-enriched suspension. Fractions 13 and 14 were pooled, tumor-infiltrating lymphocytes, TIL.

Table V. Protocol of Cell Separation—Squamous Cell Carcinoma of the Lung No. 1281[a]

Cell category	Composition of the suspension	Step 1: HSA velocity gradient				Step 2: BSA density gradient					Step 3: FI density gradient	
		Bottom 1	2% 2	1% 3	0.5% 4	Bottom 5	35% 6	31% 7	26% 8	21% 9	Bottom 10	100% 11
Viable tumor cell	83	68	63	70	<1	<1	1	±	89	93	±	±
Lymphoid cell	46	<1	1	96	271	2	M	M	<1	0	0	M
Macrophage	29	23	7	<1	0	<1	0	0	0	0	0	0
Erythrocyte	77	<1	<1	318	966	M	113	<1	0	0	M	0
Other (probably not tumor cell)	9	<1	17	3	0	15	<1	0	0	0	0	0
Use of fractions[b]:		Incubated on plastic surface, for exp.	Pooled to step 3			Disc.	To step 3	Exp. lymphocyte	Exp. tumor cell		Disc.	Exp. lymphocyte

[a] Weight, 43 g; yield, tumor cells 8.3×10^6/g; Ly, 0.12×10^6/g.
[b] Fractions 1, 2, 8, and 9 were pooled for experiment, tumor-cell-enriched suspension, fraction 11 lymphocytes, TIL.

Table VI. Protocol of Cell Separation—Adenocarcinoma of the Lung No. 1246[a]

		Fractions						
		Step 1: FCS velocity gradient				Step 2: FI density gradient		Step 3: Adherence on plastic surface
Cell category	Composition of the suspension	Bottom 1	75% 2	50% 3	25% 4	Bottom 5	100% 6	7
Viable tumor cell	93	90	97	0	0	13	<1	89
Lymphoid cell	45	<1	1	1022	0	0	M	>1
Macrophage	37	19	2	<1	0	0	0	>1
Erythrocyte	271	<1	2	M	0	M	0	0
Other (probably not tumor cell)	17	2	11	<1	0	0	0	3
Use of fractions:		Pooled to step 3		To step 2	Disc.	Disc.	Exp. lymphocytes	Exp. tumor cells

[a]Weight, 17.7 g; yield, 3.3×10^6 tumor cells/g.

Table VII. Protocol of Cell Separation—Osteosarcoma No. 1021[a]

	Composition of the suspension	Fraction											
		Step 1: FCS velocity gradient				Step 2: FI density gradient			Step 3: BSA density gradient				
Cell category		Bottom 1	75% 2	50% 3	25% 4	Bottom 5	100% 6	75% 7	Bottom 8	35% 9	31% 10	26% 11	21% 12
Viable tumor cell	95	63	93	53	<1	2	85	<1	2	<1	5	86	93
Lymphoid cell	3	0	0	14	11	<1	5	0	3	75	38	2	0
Macrophage	<1	<1	0	<1	0	2	<1	<1	0	0	0	0	0
Erythrocyte	9	0	0	64	197	M	0	<1	0	0	0	0	0
Other (probably not tumor cell)	50	84	3	0	0	13	0	0	0	0	0	0	0
Use of fractions[b]:		To step 2	Exp.	To step 2	To step 2	Disc.	To step 3	Disc.	Disc.	Pooled for exp. lymphocytes		Pooled for exp. tumor cells	

[a]Weight, 26 g; yield, 3 × 10^6 tumor cells/g.
[b]Fractions 11 and 12 were tumor cells; fractions 9 and 10 were lymphocytes.

Table VIII. Protocol of Cell Separation—Osteosarcoma No. 1010[a]

Cell category	Composition of the suspension	Fractions									
		Step 1: FCS velocity gradient				Step 2: FI density gradient			Step 3: FCS velocity gradient		
		Bottom 1	75% 2	50% 3	25% 4	Bottom 5	100% 6	75% 7	Bottom 8	50% 9	25% 10
Viable tumor cell	88	95	89	27	<1	7	93	6	96	5	3
Lymphoid cell	15	1	<1	29	18	<1	86	3	1	73	539
Macrophage	7	9	2	0	0	16	0	9	0	0	0
Erythrocyte	22	<1	0	51	478	533	0	0	0	0	0
Other (probably not tumor cell)	27	29	<1	0	0	31	3	0	0	0	0
Use of fractions[b]:		To step 2	Exp.	To step 2	To step 2	Disc.	To step 3	Disc.	Exp. tumor cells	Pooled for exp. lymphocytes	

[a]Weight, 37 g; yield, 9.6 × 10⁶ tumor cells/g.
[b]Fractions 2 and 8 were tumor-cells; fractions 9 and 10 were lymphocytes.

C. Suggestive Evidence That at Least Part of the Infiltrating Lymphocytes Are in the Activated State

1. DNA Synthesis

The early [^{3}H]-TdR uptake of TIL was in 9/12 cases higher than that of the blood lymphocytes collected at the same time (Table IX). No tumor cells were seen in these preparations.

2. "Stable" E Rosettes

The ability to form E rosettes at 37°C—"stable" E—is an indication of the activated state of a T cell and reflects the loss of the negative charge from the lymphocyte surface (Galili and Schlesinger, 1976). In 11 of the 14 biopsy samples varying numbers of T cells forming stable E rosettes were detected (Table X). This characteristic was not encountered with the blood-derived lymphocytes of the tumor patients. *In vitro*-activated T cells derived from mixed-lymphocyte culture (MLC) were used in each test as positive controls.

3. "Natural Attachment" to Cells of the Same Species

Thymocytes, neuraminidase-treated blood T cells, and *in vitro*-activated T cells (in MLC) were shown to conjugate with cells of human cell lines (Galili *et al.*,

Table IX. [^{3}H]-TdR Uptake of Lymphocytes during Overnight Incubation

		Lymphocytes separated from:	
Patient No.	Diagnosis	Blood (cpm)	Tumor (cpm)
	Sarcomas		
1021	Osteosarcoma	902	5514
1016	Osteosarcoma	511	3073
1020	Osteosarcoma	339	1710
1022	Osteosarcoma	435	1520
1019	Osteosarcoma	396	1674
1003	Osteosarcoma	313	243
1117	Synovial sarcoma	146	1856
	Lung tumors		
2227	Squamous cell carcinoma	244	264
2228	Squamous cell carcinoma	96	924
	Metastatic tumors		
1280	Melanoma (lung)	219	278
773	Melanoma (brain)	190	2180
765	Melanoma (brain)	358	2745

Table X. Stable E-Rosette Formation by Tumor- and
Blood-Derived Lymphocytes[a]

Patient No.	Diagnosis	Tumor	Blood
	Lung tumors		
2218	Squamous cell carcinoma	1	0
2238	Squamous cell carcinoma	30	0
2240	Squamous cell carcinoma	6	0
2241	Squamous cell carcinoma	7	0
2243	Squamous cell carcinoma	16	0
2244	Squamous cell carcinoma	20	1
2245	Squamous cell carcinoma	19	0
2247	Squamous cell carcinoma	6	0
9	Oat cell carcinoma	0	0
	Metastases in lung		
2211	Kidney carcinoma	1	0
505	Kidney carcinoma	54	1
2214	Kidney carcinoma	9	0
506	Seminoma	30	1
1019	Osteosarcoma	4	0

[a]Expressed as percentage of rosetting cells. The percentage
of rosetting cells in MLC populations run in parallel was
35 ± 4.2.

1978). In all six cases when TIL were mixed to various cultured cells, conjugates
were formed (Table XI). The phenomenon did not occur with blood-derived
T cells from the same patients. Also in these tests, activated T cells generated in
MLC were used as positive controls.

D. Stimulation of TIL by Autologous Tumor Cells

The autologous tumor stimulation (ATS) test registers the DNA synthesis of
blood lymphocytes following 6-day cultivation with mitomycin C(MMC)-treated
biopsy cells. Among 197 tumor cases 30% were positive. Recently, the procedure
was modified and the number of reactive cases increased considerably (65% of
45 tumors). The modification involved an improved methodology for separation
of tumor cells and the use of responder populations from which nylon-adherent
lymphocytes were eliminated.

In 11 cases, ATS was performed with blood- and tumor-derived lymphocytes
in parallel (Table XII). Blood lymphocytes were stimulated in 6/11 cases, TIL in
none. Unresponsiveness of the TIL was not due to a general loss of reactivity
because they reacted well to a low dose (0.1 μg/ml) of phytohemagglutinin (PHA).
In five cases, MLC was also performed, and a good response was obtained. It is

Table XI. Attachment of T Cells Derived from Tumor and Blood to a Variety of Human Cells[a]

Patient No.	Diagnosis	Target cell						
		Fibroblasts	Macrophages	K562	Daudi	SW982	SK-MES-1	AMA-1
	Lung tumors							
2238	Squamous cell carcinoma	65, 9	45, 10	28, 5	27, 4	55, 3	65, 3	–
2244	Squamous cell carcinoma	120, 2	–	–	–	45, 3	89, 19	85, 5
2245	Squamous cell carcinoma	85, 2	–	22, 2	29, 2	35, 4	–	–
2247	Squamous cell carcinoma	88, 2	35, 5	28, 1	25, 1	34, 4	30, 1	75, 2
	Metastasis in lung							
505	Kidney carcinoma	170, 6	235, 3	65, 3	31, 1	130, 5	95, 5	–
506	Seminoma	230, 6	103, 6	42, 4	43, 2	135, 6	80, 14	100, 12
	MLC (8 cultures) mean ± SE	74 ± 11	58 ± 8	46 ± 7	38 ± 9	137 ± 10	96 ± 1	63 ± 4

[a]Number of E-rosette-forming lymphocytes seen attached to 100 target cells. The first number in each case is the value for tumor, the second for blood-derived lymphocytes.

Table XII. Lymphocytes Isolated from Tumors in the Autologous Tumor Stimulation (ATS) Test

Patient No.	Diagnosis	Lymphocytes				Stimulation of DNA synthesis (reactivity index)[a]			
		E+ cells (%)		[3H]-TdR uptake of lymphocytes cultivated alone (cpm)		PHA (0.1 μg/ml)		ATS	
		Tumor	Blood	Tumor	Blood	Tumor	Blood	Tumor	Blood
	Sarcomas								
54	Osteosarcoma	54	41	750	1524	34	34	1.4	5.5
76	Osteosarcoma	58	49	231	120	106	159	1.2	4.7
	Lung carcinomas								
244	Squamous cell carcinoma	61	53	986	350	126	114	0.4	1.1
243	Squamous cell carcinoma	59	61	731	1756	78	16	0.6	0.7
245	Squamous cell carcinoma	51	56	608	754	24	44	0.9	0.3
1296	Squamous cell carcinoma	54	61	3871	1128	NT[b]	22	1.5	4.5
1281	Squamous cell carcinoma	65	57	3722	1250	9	10	1.3	1.5
1264	Squamous cell carcinoma	NT	NT	1109	1141	12	18	1.3	4.4
2205	Oat cell carcinoma	62	55	1362	2711	32	35	0.8	0.2
2202	Adenocarcinoma	67	53	1143	1626	9	5	1.1	5.4
	Metastases in lung								
2201	Colon carcinoma	56	70	8151	1337	11	NT	0.8	NT
1279	Kidney carcinoma	71	59	1863	719	39	43	1.2	7.1

[a]Reactivity index = $\dfrac{\text{cpm in the test culture}}{\text{cpm in the control culture}}$.

[b]NT, not tested.

Table XIII. Lymphocyte Subsets Isolated from Tumor in the Autologous Tumor Stimulation Test (ATS)

Patient No.	Diagnosis	Tumor-infiltrating lymphocytes									Blood lympho-cytes NCp	
		Total[a]			NCp[b]			NCa[c]				
		IL[d] (cpm)	ATS (RI)[e]	PHA (RI)	IL (cpm)	ATS (RI)	PHA (RI)	IL (cpm)	ATS (RI)	PHA (RI)	ATS (RI)	PHA (RI)
Sarcomas												
1003	Osteosarcoma	531	0.5	84	331	0.5	25	1155	0.5	16	0.5	10
1002	Osteosarcoma	627	1.3	46	106	34.4	45	–	–	–	28.9	46
Lung carcinomas												
1264	Squamous cell carcinoma	1109	1.3	10	96	1.5	12	–	–	–	4.4	18
1276	Squamous cell carcinoma	388	1.7	19	241	0.7	8	–	–	–	1.6	25
1281	Squamous cell carcinoma	3722	1.3	10	450	15.0	39	3722	1.5	98	15.0	31
1296	Squamous cell carcinoma	2871	1.5	14	447	17.1	30	976	1.5	47	0.7	31
2202	Adenocarcinoma	1443	1.1	9	612	5.7	69	–	–	–	5.4	51
2205	Oat cell carcinoma	1362	2.0	91	514	1.0	34	1365	0.6	32	7.1	30
Metastases in lung												
1285	Colon carcinoma	1443	1.1	36	157	36.1	577	5915	1.1	44	11.7	106
2201	Colon carcinoma	8151	0.8	11	611	18.9	38	–	–	–	32.1	227
	Mean cpm:	2311			356			2626				

[a] Total lymphocyte population.
[b] Nylon-column-passed lymphocytes.
[c] Cells which adhered to nylon wool, subset eluted with 0.02 M EDTA.
[d] Control cultures, lymphocyte confronted with mitomycin-treated identical lymphocytes.

[e] RI = reactivity index = $\dfrac{\text{cpm in the test culture}}{\text{cpm in the control culture}}$

possible that the low values for TIL are due to the activated state with elevated DNA synthesis, also in the absence of the antigen. Since antigen-induced DNA synthesis is dose dependent, the negative RI values also may be due to previous exposure of activated cells to the antigen. It is therefore impossible to say whether the TIL are in a state of unresponsiveness toward the putative tumor antigen or their behavior *in vitro* is influenced by having been exposed to the antigen *in vivo*.

In the next series comprising 10 tumors the TIL were divided into nylon-adherent and nylon-passed subsets (Table XIII). In the T-cell-enriched fraction, the background incorporation was considerably lower. It is thus likely that part of the activated T cells have also been removed by this procedure due to their adherent properties. The cells eluted from the nylon wool had in fact high levels of DNA synthesis.

The total TIL population was ATS negative. The NCp fraction reacted in 6/10 cases. The NCa population (comprising 25–60% E-receptor-positive cells) was ATS negative in all five cases tested.

The results with TIL and PBL agreed in seven cases, among which two were negative. There were three discordant cases with two negative TIL-positive PBL and one positive TIL-negative PBL.

E. Cytotoxicity of TIL against the Tumor Cell Fraction Separated from the Same Biopsy

Blood lymphocytes were previously shown to exert a cytotoxic effect for autologous tumor cells in 29/103 cases (28%). Results of cross tests with other targets indicated that the effect was restricted to the autologous tumor (Vánky *et al.*, 1979.)

When similar autologous tests were carried out with TIL as effectors, cytotoxicity occurred in 10/39 (26%) cases. Positive results were obtained with 3/12 (27%) nasopharyngeal carcinomas, 3/15 (14%) lung carcinomas, 2/4 kidney carcinomas, 1/4 sarcomas, 1/3 metastatic tumors, and 0/1 astrocytoma. Five TIL populations were tested after passage through nylon wool columns and their reactivity was not changed; one was positive both before and after passage.

The lymphocyte population separated from the biopsy did not have natural killer activity as judged by the lack of effect against the highly sensitive K562 cells. Only 1/14 tests were positive (Vose *et al.*, 1977*b*).

Parallel tests with blood- and tumor-derived lymphocytes were performed in 20 cases (Table XIV). The results correlated in 17/20 tests. Among these, 4 were positive and 13 were negative with both effectors. In 2 cases the target cells were also exposed to blood lymphocytes of healthy donors; these tests were negative. In 2 of these 7 tests the autologous lymphocytes were cytotoxic.

Table XIV. Parallel Cytotoxic Tests with Lymphocytes
Separated from Blood and Tumor[a]

Patient No.	Diagnosis	Specific cytotoxicity (%) of lymphocytes separated from:	
		Tumor	Blood
	Sarcomas		
1010	Osteosarcoma	10 (27)[b]	29
1016	Osteosarcoma	0 (38)	0
1118	Fibrosarcoma	27 (31)	2
	Lung tumors		
1253	Adenocarcinoma	3 (47)	2
1262	Adenocarcinoma	8 (22)	8
1287	Adenocarcinoma	1 (10)	19
2202	Adenocarcinoma	0 (42)	0
1269	Squamous cell cancer	1 (40)	13
1277	Squamous cell cancer	0 (35)	5
1281	Squamous cell cancer	53 (46)	24
1252	Squamous cell cancer	0 (25)	0
2225	Squamous cell cancer	0 (34)	0
2234	Squamous cell cancer	0 (44)	0
	Metastases in lung		
504	Kidney cancer	0 (17)	0
1279	Kidney cancer	43 (30)	24
2214	Kidney cancer	25 (11)	26
1280	Melanoma	3 (33)	3
	Brain tumor		
782	Astrocytoma	0 (41)	28
	Other types		
7	Nasopharyngeal cancer	56 (34)	45
473	Nasopharyngeal cancer	0 (38)	0

[a]Four-hour ^{51}Cr release test; effector:target ratio, 50:1.
[b]Spontaneous ^{51}Cr release (%).

F. Relationship between the Reactivity of Blood Lymphocytes in ATS and ALC Assays with Autologous Tumor Biopsy Cells and the Presence of Lymphocytic Infiltration in the Tumor

If the presence of lymphocytes in a tumor is a manifestation of an immunologic recognition, it may be assumed that the cases in which this occurs were among the ones with a positive result in the *in vitro* assays performed with the tumor cell-enriched populations. There were indeed indications for such correlations (Table XV). Grouping the tumors according to the presence of lymphocytes in the primary suspension (>1%), ATS occurred in 96% of the cases with and in 40% of the cases without lymphocytic infiltration. Primary ALC was obtained in

**Table XV. Reactivity of Blood Lymphocytes in ATS and ALC
Related to the Presence of Lymphocytes in the Biopsy**

Presence of lymphocytes in the biopsy suspension	Reactivity of blood lymphocytes in:		
	ATS	Primary ALC	Secondary ALC
Yes[a]	22/23 (96)[b]	14/25 (58)	10/15 (67)
No	4/10 (40)	0/25 (0)	6/16 (38)
Total:	26/33 (79)	14/50 (28)	16/31 (52)

[a]More than 1% of the cells in the parimary suspension were lymphocytes.
[b]Number of positive/number of cases; in parentheses is percentage of positive cases.

58% of the cases with and in no cases without lymphocytic infiltration. Secondary cytotoxicity was detected in 67% of the cases with and 38% of the cases without infiltration. The generation of a secondary cytotoxicity occurred only in cases in which the lymphocytes were stimulated in the ATS test.

IV. DISCUSSION

Lymphocyte infiltration is regarded as evidence for *in situ* tumor-related autoreactivity (Cochran, 1968; MacCarty, 1922; Lauder and Ahrene, 1972; Black *et al.*, 1975; Ioachim *et al.*, 1976). We only assume, however, that the infiltration is the consequence of immunologic recognition of tumor cell surface antigens and do not know whether the lymphoid cells influence the tumor growth. In fact, the majority of pathologists find no prognostic significance in the extent of lymphoid infiltration seen in the tumor (Tanaka *et al.*, 1970; Champion *et al.*, 1972; Morrison *et al.*, 1973).

The task of determining the functional characteristics of the lymphoid infiltration, especially with regard to their antitumor cell reactivity, is difficult and is burdened with a number of technical problems. The first difficulty is encountered when the disaggregation of the tumor into a cell suspension and the separation of the various cell components takes place. Disaggregation yielding viable suspensions of good quality can be achieved with the help of enzymes. Such a procedure alters the plasma membrane properties both on the tumor and on the lymphoid cells. A period of recovery under culture conditions is therefore necessary before the cells can be used for experiments (Vánky *et al.*, 1978*b*). Enzyme treatment has to be avoided when the studies are aimed at elucidating certain features which characterize the state of the tumor cells *in vivo*, such as attachment of antibodies to their surface and contacts between tumor cells and lymphocytes.

Experiments with the use of enriched tumor or lymphocyte suspensions of good purity involve several manipulations during which considerable cell loss occurs. Because this may be selective the resulting populations are hardly representative for the whole tumor.

T cells represent the predominant lymphoid infiltration at the site of auto-immune reactivity, such as the synovial fluid and membrane in patients with rheumatoid arthritis (Frøland *et al.*, 1973; Abrahamsen *et al.*, 1975), the thyroid tissue in Grave's disease (Sköldstam *et al.*, 1978), or in thyroiditis (Tötterman *et al.*, 1978). In some tumor types such as nasopharyngeal carcinoma (Jondal and Klein, 1975) and seminoma (Häyry and Tötterman, 1978), most of the infiltrating cells are T lymphocytes. In thyroid and mammary carcinomas Häyry and Tötterman (1978) detected mainly null cells, and in ovarian and uterine carcinomas about equal populations of T, B, and null cells. We have detected variable proportions of T cells and only a few B cells in the dispersed tumor specimens. In the lymphocyte-enriched suspensions the proportion of T cells was higher than in the primary tumor cell suspension, indicating that in this early step of the separation procedure a selective loss of certain lymphocyte types had already occurred.

Attachment of lymphoreticular cells to tumor cells has been observed in pleural and in ascitic malignant effusions (Sulitzeanu *et al.*, 1974). We have detected similar conjugates in suspensions of the solid tumors and by means of E rosetting showed that the attached lymphocytes were T cells.

Our experiments indicated that a proportion of the tumor-infiltrating T cells are in an activated state because they formed stable E rosettes, i.e., E rosettes at $37°C$ (Galili and Schlesinger, 1976), and when admixed they attached to a variety of normal and malignant human cells. This latter phenomenon, designated natural attachment (NA), was shown to be the property of thymocytes, neuraminidase-treated blood T cells, and *in vitro*-activated T cells (Galili *et al.*, 1978). An additional sign for activation was their relatively high DNA synthesis in comparison to the blood lymphocytes. T cells with these signs of the active state were absent from the blood of the patients.

The biological significance of the few tumor cell–T lymphocyte conjugates seen in the suspensions is unknown. It may be the manifestation of the recognition of cell surface antigen in the tumor by T cells equipped with specific receptors and/or it may represent the NA phenomenon. As demonstrated in the mouse system, the consequence of the former interaction is target killing (Berke, 1976). While not cytotoxic *per se*, NA interaction may lead to cytotoxicity through enhancement of the effect of other killer cells (Galili *et al.*, 1979).

The number of cases with positive blood ALC was low. In some cases the TIL were also positive. The experience with animal systems would predict that cytotoxicity with blood lymphocytes should be detected more often after *in vitro* sensitization. Therefore, we have cocultivated blood lymphocytes with tumor cells. In some cases in which direct or primary ALC did not occur secondary ALC was generated (Vose *et al.*, 1978). The experience obtained in model systems for the optimal conditions in the generation of specific cytotoxicity is still waiting to be employed in the human tumors. However, the possibilities with the lymphocytes isolated from the tumor are limited because of the scarcity of the material. One possibility presently under investigation is establishment of T-cell cultures with the help of blastogenic factors and testing their reactivity toward frozen preserved autologous tumor cells.

In the two human tumors in which Epstein–Barr virus (EBV) is involved as an etiologic factor, cellular response can be studied with more exactness because EBV-positive lymphoblastoid lines can be used as specific targets. Healthy individuals who are infected with the virus, as judged by the presence of EBV antibodies in the serum, have EBV-specific memory T cells (Moss *et al.*, 1978).

Burkitt's lymphoma is a monoclonal proliferation of B cells and can easily be dispersed mechanically. Thus, isolation of infiltrating T cells did not present technical problems. Their proportion was low, however, in our hands lower than 1%. In the report of Gross *et al.* (1975) the proportion varied between 4 and 38%. Because of the lack of a sufficient number of T cells we have tested the cytotoxicity of such cells in only three cases. In one experiment the biopsy cells were also included as target. These results indicated an EBV-related reactivity, because EBV-positive but not EBV-negative lymphoblastoid cell lines were killed (Jondal *et al.*, 1975). Further experiments are badly needed. Because of the decrease of the number of Burkitt's lymphoma patients admitted to the city hospitals (they are treated mainly at local hospitals), we presently receive very few biopsies.

Nasopharyngeal carcinoma (NPC) is the other tumor in which the EBV has an etiological role. Its cells carry the viral genome (Wolf *et al.*, 1973*a,b*). Usually the tumor is heavily infiltrated with lymphocytes. Among these, a proportion of T cells were shown to have the above mentioned characteristics of the activated state (Galili *et al.*, 1980). In 3/8 cases cytotoxicity was registered against autologous biopsy cells in the short-term ^{51}Cr release test (Vose *et al.*, 1978).

Application of the ATS for the demonstration of specific reactivity of TIL is complex. Because at least part of the lymphocytes are activated when separated from the tumor, reactivity under the conditions performed with the blood lymphocytes is not necessarily expected nor found. It is possible that the test has to be carried out with different kinetics and antigen doses because a secondary response may be expected. Another possibility is that the population contains suppressor cells. This is suggested by the finding that ATS was positive with the nylon fiber column-passed TIL population. This population had lower background DNA synthesis.

In our initial series the ATS-positive cases were fewer (30%). Modification of the procedure was introduced both in the treatment of blood lymphocytes and the tumor cells. The former were passed through nylon fiber columns. In separation of the tumor cells we have sharpened our criteria for the suitable suspensions; experiments were only performed with highly purified viable tumor cell populations and the cells were incubated overnight in culture conditions before the experiments were initiated. The decisive factor is unknown. Putative cell surface antigen(s) affected during the separation procedure may have been resynthesized. Another possibility is that antibodies attached to the cell surface may have been eliminated through shedding (Yefenof *et al.*, 1976). Support for the significance of this event may be provided by our earlier series of experiments in which we measured the amount of immunoglobulin in mechanically dispersed tumor biopsy suspensions (Vánky *et al.*, 1975). This was found to vary. The same biopsies were used in ATS and except for one, all the positive ATS results were obtained with the immunoglobulin-negative tumors. Antibody-coated cells may not be recognized by the T lymphocytes. Support for this is given by another series of experiments in which we have shown that ATS does not occur or is weaker in the presence of autologous serum. The result of interaction of antibodies and immunocompetent cells with regard to the fate of the tumor cell is complex. It could be expected that the majority of the antibody-coated cells should be eliminated by the mechanism of ADCC. Still, cells of growing tumors have been shown to have antibody coat in experimental systems (Witz, 1973).

With the present methodology the ATS-positive cases are twice as frequent (68%) than in the initial series. A high proportion of the patients thus recognize their own tumor cells immunologically. Because we receive material only from cases judged suitable for operation the patients are selected. It is an open question whether or not the other category of patients—the inoperable ones—would present a similarly high frequency of positive ATS.

Our experiments focused on the characteristics of the T cells in the tumor. However, these represent only part of the immunologic orchestra. T cell response shares one aspect with serology in that when properly analyzed it also reveals specificity. At the level of effector mechanisms, monocyte macrophages are also of great importance. Their presence may be of more significance for an efficient tumor response (Lauder *et al.*, 1977).

Another aspect which is not dealt with in our experiments is the possible growth stimulatory effect of lymphocytes shown to occur both *in vitro* and *in vivo* (Prehn, 1976). In a recent series of experiments evidence was obtained for the *in vitro* growth-promoting effect of TIL on explanted tumor cells in a mouse mammary tumor system (Blazar *et al.*, 1980).

ACKNOWLEDGMENTS

This work was supported by Contract NO1 CB 74144 with the Division of Cancer Biology and Diagnosis, National Cancer Institute, U.S. Department of

Health Education and Welfare, and by the Swedish Cancer Society. F. Vánky was supported by the Stanley Thomas Johnson Foundation, Bern, Switzerland; U. Galili by the International Agency for Research on Cancer; B. M. Vose by the Cancer Research Campaign and the Medical Research Council of Great Britain; and M. Fopp by the Schweizerische Akademie der Medicinischen Wissenschaften.

V. REFERENCES

Abrahamsen, T. G., Frøland, S. S., Natvig, J. B., and Pahle, J., 1975, Elution and character-
    ization of lymphocytes from rheumatoid inflammatory tissues, *Scand. J. Immunol.*
    22:823–830.
Bakács, T., Klein, E., and Ljungström, K. K., 1978, Search for disease-related cytotoxicity
    in mammary tumor patients, *Cancer Lett.* 4:191–197.
Bansal, S. C., Hargreaves, R., and Sjögren, H. O., 1972, Facilitation of polyoma tumor growth
    in rats by blocking sera and tumor eluate, *Int. J. Cancer* 9:97–108.
Berke, G., 1976, Lymphocyte–target cell conjugation: Membrane receptors for alloantigens,
    Adv. Exp. Med. Biol. 65:483–488.
Black, M. M., Barclay, T. H. C., and Hankey, B. F., 1975, Prognosis in breast cancer utilizing
    histologic characteristics of the primary tumor, *Cancer* 36:2048–2055.
Blazar, B., Galili, N., and Klein, E., 1980, *In vitro* growth of murine mammary tumor cells.
    The effect of lymph node, spleen and tumor associated lymphocytes alone and in
    combination, *Int. J. Cancer*, submitted.
Bøyum, A., 1974, Separation of blood leukocytes, granulocytes and lymphocytes, *Tissue
    Antigens* 4:269–274.
Champion, H. R., Wallace, I. W., and Prescott, R. J., 1972, Histology in breast cancer
    prognosis, *Br. J. Cancer* 26:129–138.
Cochran, A. J., 1968, Histology and prognosis in malignant melanoma, *J. Pathol.*
    97:459–468.
Eccles, S. A., and Alexander, P., 1974, Sequestration of macrophages in growing tumors and
    its effect on the immunological capacity of the host, *Br. J. Cancer* 30:42–49.
Frøland, S. S., Natvig, J. B., and Husby, G., 1973, Immunological characterization of lym-
    phocytes in synovial fluid from patients with rheumatoid arthritis, *Scand. J. Immunol.*
    2:67–73.
Galili, U., and Schlesinger, M., 1976, The formation of stable E rosettes by human T-lympho-
    cytes activated in mixed lymphocyte reactions, *J. Immunnol.* 117:730–735.
Galili, U., and Schlesinger, M., 1978, Regulation of the cytotoxic effect of human killer cells
    and tumor cell lines by neuraminidase-treated T-lymphocytes, *Cancer Immunol. Immu-
    nother.* 4:33–39.
Galili, U., Galili, N., Vánky, F., and Klein, E., 1978, Natural species restricted attachment of
    human and murine T lymphocytes to various cells, *Proc. Natl. Acad. Sci. USA* 75:2396–
    2400.
Galili, U., Rosenthal, L., Galili, N., and Klein, E., 1979, Activated T cells in the synovial fluid
    of arthritic patients: Characterization and comparison with *in vitro* activated human and
    murine T cells in cooperation with monocytes in cytotoxicity, *J. Immunol.* 122:828–883.
Galili, U., Klein, E., Klein, G., Singh, S., and Bal, I., 1980, Activated T lymphocytes in in-
    filtrates and draining lymph nodes of nasopharyngeal carcinoma, *Int. J. Cancer*, in press.
Gross, R. L., Steel, C. M., Levin, A. G., Singh, S., and Brubaker, G., 1975, In vitro immuno-

logical studies on East African cancer patients. III. Spontaneous rosette formation by cells from Burkitt lymphoma biopsies, *Int. J. Cancer* 15:139-143.

Háyry, P., and Tötterman, T. H. 1987, Cytological and functional analysis of inflammatory infiltrates in human malignant tumors. I. Composition of the inflammatory infiltrates, *Eur. J. Immunol.* 8:866-871.

Holden, H. J., Haskill, J. S., Kirchner, H., and Herberman, R. B., 1976, Two functionally distinct anti-tumor effector cells isolated from primary murine sarcoma virus-induced tumors, *J. Immunol.* 117:440-446.

Ioachim, H. L., Dorsett, B. H., and Paluch, E., 1976, The immune reponse at the tumor site in lung carcinoma, *Cancer* 38:2296-2309.

Jondal, M., and Klein, G., 1975, Classification of lymphocytes in nasopharyngeal carcinoma (NPC) biopsies, *Biomedicine* 23:163-165.

Jondal, M., Svedmyr, E., Klein, E., and Singh, S., 1975, Killer T cells in a Burkitt's lymphoma biopsy, *Nature (London)* 255:405-407.

Julius, M. H., Simpson, E., and Herzenberg, L. A., 1973, A rapid method for the isolation of functional thymus-derived murine lymphocytes, *Eur. J. Immunol.* 3:645-649.

Klein, E., Klein, G., Nadkarni, J. S., Nadkarni, J. J. Wigzell, H., and Clifford, P., 1968, Surface IgM-kappa specificity on a Burkitt lymphoma cell *in vivo* and in derived culture lines, *Cancer Res.* 28:1300-1310.

Lauder, I., and Ahrene, W., 1972, The significance of lymphocytic infiltration in neuroblastoma, *Br. J. Cancer* 26:321-330.

Lauder, I., Ahrene, W., Steward, J., and Sainsbury, R., 1977, Macrophage infiltration of breast tumors: A prospective study, *J. Clin, Pathol.* 30:563-568.

Lozzio, C. P., and Lozzio, B. B., 1975, Human chronic myelogenous cell line with positive Philadelphia chromosome, *Blood* 45:321-328.

MacCarty, W. C., 1922, Factors which influence longevity in cancer, *Ann. Surg.* 76:9-12.

Morrison, A. S., Black, M. M., Lowe, C. L., MacMahon, B. and Yuasa, S., 1973, Some international differences in histology and survival in breast cancer, *Int. J. Cancer* 11:261-267.

Moss, D. J., Rickinson, A. B., and Pope, J. A., 1978, Long term cell-mediated immunity to Epstein-Barr virus in man. I. Complete regression of virus induced transformation in cultures of seropositive donor leukocytes, *Int. J. Cancer* 22:662-668.

Prehn, R. T., 1976, Tumor progression and homeostasis, *Adv. Cancer Res.* 23:203-236.

Quan, P. C., and Burtin, P., 1978, Demonstration of nonspecific suppressor cells in the peripheral lymphocytes of cancer patients, *Cancer Res.* 38:288-296.

Sköldstam, L., Anderberg, B., and Norrby, K., 1978, B and T lymphocytes in toxic diffuse goiter, *Clin. Exp. Immunol.* 31:524-525.

Sulitzeanu, D., Gorsky, Y., Paglin, S., and Weiss, D., 1974, Morphologic evidence suggestive of host-tumor cell interactions *in vivo* in human cancer patients, *J. Natl. Cancer Inst.* 53:603-604.

Tanaka, T., Cooper, E. H., and Anderson, C. K., 1970, Lymphocyte infiltration in bladder carcinoma, *Rev. Eur. Etudes Clin. Biol.* 15:1081-1089.

Ting, C. C., Tsai, S. C., and Rogers, M. J., 1977, Host control of tumor growth, *Science* 197:571-573.

Tötterman, T. H., Gordin, A., Häyry, O., Andersson, L. C., and Makinen, T., 1978, Accumulation of thyroid antigen reactive T lymphocytes in the gland of patients with subacute thyroiditis, *Clin. Exp. Immunol.* 32:253-258.

Underwood, J. C. E., 1972, Lymphoreticular infiltration in human tumors—Prognostic and biological implications—A review, *Br. J. Cancer* 30:538-547.

Vánky, F., and Stjernswärd, J., 1976, Lymphocyte stimulation test for detection of tumor-host interaction in humans, in: *In Vitro Methods in Cell Mediated and Tumor Immunity*, Vol. II (B. Bloom and J. R. David, eds.) pp. 597-606, Academic Press, New York.

Vánky, F., Trempe, G., Klein, E., and Stjernswärd, J., 1975, Human tumor–lymphocyte interaction *in vitro:* Blastogenesis correlated to detectable immunoglobulin in the biopsy, *Int. J. Cancer* **16**:113–124.

Vánky, F., Klein, E., Stjernswärd, J., Rodriguez, L., Péterffy, Á., Steiner, L., and Nilsonne, U., 1978*a*, Human tumor–lymphocyte interaction *in vitro*. III. T-lymphocytes in autologous tumor stimulation (ATS), *Int. J. Cancer* **22**:679–686.

Vánky, F., Klein, E., Stjernswärd, J., Nilsonne, U., Rodriguez, L., and Péterffy, Á., 1978*b*, Human tumor–lymphocyte interaction *in vitro*. II. Conditions which improve the capacity of biopsy cells to stimulate autologous lymphocytes, *Cancer Immunol. Immunother.* **5**:63–69.

Vánky, F., Vose, B. M., Fopp, M., and Klein, E., 1979, Human tumor–lymphocyte interaction *in vitro*. VI. Specificity of primary and secondary autologous lymphocyte mediated cytotoxicity, *J. Natl. Cancer Inst.* **62**:1407–1413.

Vose, B. M., Vánky, F., and Klein, E., 1977*a*, Lymphocyte cytotoxicity against autologous tumor biopsy cells in humans, *Int. J. Cancer* **28**:512–519.

Vose, B. M., Vánky, F., Argov, S., and Klein, E., 1977*b*, Natural cytotoxicity in man: Activity of lymph node and tumor infiltrating lymphocytes, *Eur. J. Immunol.* **7**:753–757.

Vose, B. M., Vánky, F., Fopp, M., and Klein, E., 1978, *In vitro* generation of cytotoxicity against autologous tumor biopsy cells, *Int. J. Cancer* **21**:588–593.

Witz, I. P., 1973, The biological significance of tumor bound immunoglobulins, *Curr. Topics. Microbiol. Immunol.* **61**:151–171.

Witz, I. P., 1977, Tumor bound immunoglobulins, *in situ* expression of humoral immunity, *Adv. Cancer Res.* **25**:95–141.

Wolf, H., zur Hausen, H., and Becker, V., 1973*a*, EB viral DNA in epithelial nasopharyngeal carcinoma cells, *Nature (London)* **244**:245–247.

Wolf, H., zur Hausen, H., Klein, G., Becker, V., Henle, G., and Henle, W., 1973*b*, Attempt to detect virus-specific DNA sequences in human tumors. III. Epstein–Barr viral DNA in non lymphoid nasopharyngeal carcinoma cells, *Med. Microbiol. Immunol.* **161**:15–21.

Yefenof, E., Witz, I. P., and Klein, E., 1976, Interaction of antibody and cell surface localized antigen, *Int. J. Cancer* **17**:633–639.

Chapter 5

Intratumor Host Cells of Experimental Rat Neoplasms: Characterization and Effector Function

M. Moore and K. Moore*

Paterson Laboratories
Christie Hospital and Holt Radium Institute
Manchester M 20 9BX, England

I. INTRODUCTION

That host resistance against experimental neoplasms is a biological reality has long been sustained by the plethora of tumor–host systems in which immunological reactions have been demonstrated. The evidence has been derived principally from the unequivocal demonstration of tumor rejection *in vivo* and of serological and antitumor cellular reactivity *in vitro* (reviewed by Herberman, 1974). Considerable progress has been made toward the identification of the principal cellular components involved which, depending on the tumor–host system, include cytolytic thymus-derived lymphocytes (CTL), antibody-dependent killer (K) cells, and natural killer (NK) cells (reviewed by Levy and Leclerc, 1977), and macrophages acting alone, or in concert with other cell types (Evans and Alexander, 1976; Keller, 1977). In the majority of these studies, effector function has been demonstrated at a systemic level, in populations variously derived from regional lymph nodes, spleen, peripheral blood, and the peritoneal cavity (Cerottin and Brunner, 1974). The interpretation of these reactions in relation to actual *in vivo* events governing tumor progression or regression is difficult in the absence of comparable data on the activity of effector cells from within the tumor itself. Information on the nature of the tumor–host inter-

*Present address: Department of Bacteriology, University of Edinburgh Medical School, Teviot Place, Edinburgh, Scotland.

action which occurs *in situ*, and is probably critical to the balance of the tumor-host relationship, is just beginning to emerge.

The demonstration by Evans (1972) that certain intratumor host cells (macrophages) could be recovered from solid experimental neoplasms by enzymatic disaggregation without apparent loss of morphological or functional integrity opened up the prospect that other cellular components of the *in situ* host response could be isolated and similarly analyzed. Primary and transplanted experimental neoplasms are now known to contain a diversity of host cells including T cells (Plata *et al*, 1976; Russell *et al.*, 1976*b*; Holden *et al.*, 1976; Pross and Kerbel, 1976; Blazar and Heppner, 1978), B cells (Russell *et al.*, 1976*a*; Pross and Kerbel, 1976), cells with receptors for the third component of complement (C3), or the Fc portion of IgG (FcR) (Kerbel *et al.*, 1975; Kerbel and Pross, 1976; Wood *et al.*, 1975; Haskill *et al.*, 1975*b*; Szymaniec and James, 1976; Pross and Kerbel, 1976), macrophages (Evans, 1973; Van Loveren and Den Otter, 1974; Haskill *et al.*, 1975*a*), and other minority populations (neutrophils, eosinophils, mast cells) (Russell *et al.*, 1976*b*) which frequently differ qualitatively and quantitatively for each tumor. In some situations there are functional differences in the activity of intratumor host cells of regressors and progressors (Russell and McIntosh, 1977; Gillespie *et al.*, 1977; Lill and Fortner, 1978); while in others, where spontaneous regression occurs only rarely, if at all, a correlation exists between the degree of host cell infiltration and the biological properties of the tumor in terms of growth rate and/or propensity to metastasize (Eccles and Alexander, 1974*a*; Wood and Gillespie, 1975).

From these and other studies it is apparent that a tumor is a complex structure consisting of neoplastic cells, supported by stromal and vascular elements that, together with the inflammatory infiltrate, contribute to a host cell compartment which in some instances numerically exceeds that of its malignant counterpart. The factors that influence tumor growth are therefore likely to be multifarious and include nonimmunological mechanisms. Even so, circumstantial evidence attributes at least a partial role to infiltrating leukocytes, and in some tumor-host systems to identifiable leukocyte populations, e.g., macrophages, in the process of tumor restraint. Evidence from some laboratories indicates that macrophages in turn enter a neoplasm as part of an immune reaction against tumor antigens, in a manner comparable to their entry into delayed hypersensitivity sites (Eccles *et al.*, 1976). The proportion of macrophages is thus diminished in tumors of weak immunogenicity in normal syngeneic hosts and in tumors of strong or moderate immunogenicity in immunodeficient hosts (Eccles and Alexander, 1974*a*).

Four years ago, studies were initiated on a series of five tumors passaged in syngeneic recipients (W/Not rats) to ascertain the relationship between the pattern of cellular infiltration, immunogenicity, and growth rate (K. Moore and Moore, 1977*a*). These comprised two immunogeneic sarcomas (Mc40A and Mc57) originally induced by methylcholanthrene (MC) and three nonimmunogenic tumors of which one, a mammary tumor (AAF57), was originally induced by N-hydroxy-2-acetylaminofluorene, and two, a squamous cell carcinoma (SP1) and a mammary carcinoma (SP22), arose spontaneously (Baldwin et al., 1979).

The finding that the pattern of infiltration bore a potentially meaningful relationship to the course of tumor growth required the extension of these studies to an analysis of effector function in an attempt to identify which cell types might be important for tumor rejection (M. Moore and Moore, 1977b; K. Moore and Moore, 1979). To this end, one of the immunogenic sarcomas, Mc40A, characterized by a heterogeneous cellular infiltrate comprising principally T cells, macrophages and nonphagocytic FcR+ cells, was selected for further investigation.

II. CHARACTERISTICS OF TUMOR INFILTRATION BY HOST LEUKOCYTES

A. Tumor Disaggregation

The identification, quantitation, and functional assessment of the tumor-infiltrative component of inflammatory host cells is dependent upon several major requirements. First, tumor cell suspensions should be representative of the intact tissues from where they are derived. Second, the techniques for the differential characterization of the various cellular components should not be adversely affected by the disaggregation procedures. Third, isolated components of the inflammatory response should retain their functional integrity. In our experience, mechanical disruption invariably resulted in preparations of low viability so that recourse to enzymes was unavoidable. No satisfactory technique is available for estimating the yield of cells recovered after total enzymatic dissociation; hence, the composition of the tumor tissue can be represented only by those cells surviving disaggregation in the viable state. Tumor cells which are rendered moribund in vivo by host responses or by other means are presumably degraded by enzyme. Determination of the extent to which the tumor cell suspensions were representative of the undigested tumor was attempted by estimating the release of a given cell type (macrophage) under conditions of different enzyme substrate specificity. For this purpose, macrophages were enumerated after intracytoplasmic uptake of polystyrene latex. Little difference was observed in the relative proportions of macrophages released from tumors using trypsin, collagenase, papain, elastase, or hyaluronidase, and it was concluded that selective release of cells other than macrophages would be unlikely to occur (K. Moore and Moore, 1977a).

Trypsin was the most efficient of the enzymes tested. Although we observed no adverse effects of this enzyme on the functional tests or surface markers under study, we acceded to the caveat of Werb (1975) that trypsin might affect the "macrophage non-immunologic phagocytic receptor," and used papin, collagenase, and DNase (PCD) instead. This mixture induced no inhibitory effect on the phagocytosis of polystyrene particles by starch-stimulated peritoneal macrophages, even after prolonged exposure, an observation which virtually eliminated the possibility that tumor macrophages could be underestimated when released by milder enzymatic treatment.

B. Identification of Intratumor Host Cells

Infiltrating cells were identified in freshly disaggregated tumor cell suspensions by several techniques, schematically summarized in Fig. 1. Total host cell content was estimated by immunofluorescence analysis of tumors developing in $(W/Not \times PVG/c)F_1$ hybrids from a subcutaneous injection of 5 million tumor cells previously cultivated to eliminate contaminating donor leukocytes. The tumor cells, having originated in W/Not rats, express antigens of the W/Not genotype *(AgB-2)*, whereas host cells present in W/Not tumors growing in F_1 hybrids express antigens of both W/Not and PVG/c *(AgB-5)* genotypes. Tested against spleen, lymph node cells, and peripheral blood leukocytes, this allo-antiserum stained 99% of all cells. The extent of host cell infiltration (comprising leukocytes and cellular elements of stroma and vasculature) could thus be estimated using this reagent.

Cells with receptors for the Fc portion of immunoglobulin (FcR) were identified and quantitated by formation of erythrocyte–antibody (EA) rosettes. The rationale for using EA-rosette formation as a principal marker of infiltrating leukocytes is the virtual ubiquity of FcR on cells in this category (Kerbel and Davies, 1974). They are present on monocytes, macrophages, and lymphocytes (K and NK cells) as well as polymorphonuclear leukocytes. They are also present on a subpopulation of "activated" T cells (Rubin and Hertel-Wolff, 1975). Ea-rosette-forming cells (Ea-RFC) accounted for $31 \pm 1\%$ (SE) of W/Not spleen cells using sheep erythrocytes plus amboceptor.

Cells with receptors for the third component of complement (C_3R) were identified and quantified by formation of erythrocyte-antibody-complement (EAC) rosettes, C_3R^+ cells (mainly B lymphocytes and macrophages) accounted for $33 \pm 1\%$ (SE) of EAC-RFC in W/Not spleen. The capacity of spleen cells to form EA or EAC rosettes was unaffected by exposure to PCD. Thus, the techniques available for the characterization of leukocytes in nontumor tissues could also be used to identify and enumerate similar cells in disaggregated tumor suspensions.

Phagocytic cells were identified in Jenner–Giemsa-stained cytocentrifuge preparations by their ability to phagocytose membrane-bound EA complexes after formation of rosettes. Mononuclear phagocytes were identified by their greatly enlarged cytoplasm containing erythrocytes and numerical correspon-

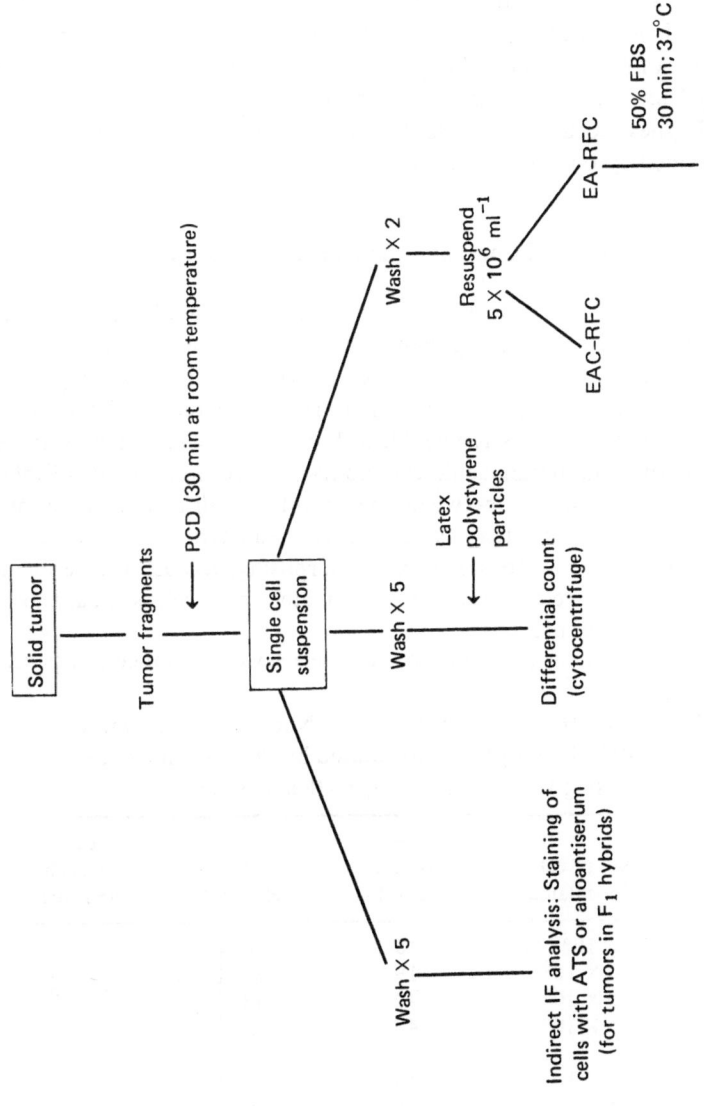

Figure 1. Scheme for identification of intratumor host cells. PCD, papain (0.1 mg/ml⁻¹), collogenase (0.1 mg/ml⁻¹), DNase (0.001 mg/ml⁻¹); ATS, rabbit anti-rat thymocyte serum; EAC-RFC, erythrocyte-antibody-complement rosette-forming cells; EA-RFC, erythrocyte-antibody rosette-forming cells.

dence with cells routinely estimated by polystyrene uptake (Section II.A) was within 10%. Neutrophils phagocytosed polystyrene but could be readily distinguished from macrophages by their characteristic nuclear structure.

Thymus-derived lymphocytes were enumerated in single cell suspensions of tumors by an indirect immunofluorescence assay using rabbit anti-rat thymocyte serum (ATS). This antiserum stained 96% of thymocytes, 49% of splenic leukocytes, 38% of lymph node leukocytes, and 10% of bone marrow cells, values which remained unchanged by exposure to PCD.

Other cell types (eosinophils, basophils, mast cells) were identified morphologically on stained cytocentrifuge films.

C. Host Cell Content of Tumors in F_1 Hybrids

The proportion of intratumor host cells determined by serological analysis of two of the tumors (Mc40A, SP22) grown from tissue cultures on transplantation to F_1 hybrids was similar to that obtained on serial transplants using surface marker techniques and functional assays. Forty-one percent of the cellular content of the immunogenic sarcoma Mc40A consisted of nonmalignant cells, whereas that of the nonimmunogenic carcinoma SP22 comprised 14% (Table I). The degree of correspondence between the total host cell content determined with the alloantiserum and that concurrently estimated by surface marker analysis (Section II.D) was to some extent surprising because the serological procedure should also have detected noninflammatory host cells such as those of the tissue stroma and vasculature.

It is possible that under the conditions of the assay on tumor cell suspensions

Table I. Total Host Cell Content of W/Not Tumors Grown in (W/Not $\times$ PVG/c) F_1 Hybrids, Estimated by Immunofluorescence Using W/Not Anti-PVG/c Alloantiserum

Tumor	No. of cells inoculated	Time of excision (days)	Stained cells[a] (%)	Mean % host cells (± 1 SE)
Mc40A	10^6	16	36 ⎫	
	5×10^6	19	38 ⎬	
	5×10^6	40	43	41 ± 3
	5×10^6	40	47 ⎭	
SP22	5×10^6	18	13 ⎫	
	5×10^6	18	13 ⎬	14 ± 1
	5×10^6	24	15 ⎭	

[a]Values given are corrected for staining with normal (control) W/Not rat serum.

certain nonlymphoid host cells escaped detection, either through preferential loss or failure to separate into single cells during the disaggregation procedure. However, these estimates are not strictly comparable because tumors in F_1 hybrids originated from tissue culture lines of neoplastic cells, whereas surface marker analyses were performed on transplants initially contaminated with donor inflammatory cells. Since double-marker tests were not performed, we have no *direct* evidence that the fluorescing cells in the F_1 hybrid tumors were identical with those detected by the other procedures. However, in a similar study Kerbel *et al.* (1975) showed that FcR^+ cells in murine neoplasms resulting from the injection of FcR^--cultured tumor cells in F_1 hybrids, where host cells could be distinguished by anti-H-2 antisera, were virtually all of host origin.

D. Leukocytes within Tumors Serially Transplanted in Syngeneic Hosts

Estimates of the proportion of the different leukocytes were based on serially transplanted tumors selected at random. With the exception of SP1, wherein markedly diminished infiltration occurred with tumor enlargement, such variations as occurred in the number and type of inflammatory cells were unrelated to tumor mass or time after implantation. The infiltrating population consisted of three principal components; two of these (macrophages and thymus-derived lymphocytes) were estimated directly while the third (nonphagocytic EA-RFC) was calculated by subtraction of the macrophage component from the total EA-RFC (Fig. 2). Because most leukocytes express FcR, the total infiltrating leukocyte population could thus be approximately represented by the summation of values for EA-RFC and ATS-positive cells. In this respect our assessment differed slightly from that of Kerbel and Pross (1976) who proposed that FcR^+ cells alone provided quantitative indication of infiltration in transplanted murine tumors. In their initial studies the T-cell component (measured by susceptibility to anti-theta serum) scarcely exceeeded 10% for any tumor, but more detailed examination of primary tumors and early generation transplants disclosed more variable and frequently greater T-cell infiltration (Pross and Kerbel, 1976).

The total inflammatory infiltrate was greatest in the immunogenic sarcomas Mc40A and Mc57 (42 and 45%, respectively) with the three major components present in roughly equivalent proportions. The degree of infiltration of the nonimmunogenic tumors was low by contrast, and did not exceeed 15%. Also, the EA-RFC were virtually all macrophages, i.e., nonphagocytic EA-RFC were minimally present. There was thus a significant difference (by Student's t-test) between the immunogenic sarcomas (Mc40A, Mc57) and the nonimmunogenic carcinomas (AA57, SP1, SP22) in respect to all three inflammatory components: EA-RFC ($p < 0.01$), macrophages ($p < 0.01$), and thymus-derived lymphocytes ($p < 0.005$).

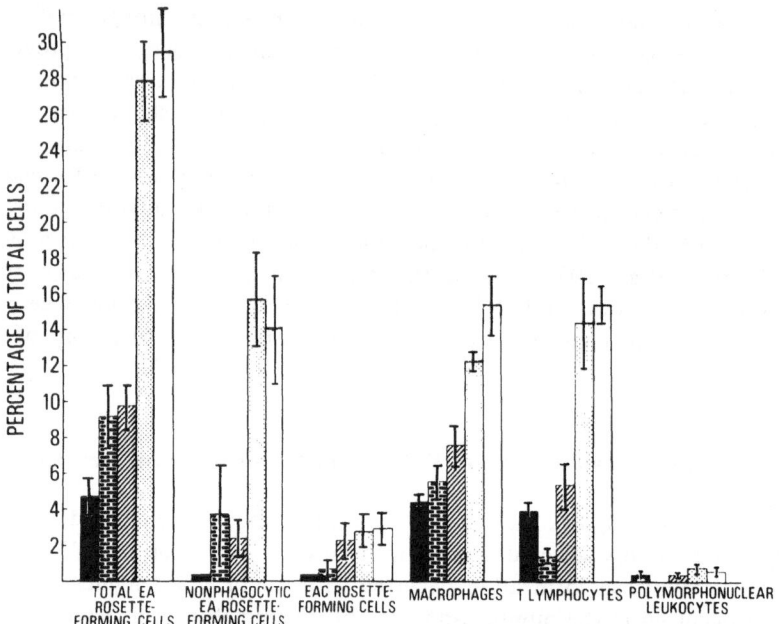

Figure 2. Numbers of inflammatory cell types identified within five serially transplanted tumors of differing immunogenicity. Tumors were selected at random from those developing after serial transplantation of tumor tissue into syngeneic rats. Two immunogenic tumors, Mc57 (☐) and Mc40A (▨), and three nonimmunogenic tumors, SP1 (▨), SP22 (▨), and AAF/57 (■) were analyzed. Error bars, ±1 SE.

The fact that macrophage content was not also reflected by infiltrating EAC-RFC, which were low in all of the tumors, was unexpected (Lay and Nussenzweig, 1968). If PCD had exerted a deleterious effect on the macrophage complement receptor, then it was preferential inasmuch as the enzyme mixture had no such effect on C-reactive spleen cells (Section II.B). It seems more likely that macrophages have their receptors blocked by a C_3-containing complex which remains bound throughout the incubation period, or unlike the FcR is lost through activation. Our observations have a parallel in acutely rejecting rat cardiac allografts where neither B lymphocytes nor macrophages formed EAC rosettes (Tilney *et al.*, 1975).

Neutrophils and basophils were present to a negligible extent ($< 2\%$) in all tumors tested and eosinophils were rarely detectable.

A correlation between the degree of infiltration and tumor immunogenicity was suggested earlier by Evans (1972) and was subsequently related to the biological behavior of a range of tumors (Eccles and Alexander, 1974*a*), but with reference to the tumor macrophage population only. It should be realized that, although important, macrophages are not the only infiltrating cells and in the

Table II. Intratumor Host Cells of Three Primary MC-Induced Rat Sarcomas

Tumor	Weight (g)	Host leukocytes as percentage of total tumor cell population[a]				
		EA-RFC	Macrophages	PMN	E	B
MC2	22	41	40	4	0	0
MC3	3	33	21	0	2	0
MC5	17	44	39	0	0	0

[a]PMN, polymorphonuclear leukocytes; E, eosinophils; B, basophils.

mature form may account by our criteria for little more than a third of the total inflammatory infiltrate. The macrophage content of three primary tumors induced by MC was between 20 and 40% of the total tumor cell population (Table II).

In situ lymphocytes reactive with ATS were not unexpected in immunogenic tumors, but the concurrent presence of a significant nonphagocytic FcR^+ population was less readily interpretable. Several cell types could be involved, e.g., B lymphocytes, "activated" T lymphocytes, lymphocytes of neither B- or T-cell lineage (NK cells?), or even cells of the mononuclear phagocytic system in which phagocytosis is actively inhibited or unexpressed (Nathan *et al.*, 1976). In the interpretation of such data where surface marker techniques lack specificity for any one cell type, due allowance must be made for "overlap" among some populations. This is true of serological identification as well as rosetting techniques. For instance, antithymocyte antisera prepared by procedures very similar to our own, notwithstanding their apparent specificity for thymocytes, may react with minority populations of non-T-lymphocytes, e.g., those expressing NK activity (Section III.B) (Shellam, 1977). Also, deployment of unfractionated antisera, unless IgG is digested to the $F(ab')_2$ fragment, may lead to nonspecific attachment to a variety of FcR^+ cells.

E. Kinetics of Leukocyte Infiltration

Studies on the time course of infiltration of tumors arising from previously cultivated cells amplified the data obtained on serial transplants in several respects. The macrophage content of each neoplasm, regardless of immunogenicity, was significantly greater 7–8 days after injection (when tumors were first clinically manifest) than at any time in their subsequent development (Figs. 3 and 4), a feature which was also apparent on histological examination. Thus, macrophages accounted for 17% of cells in AAF57 (compared with 5% from day 14 onward, $p < 0.05$, by Student's *t*-test), 24% in SP22 (cf. 5% from day 14,

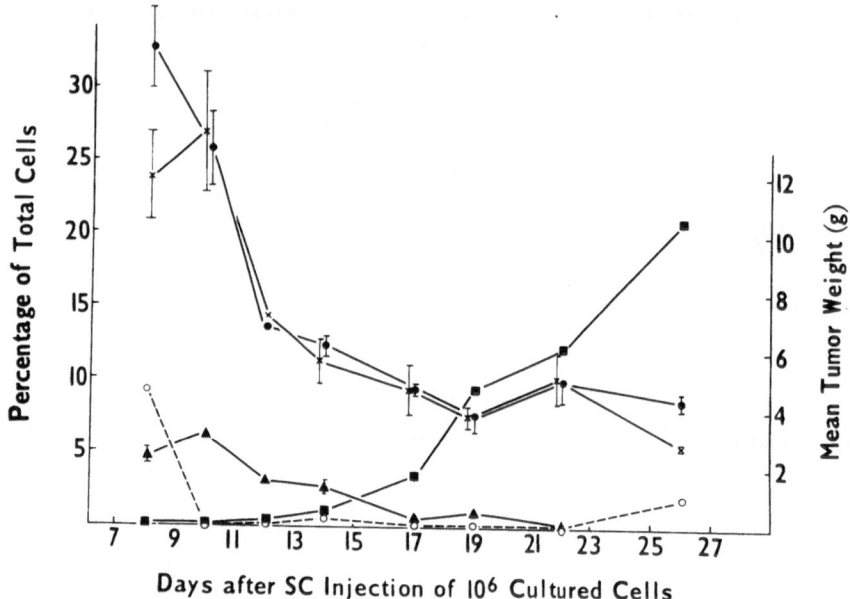

Figure 3. Time course of infiltration of inflammatory cells into tumors derived from cultured SP22 tumor cells. Tumors were induced by SC inoculation of 10^6 *in vitro*-cultured tumor cells on day 0. Points at days 8 and 10 represent the mean of six analyses each of a pool of three tumor nodules, that at day 12 a single analysis of a pool of three tumor nodules, and those from day 14 onward the mean of analyses of three tumors. EA-RFC, ●—●; macrophages, ×—×; nonphagocytic EA-RFC, o---o; EAC-RFC, ▲—▲; tumor weight, ■—■. Error bars, ±1 SE.

$p < 0.01$), and 24% in Mc40A (cf. 12% from day 14, $p < 0.005$). Essentially similar data were obtained by Haskill *et al.* (1975*a*) for murine MC sarcomas. Also, Mc40A differed from AAF57 and SP22 in respect to the nonphagocytic EA-RFC population (Fig. 4). In the latter tumors EA-RFC were virtually all phagocytic, but in Mc40A initial EA-RFC levels were maintained throughout the time course by ingress of nonphagocytic EA-RFC, the numbers of which were related inversely to those of the phagocytic EA-RFC (macrophages).

Delineation of the nature of the early host response to a tumor nidus requires characterization of the cellular infiltrate before the tumors become clinically apparent, an approach which has to date proven elusive. The almost total absence of polymorphonuclear leukocytes from the tumors studied suggests that at no time was the host reaction one of classical inflammatory type. This conclusion is consistent with the fact that indomethacin, administered according to a regime (Winter *et al.*, 1962; Hall and Hallet, 1975) in which it was demonstrably anti-inflammatory, was without discernible effect on the leukocyte infiltration profiles of Mc40A and SP22 (M. Moore and Moore, 1977*b*).

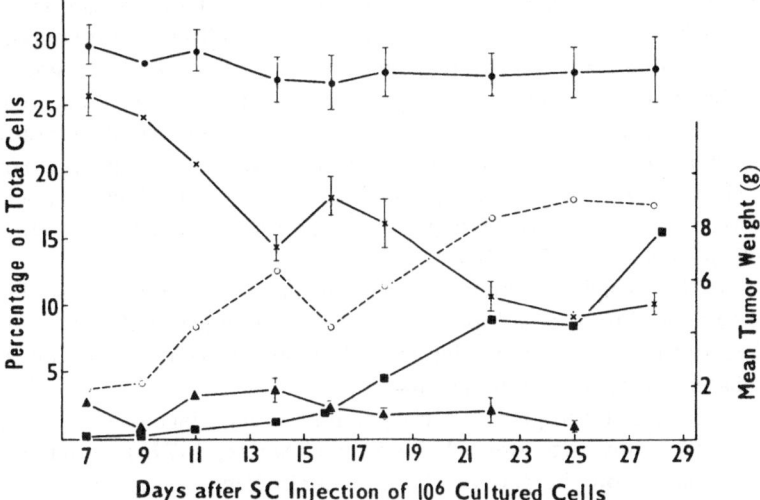

Figure 4. Time course of infiltration of inflammatory cells into tumors derived from cultured Mc40A tumor cells. Tumors were induced by SC inoculation of 10^6 *in vitro*-cultured tumor cells on day 0. From day 14 onward each point represents the mean of analyses of six tumors. Points at days 7 and 11 (EA-RFC only) represent the mean of three analyses each of a pool of three tumor nodules and the points at days 9 and 11 (macrophages and EAC-RFC) represent the mean of two analyses, each of a pool of three tumor nodules. EA-RFC, ●—●; macrophages, X—X; nonphagocytic EA-RFC, ○---○; EAC-RFC, ▲—▲; tumor weight, ■—■. Error bars, ±1 SE.

However, it is conceivable that initial infiltration by polymorphonuclear leukocytes may have occurred at the injection site and that such a reaction could have already waned by the time the tumors became palpable.

F. Factors Controlling Leukocyte Infiltration

It is apparent from the foregoing data that the appearance of leukocytes within a developing neoplasm is a predictable phenomenon, largely characteristic for each transplanted tumor. However, the regulatory mechanisms that such data subsume have not been elucidated, a situation complicated by the only partial characterization of some of the cell types involved. Necrosis is clearly not a factor (Evans, 1972), and the almost total absence of polymorphonuclear leukocytes eliminates infection as an explanation of our findings. As already discussed, leukocyte infiltration appears to be associated primarily with the generation of an immune response to tumor-associated antigens (Section II.D). Even so, the features of infiltration observed for different experimental tumors are too varied to allow much generalization.

The presence of cells reactive with ATS of which at least a significant proportion are T cells (Section II.D) is not inconsistent with the above hypothesis, although the subsequent detection of specifically cytotoxic T cells *in situ* proved elusive (Section III.B). Even in allografts the proportion of committed cells which ingress is small; the majority are probably unsensitized, appearing at random from the circulation by attraction into the graft via signals emanating from the sensitized population. In rat cardiac allografts, however, selective accumulation occurred to the extent that allospecific cytotoxicity was detectable *in situ* (Tilney *et al.*, 1975, 1978).

The level at which macrophages are maintained within tumors may be considered to depend upon a multiplicity of factors favorable or unfavorable to continued recruitment from circulating monocyte precursors and upon the flux of macrophages within the tumor mass itself.

The decline of macrophages in progressive tumors, which received particular emphasis in our investigations (M. Moore and Moore, 1977*b*), could reflect a reduced capacity on the part of the host confronting a developing tumor to furnish sufficient macrophages, a failure of the immune response, or of monocyte sequestration. Experiments in which the initial inoculum of Mc40A cells was increased by 5- or 10-fold, so as to produce tumors of disparate size for analysis at similar times after injection, provided no evidence of an association with a deficiency in macrophage production. Indeed, Eccles *et al.* (1976) reported that tumor-bearing rats frequently exhibit a marked monocytosis. The same investigators (Eccles and Alexander, 1974*a*) have also demonstrated that macrophages enter tumors growing in T-cell-deficient rats, but with otherwise normal bone marrow function, less readily than their normal immunocompetent counterparts, again suggesting that immunity and macrophage ingress are closely linked (Section I).

However, others (e.g., Szymaniec and James, 1976) have reported that the content of FcR+ host cells in murine tumors was similar whether the recipient mice were immunologically intact or T-cell deprived. These findings are difficult to relate to those of Eccles and Alexander (1974*a*) because in the mouse studies the extent to which the FcR+ cells comprised macrophages was not delineated. Even so, the data suggest that there are stimuli other than immunological factors which determine, at least in part, the characteristics of cellular infiltration. On a similar theme, S. Haskill and Parthenais (1978) demonstrated that although the *in situ* inflammatory reaction against the TC1699 mammary carcinoma appeared to be dependent on an immunocompetent host, neither the delayed hypersensitivity response nor the antibody response was solely responsible for the localization of ADCC effector cells in this tumor.

Although some impairment of immune responsiveness in the tumor-bearing host cannot be excluded, where the tumor macrophage is concerned other limiting factors may operate at the level of the circulating monocyte. The nature of the stimulae by which monocytes enter a tumor, and the extent to which such factors might be modified by the presence of antichemotactic (Snyderman and Pike, 1976) or antiinflammatory factors (Fauve *et al.*, 1974) and chemotactic inhibitors (Brozna and Ward, 1975), are still unknown. Peripheral blood monocytes of tumor-bearing rodents respond poorly to chemotactic and inflammatory stimuli *in vivo* (Eccles and Alexander, 1974*b*; Eccles *et al.*, 1976; Snyderman *et al.*, 1976) and soluble tumor products (Snyderman and Pike, 1976). Also, immune complexes known to be present in the circulation of rats bearing tumors with a high macrophage content (Thomson *et al.*, 1973) may bind to monocytes via FcR to influence their extravasation and/or migration. In summary it seems likely, as emphasized by Evans (1977), that infiltration of tumors by leukocytes may be largely controlled by the interaction of protagonists and antagonists of chemotaxis, which in turn are under the control of the immune response. An antigenic tumor may thus be regarded as a putative chemotactic stimulus, but the relative importance of antigen, immune complexes, complement factors (Snyderman and Mergenhagen, 1976), or products of neoplastic cells (Meltzer *et al.*, 1977) in this multifactorial process has yet to be evaluated.

G. Implications for Tumor Growth *in Vivo*

The rate of growth of Mc40A, AAF57, and SP22 following the subcutaneous injection of 1 million cultured cells is shown in Fig. 5. By day 22 there was more than a threefold difference in weight between AAF57 on the one hand and Mc40A ($p < 0.001$ by Student's *t*-test) and SP22 ($p < 0.01$) on the other, but the apparent increased growth rate of SP22 over Mc40A was not statistically significant. In the present context, the important question is whether the *in vivo* behavior of a neoplasm determines, or is determined by, the degree of cellular infiltration. Despite the rapacious character of AAF57, the possibility that its growth was so rapid as to completely outflank the host immune response is difficult to envisage. It is more likely that the absence of a significant antigenic stimulus is the critical factor limiting the ingress of host leukocytes, which in turn is reflected in a rapid growth rate. In this view, the presence of intratumor leukocytes would then be indicative of antitumor reactivity *in situ*.

However, the comparability of the growth rates of Mc40A and SP22 emphasizes that the relationship between immunogenicity, infiltration, and *in vivo* behavior is complex. Thus the differences in infiltration between SP22 and AAF57 are probably too small to account for the disparity in growth rate of these tumors, although the macrophage content of the former was greater than that of the latter in the early phases of tumor growth.

Since the growth of most tumors is inexorable, even when infiltrating leukocytes outnumber the neoplastic cells (Evans, 1972), there is the possibility

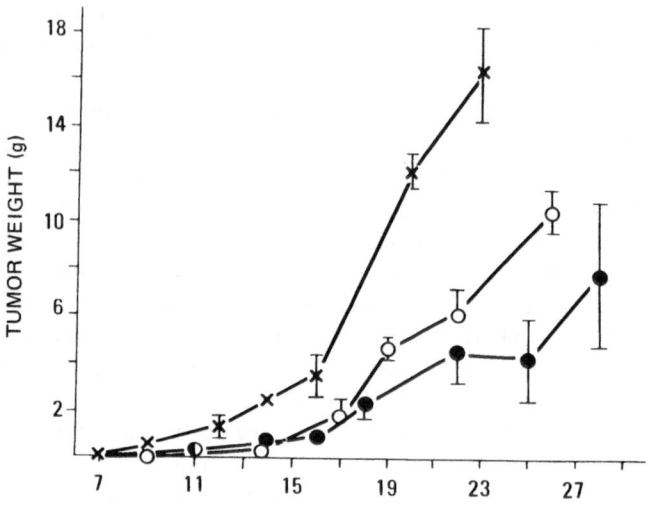

Figure 5. Relative growth rates of tumors derived from a SC inoculation of 10^6 *in vitro* cultured tumor cells. Mc40A, ●—●; SP22, ○—○; AAF57, ×—×.

that certain host cells may facilitate the processes of tumor initiation and development. Generalizations about the possible dependency of malignant cells on host cells are impossible because in some tumors the latter constitute a very small minority population. However, recent reports that macrophages, for instance (whose role in a multiplicity of other phenomena is well recognized), may also stimulate proliferation or maturation of various normal and neoplastic cells by the release of soluble mediators (Nelson, 1976; Evans, 1976), suggest that in some circumstances macrophages may be a requirement for tumor growth. Under the complex dynamic conditions of tumor development it is even possible to envisage the coexistence of opposing reactions in which different properties of similar cells serve mutually antagonistic ends.

Further discussion of this topic is beyond the scope of this article. The circumstantial evidence that is available suggests that, notwithstanding other possible effects of a nonimmunological nature, certain infiltrating leukocytes, alone or in concert, are growth-inhibitory *in situ,* and this function is reflected at a systemic level where the incidence of metastases is primarily determined by the macrophage content of the primary neoplasm. This potentially meaningful relationship provided the rationale for an extension of our studies to an analysis of the effector functions associated with tumor-infiltrating leukocytes. Because this phase of the investigation necessitated the isolation of these cells, the immunogenic sarcoma Mc40A, in which the host cell compartment numerically approaches that of the neoplastic cells, was selected for further study. If effector functions relevant to biological behavior could not be demonstrated for this tumor, it is highly unlikely that they would be for tumors such as AAF57, SP22, or SP1 in which leukocyte infiltration was relatively minimal.

The experimental approach was based on the presumption that systemic activity in tumor bearers and that of infiltrating cells might consist of at least three components: a specific component in which the effector cells are cytotoxic T lymphocytes (CTL) generated by immunization against specific tumor-rejection antigens; a nonspecific component where the properties of the effector cells [natural killer (NK) cells] include rapid lysis of certain susceptible cell lines, possession of FcR, absence of T- and B-cell-surface markers, and a characteristic anatomical distribution (Oehler *et al*, 1978*a*; Potter and M. Moore, 1978); and a macrophage component which with reference to analogous tumor–host systems might constrain tumor growth in an immunologically specific (Van Loveren and Den Otter, 1974; Haskill and Fett, 1976) or nonspecific manner (Evans and Alexander, 1976).

III. TUMOR-INFILTRATING LYMPHOCYTES

A. Isolation

In the assessment of antitumor leukocyte reactivity *in vitro*, the recovery of viable and functionally active leukocytes essentially free from other cellular contaminants is obligatory. Tumor-infiltrating lymphocytes (TIL) were isolated from disaggregated suspensions by a modified Sephadex G-10 column fractionation procedure based on the method described by Ly and Mishell (1974) for separation of antibody-forming cells from immune spleen cell populations. Applications of the original method have proven effective for the removal of adherent phagocytic cells (Pollack *et al.*, 1976) and tumor cells (Hansen *et al.*, 1977) and have yielded an almost exclusively lymphocytic eluate retaining the functional attributes of T lymphocytes and K and NK cells (Wolfe *et al.*, 1976). The purity of the eluates originating from the disaggregated Mc40A suspensions was essentially similar to the MSV system (Gillespie *et al.*, 1977) using a comparable technique, provided that two columns were used in succession (Table III); even so, a small degree of tumor cell contamination was unavoidable (K. Moore and Moore, 1979). Probably the greatest limitation, however, was the recovery of lymphocytes which amounted on the basis of reactivity with ATS to only 30% of the prefractionation population. The adventitious removal of cells of potential importance in cytotoxic reactions is thus a possibility which must be considered in the interpretation of our data, and represents a pervasive problem in the functional elucidation of leukocytes recovered from tumors, both human and experimental.

Table III. Differential Composition of Sephadex G-10 Eluates of Enzyme-Disaggregated Mc40A Tumor Cell Suspensions[a]

Cell type	Mean % cells[b] (±1 SE)
Total lymphocytes	92.0 ± 2.6
ATS-stained lymphocytes[c]	84.0 ± 4.2
Macrophages	1.7 ± 1.6
Neutrophils	0.8 ± 0.8
Eosinophils	0.6 ± 0.8
Basophils	0.4 ± 0.5
Tumor cells	4.7 ± 2.7

[a] Differential counts were made on Jenner–Giemsa-stained cytocentrifuge films prepared from cell suspensions incubated with polystyrene latex for 45 min at 37°C prior to centrifugation.
[b] Based on 14 independent separations.
[c] Determined by immunofluorescent staining with rabbit anti-rat thymocyte antiserum (Moore and Moore, 1977a).

B. Cytotoxic Activity

Initially, evidence for CTL was sought using a short-term ^{51}Cr release assay employing Mc40A targets. Further application was limited by the unpredictable extent of spontaneous isotopic release (28–60% over 18 h) but more particularly by the failure of the test to disclose increased cytotoxicity in the lymphoid tissues of tumor bearers compared with those from normal controls. Naturally occurring (spontaneous) cytotoxicity could thus be readily monitored in short-term ^{51}Cr release assays using Mc40A and especially the human cell line K562 as targets, but the detection of activity against the former which might be attributable to CTL was not unequivocal (Fig. 6). Such variations that did occur were probably attributable to the inherent variability of the test. Thus, the cytotoxicity of both TIL and tumor-bearer spleen cells was found to be no greater than that of normal spleen cells. In these circumstances tumor-directed activity was sought by the method of Brooks *et al.* (1978) in which surviving tumor target cells were quantified by incorporation of the γ-emitting analogue of methionine, Selenomethionine-75 (^{75}Se), in an assay of 48-h duration (K. Moore and Moore, 1979). The term "cytotoxicity" used in the context of this long-term assay thus refers to the extent of damage or disturbance induced in a target cell after interaction with an effector cell and embraces both growth inhibition and lysis (Evans and Alexander, 1976).

(a) Lymph Node and Splenic Lymphocytes. Analysis of the cytotoxicity of TIL was preceded by studies on splenic and lymph node lymphocytes from

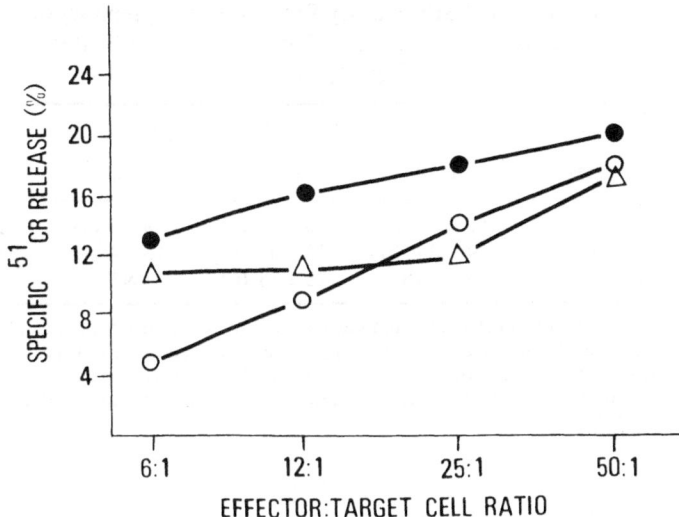

Figure 6. Cytolysis of Mc40A targets in short-term ^{51}Cr release assay following exposure to spleen cells and tumor-infiltrating lymphocytes (TIL). Tumor-bearer rats were killed 21 days after trocar implantation of Mc40A tumor tissue. Lymphoid cells from rats killed on days 17 and 20 gave similar results. Normal W/Not spleen cells (adherent cell depleted), o—o; tumor-bearer spleen cells (adherent cell depleted), △—△; Mc40A TIL, •—•.

normal and tumor-bearing rats. Here a significant distinction was disclosed in the activity of cells from the different lymphoid organs and in the susceptibility of different tumor targets to active effector populations. Normal lymph node lymphocytes were stimulatory for all the tumor cell lines, with the exception of Mc40A against which they were minimally cytotoxic. By contrast, spleen cells were consistently cytotoxic against Mc40A whereas the other cell lines displayed only limited sensitivity (Table IV). Treatment of normal spleen cells by the Sephadex G-10 procedure for isolating TIL significantly reduced their cytotoxicity against Mc40A targets. Their precolumn cytotoxicity fell from 59 ± 6 to a postcolumn value of 27 ± 5, a reduction of $46 \pm 9\%$ ($p < 0.005$ by Student's t-test) in cytotoxic capacity. This observation, based upon a series of seven replicate experiments, is important for the interpretation of cytotoxicity data in that it implicates a second (adherent) population of effector cells which is active in the ^{75}Se assay. This population, putatively consisting primarily of macrophages, may be similar to the phagocytic, nonspecifically cytostatic population identified in the spleens of tumor-bearing mice (Mantovani *et al.*, 1977). In that study the presence of tumor was a prerequisite for demonstration of this activity, in contrast to our findings where it was also detected in normal spleen. The involvement of such a cell, being cytostatic as opposed to cytolytic, would not be expected in ^{51}Cr release assays, a conclusion subsequently justified by the

Table IV. Cytotoxic and Stimulatory Properties of Lymphocytes from
Normal W/Not Rats against Cultured Tumor Targets Estimated by the
^{75}Se Assay

Source of lymphocytes	Tumor targets[a]			
	Mc40A	Mc57	SP22	AAF57
Spleen	58 ± 5 (13)	5 ± 7 (8)	9 ± 9 (4)	−11 ± 11 (4)
Cervical lymph node	14 ± 3 (12)	−33 ± 4 (8)	−13 ± 4 (4)	−25 ± 8 (3)
Axillary lymph node	13 ± 3 (8)	−28 ± 11 (6)	NT	NT

[a]Figures quoted represent cytotoxicity indices (±1 SE), calculated with respect to control targets incubated in the absence of lymphocytes. Negative values denote growth stimulation. The number of determinations against each target are given in parentheses. NT, not tested. All lymphocyte preparations were depleted of adherent cells and used at a constant E:T ratio of 100:1.

finding that Sephadex G-10 filtration of spleen cells actually enhanced ^{51}Cr release from K562 cells (see below).

Reactivity in the lymphoid tissues of tumor bearers was monitored over a period of 28 days after trocar implantation of Mc40A. The cytotoxicity of tumor-draining axillary lymph node and cervical lymph node lymphocytes did not consistently exceed 10% of that in the corresponding populations from normal donors. However, between days 15 and 28 of tumor growth, tumor-bearer spleen cells were consistently more cytotoxic than their normal counterparts (Table V). That this represented a real increase in cytotoxicity was apparent from Sephadex G-10 treatment, after which the population still retained cytotoxic capacity equivalent to that of untreated normal spleen, i.e., there was a significant difference in cytotoxicity between tumor-bearer and normal spleen cell popula-

Table V. Cytotoxic and Stimulatory Properties of Lymphocytes from
Tumor-Bearer Rats against Mc40A Targets, Estimated by the ^{75}Se Assay

Effector cells	Percent cytotoxicity with respect to control lymphocytes on day[a]					
	4	7	11	15	22	28
Spleen	4 ± 4	1 ± 5	3 ± 7	16 ± 2	19 ± 1	15 ± 6
Spleen (Sephadex G-10 treated)	10 ± 7	9 ± 5	−3 ± 5	−7 ± 5	10 ± 10	−4 ± 6
Cervical lymph node	−14 ± 5	5 ± 4	−3 ± 3	6 ± 4	7 ± 6	4 ± 4
Axillary lymph node	−26 ± 4	12 ± 1	1 ± 7	−2 ± 4	5 ± 4	ND

[a]Day after implantation of trocar graft. Figures quoted represent cytotoxicity indices (±1 SE) calculated with respect to normal lymphocyte control. Negative values denote growth stimulation. All lymphocyte preparations were depleted of adherent cells and used at a constant E:T ratio of 100:1. ND, not determined.

tions after each had been passed over Sephadex G-10. The activity in this population was most probably mediated by lymphocytes inasmuch as the preparations were virtually devoid of macrophages, and therefore implies the involvement of a third cell type in the mediation of cytotoxicity at certain stages of tumor growth. Insofar as Sephadex G-10 eluates consist predominantly of T lymphocytes and comparable cytotoxicity could not be demonstrated against an antigenically unrelated target (Mc57), the data are consistent with a tumor-related (specific?) component. However, this interpretation must be considered in light of the greater inherent susceptibility to NK cells of Mc40A targets compared with Mc57 targets. In this view, excess cytotoxicity in tumor-bearing splenic lymphocytes could be attributable to elevated NK activity.

(b) Tumor-Infiltrating Lymphocytes (TIL). Because there is no adequate control for TIL in the normal host, the cytotoxicity of this population was compared with that of normal spleen cells. The susceptibility of Mc40A targets to cytotoxicity by splenic lymphocytes and TIL was essentially comparable in these experiments. In reciprocal tests reactivities of TIL isolated from Mc40A and Mc57 were virtually identical against the same targets (i.e., high against Mc40A and low against Mc57) (Table VI), indicating that target cell susceptibility, as distinct from antigenic specificity, influenced the outcome of the cytotoxicity assays.

These patterns of selective cytotoxicity among TIL and spleen cells against tumor targets and the absence of comparable activity in lymph nodes suggested that the lymphocyte-mediated component of the cytotoxic reactions monitored using the ^{75}Se assay was attributable for the most part, if not wholly, to NK cells.

Because it is likely that specific CTL are present in the tumor-bearing host, these findings raise questions about the validity of the ^{75}Se assay for the detection of tumor-specific lymphocyte-mediated cytotoxicity. One possible limitation is that the small minority ($<5\%$) of contaminating tumor cells competitively inhibit cytotoxicity against the cultured target cells in the test. While this is

Table VI. Cytotoxicity of Spleen Cells and Tumor-Infiltrating Lymphocytes (TIL) Derived from Mc40A and Mc57 against the Respective Targets, Estimated by the [75]Se Assay

	Percent cytotoxicity (±1 SE)	
Effector cells[a]	Versus Mc40A	Versus Mc57
Normal splenic lymphocytes (8)	64 ± 6	17 ± 15
Mc40A TIL (8)	60 ± 8	23 ± 9
Mc57 TIL (4)	53 ± 10	15 ± 19

[a]The E:T ratio was 100:1 in all instances. Numbers of determinations are given in parentheses.

undoubtedly an important and pervasive problem in short-term assays utilizing TIL (Gillespie *et al.*, 1977, and below) it is probably not relevant in the longer term ^{75}Se assay, wherein the TIL activity was comparable with that of splenic lymphocytes regardless of the degree of tumor cell contamination and of the tumor of origin of TIL. Our data thus justify the conclusion that although specific CTL may be present in the tumor-bearing host, this component is relatively weak compared with the natural killer element. Although association with a minority population within the TIL compartment cannot be excluded, it is likely that the effectors belong to the predominant population which stains with ATS. Antisera prepared by conventional procedures, like our reagent, have been shown to react with NK cells (Shellam, 1977). Such reactivity is removed by an additional absorption step using spleen cells from thymectomized, irradiated, and bone-marrow-reconstituted rats and leaves anti-T-cell activity intact.

The presence of NK cells in the TIL population was consolidated in cyto-toxicity experiments using the human cell line K562, which is sensitive to spontaneous killing by normal rat lymphoid cells (Oehler *et al.*, 1978a; Potter and M. Moore, 1978), in common with those of mouse (Haller *et al.*, 1977a) and man (West *et al.*, 1977).

The levels of NK activity in the lymphoid tissues of normal W/Not rats were as previously reported from this laboratory (Potter and M. Moore, 1978) in that the activity of spleen cells significantly exceeded that of lymph nodes, which was minimal, a pattern of distribution also observed in tumor bearers. However, the reactivity of the TIL population separated from a 15-day Mc40A implant was lower than that of normal spleen (Fig. 7), an observation which was reproduced in similar experiments upon tumors obtained at 20 and 21 days. Selective loss of NK cells by the TIL separation procedure was excluded by the finding that passage of normal and tumor-bearing spleen cell populations over Sephadex G-10 columns actually enhanced NK activity against K562 and Mc40A, presumably by removal of irrelevant cells from the effector population. For example, in a series of seven independent tests using K562, the mean ($\pm$ ISE) of untreated spleen cells (30 $\pm$ 2% SCR) was increased by 34% to a postcolumn value of 41 $\pm$ 3% SCR, and this difference was significant ($p < 0.05$, by Student's *t*-test). Furthermore, no deleterious effects on NK function could be attributed to the PCD enzyme mixture used for tumor disaggregation. Because as already discussed (Section III.A) the TIL populations invariably contained a small minority of tumor cells (Table III), it seemed probable in the short-term assay that these contaminants were responsible for the lower reactivity of TIL in relation to normal spleen. This was investigated by quantitative assessment of the inhibitory effect of third-party Mc40A cells on K562 killing by normal splenic lymphocytes. Under these conditions, inhibition of specific ^{51}Cr release from K562 cells was found to be Mc40A cell dose-dependent and detectable at ratios of less than 1:1 (Fig. 8). It was clear from this experiment that the

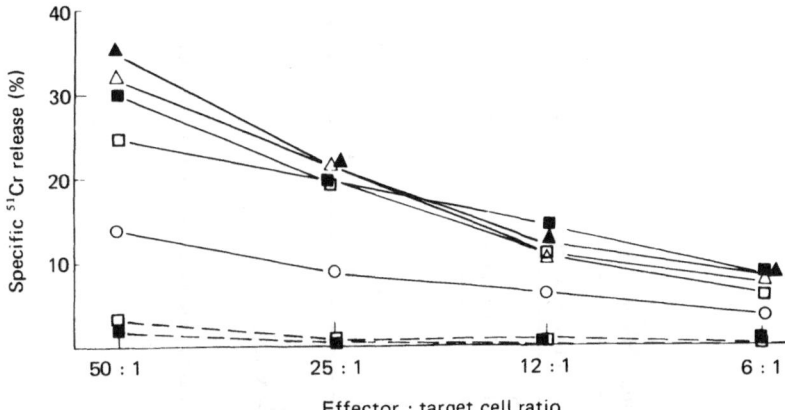

Figure 7. Natural killer (NK) activity of lymphocytes from a normal and a tumor (Mc40A)-bearing rat estimated by ^{51}Cr release from K562 target cells. The tumor-bearing rat was killed 15 days after trocar implantation. All preparations from lymphoid tissues were depleted of adherent cells. Tumor-infiltrating lymphocytes (TIL), o—o; tumor-bearer spleen, □—□; tumor-bearer spleen after passage over Sephadex G-10, △—△; tumor-bearer axillary lymph nodes, □---□; normal spleen, ■—■; normal spleen after passage over Sephadex G-10, ▲—▲; normal axillary lymph nodes, ■---■.

presence of tumor cells in excess of 2% of the TIL population would give rise to dose-dependent inhibition of NK function. The phenomenon was confirmed to be one of cold inhibition, as distinct from steric interference, inasmuch as fixed extraneous Mc40A cells were without effect.

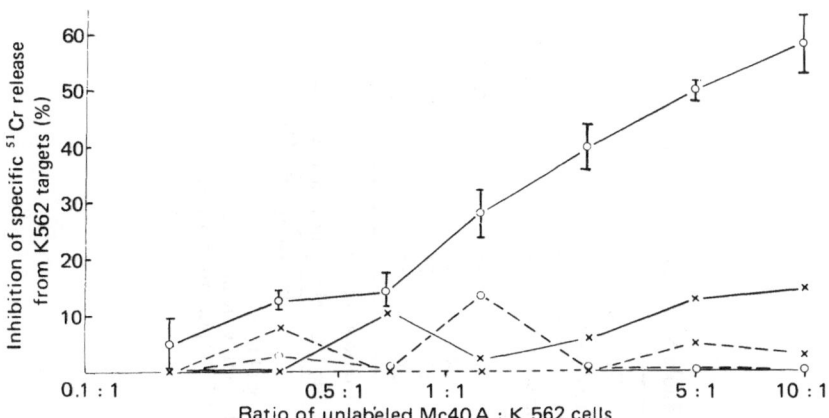

Figure 8. Effect of viable and nonviable unlabeled Mc40A cells on natural killer (NK) activity of normal rat spleen against K562 targets. Viable Mc40A cells, o—o (values represent mean of four experiments ±1 SE) formalin-fixed Mc40A cells, ×–×, o---o, and ×---× (values are those of three individual experiments).

Table VII. Comparison of Natural Killer (NK) Reactivity against K562 of Normal Spleen Cells and TIL[a]

Exp. No.	^{51}Cr release mediated by (%)		Actual decrease in ^{51}Cr release[b] (%)	Predicted decrease in ^{51}Cr release[c] (%)	Differential cell composition of TIL[d]				
	Spleen cells	TIL			TIL	Tumor cells	Monocytes	Polymorphs	Other
1	30	14	54	51	90	5	2	2	1
2	24	20	15	20	94	1	3	2	3
3	32	26	21	38	94	2	3	0	1
4	29	<1	99	56	88	9	1	1	1

[a] Constant E:T ratio was 50:1.

[b] Percent specific ^{51}Cr release mediated by spleen cells – percent specific ^{51}Cr release mediated by TIL

Percent specific ^{51}Cr release mediated by spleen cells × 100.

[c] Calculated from Fig. 8.

[d] Differential counts were made on Jenner–Giemsa-stained cytocentrifuge films prepared from cell suspensions incubated with polystyrene latex for 45 min at 37°C prior to centrifugation.

Assuming that the cytotoxicity of a theoretically uncontaminated TIL compartment for K562 approximated that of normal spleen cells, as was found to be the case in the ^{75}Se assay wherein tumor cells apparently did not interfere, Fig. 8 could be employed to estimate the degree of inhibition which might be expected in a contaminated TIL preparation. This calculation is shown in Table VII where the correlation between the predicted and actual decrease in specific ^{51}Cr release is as close as might reasonably be expected where the morphological identification of tumor cells in stained cytocentrifuge preparations is not unequivocal.

In summary, lymphocyte cytotoxicity determined by the long-term ^{75}Se assay reveals several of the features (lymphoid organ distribution, differential target cell susceptibility) of NK cells assessed independently against the uniquely sensitive xenogeneic cell line, K562. Whereas lysis of the latter is probably exclusively a function of lymphoid cells and is sensitive to competitive inhibition, cytotoxicity of Mc40A in the ^{75}Se assay involved the participation of at least one other population of effector cells of nonlymphoid type, but interference by contaminating tumor cells, at least at the level monitored in our TIL preparations, was minimal. Because the tumor targets used in the ^{75}Se assay displayed inherent differential susceptibility to NK cells, the excess lymphocyte cytotoxicity detected in the spleen of tumor bearers at certain stages of tumor growth could not be exclusively attributed to specific CTL or enhanced NK activity. By the assays used TIL cytotoxicity was indistinguishable from that of normal splenic lymphocytes in respect to magnitude and tumor selectivity.

IV. INTRATUMOR MACROPHAGES

A. Isolation

Adherent cells were isolated from disaggregated tumor suspensions by incubation in petri dishes at 37°C. These comprised 89 ± 1% (range: 83-94%) macrophages as determined by uptake of polystyrene latex, but the populations were heterogeneous with respect to size and degree of differentiation. Scanning electron microscopy revealed a minority subpopulation of monocytic cells. To ensure numerical uniformity in cytotoxicity tests, macrophage monolayers were harvested by exposure at 0°C to ethylenediaminetetraacetic acid (EDTA) (6×10^{-5} M), washed, and resuspended in serum-supplemented tissue culture medium. This was an efficient procedure and viability remained in excess of 80%.

B. Cytotoxic Activity

Although intratumor macrophage (ITM) monolayers were actively phagocytic, their ability to lyse sensitized human red blood cells (HRBC) in an 18-h ^{51}Cr release assay was monitored as another index of functional integrity (Holm, 1972). In five experiments with macrophages isolated from different Mc40A tumors, performed at an E:T ratio of 2:1, the mean specific ^{51}Cr release (± ISE) was 20 ± 2%, which represented more than six times the low level (~3%) of spontaneous ^{51}Cr release in the absence of the sensitizing antibody. However, these effectors were incapable of inducing significant cytotoxicity in 18-h assays using ^{51}Cr-labeled Mc40A targets (Table VIII) even at the high E:T ratio of 50:1. The mean specific ^{51}Cr release at this ratio was 8%, a value of little significance compared with the spontaneous isotopic release of 40%. This failure of ITM to accomplish lysis of tumor targets may be an intrinsic deficiency of the populations under test, or a consequence of the isolation procedure. Their ineffectiveness in this regard is clearly not attributable to a generalized state of inactivation, although cytotoxicity could conceivably depend upon the presence of arming factors (Evans and Alexander, 1972) removed by exposure to proteolytic enzymes. It is unlikely that the separation procedure favored the selection of a predominantly noncytolytic subpopulation by differential adherence. Cytolytic macrophages isolated from regressing MSV tumors were adherent within a shorter time period (10 min) (Russell et al., 1977) than that used in the present study (15 min). Nevertheless, it is noteworthy that the heterogeneity of macrophage populations is such as to encompass a range of cytotoxic capacity. For instance, Walker (1976) separated rat peritoneal macrophages into several subpopulations on the basis of size, each comprising in excess of 90% macrophages, and observed a fourfold variation in cytotoxicity against a syngeneic tumor.

Table VIII. Cytolysis of Mc40A Targets in Short-Term ^{51}Cr Release Assay following Exposure to Mc40A Tumor Macrophages

| | Specific ^{51}Cr release at E:T ratio of[a]: | | | |
Exp. No.	50:1	25:1	15:1	10:1
1	11	NT	NT	6
2	2	3	2	NT
3	8	6	6	NT
4	NT	10	10	NT
5	7	0	NT	0
6	14	13	4	NT
7	4	NT	NT	NT
Mean ± SE:	8 ± 2	6 ± 2	5 ± 2	3

[a]Each experiment was performed with macrophages isolated from different Mc40A tumors excised 20 days after trocar implantation. Duration of the assay was 18 h. NT, not tested.

A further possibility may account for these observations that macrophages isolated from progressive tumors, as in this instance, may exist in a noncytolytic state of activation analogous to that of macrophages in progressive MSV tumors (Russell *et al.*, 1977). In these tumors, ITM superficially similar in function to noncytolytic macrophages elicited from the peritoneal cavity of normal mice following i.p. injection of thioglycollate broth could be stimulated to cytolytic activity by minute doses of bacterial lipopolysaccharide (LPS), a property not shared by those from the peritoneum. Whether Mc40A ITM represent, in part, such an intermediate "primed" population, which in the absence of LPS falls short of full activation and cytolytic activity, was not investigated.

Mc40A targets surviving incubation with macrophages derived from tumors between 15 and 28 days after implantation were quantified as for lymphocytes by postlabeling with ^{75}Se. Significant growth inhibition, compared with medium controls, was observed at ratios approaching one effector cell per target cell, and at higher ratios (50:1) this inhibition was almost complete (Fig. 9). Identical tests using tumor targets other than Mc40A indicated that tumor–macrophage-induced inhibition was essentially nonspecific, revealing only minor quantitative differences in susceptibility among the various targets (Fig. 10). This absence of immunological specificity was reminiscent of macrophages activated by stimuli such as zymosan, bacterial lipopolysaccharide, or lymphokine (Alexander and Evans, 1971; Hibbs, 1976).

In murine systems, the production and release of arginase by activated mac-

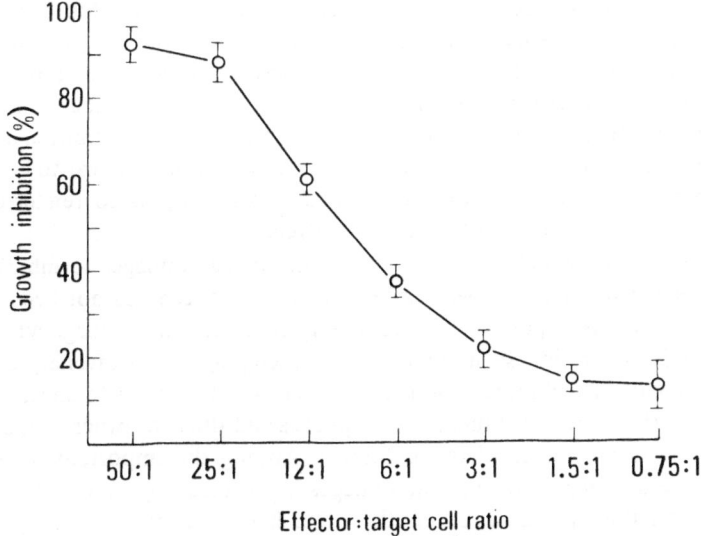

Figure 9. Mc40A-derived macrophage-mediated growth inhibition of cultured Mc40A target cells (measured by ^{75}SE assay). Values represent the means (±1 SE) of four experiments.

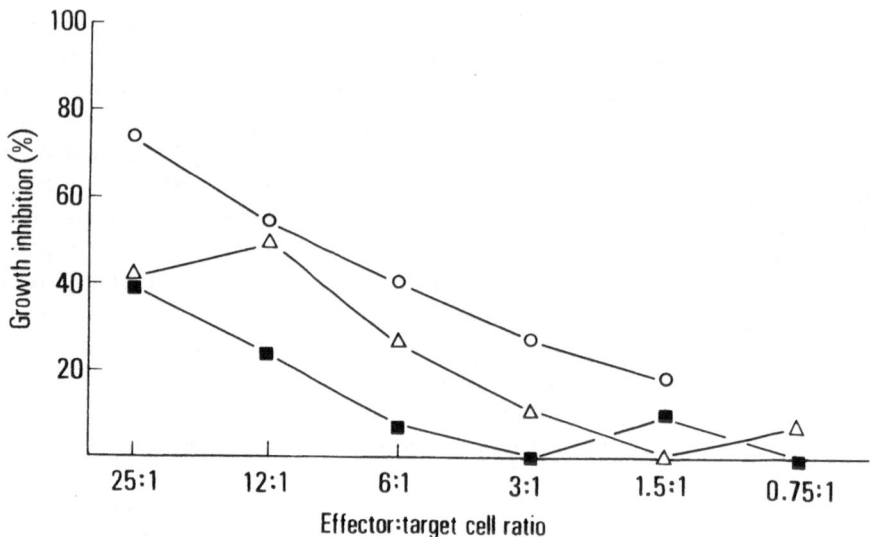

Figure 10. Mc40A-derived macrophage-mediated growth inhibition of cultured Mc40A cells and unrelated (Mc57, SP22) tumor targets (measured by ^{75}Se assay). Macrophages were isolated from a single tumor and tested simultaneously against all three targets: Mc40A, o—o; Mc57, △—△; SP22, ■—■.

rophages have been shown to have deleterious effects on lymphocytes (Kung *et al.*, 1977) and tumor cells (Currie, 1978), as a consequence of arginine deprivation of the tissue culture media. The possibility that growth inhibition might be a consequence of a deficit in arginine or of other component(s) because of the high biosynthetic capability of the isolated macrophages was tested by replenishment of 50% of the culture medium after 18, 24, and 42 h of incubation, successively. Under these conditions little difference in the growth inhibition of Mc40A targets was observed (Fig. 11). This mechanism would not appear to be relevant to the present study unless depletion occurs so rapidly as to render even the maneuver of medium replenishment to no effect.

The extent to which the capacity of tumor macrophages to inhibit tumor growth relates to macrophages resident in normal tissue has not been studied. Keller (1978) has reported that adherent, predominantly phagocytic mononuclear cells expressing spontaneous cytotoxicity against a diversity of targets *in vitro* are virtually ubiquitous in the organism, so that any differences in growth inhibitory effects between tumor macrophages and those of other sites are likely to be quantitative, rather than qualitative. Among the important questions is whether the activity of tumor macrophages is enhanced by an ongoing immune response, on the one hand, or on the other hand is compromised by hitherto undefined inhibitory factors in the microenvironment of the tumor (James, 1977).

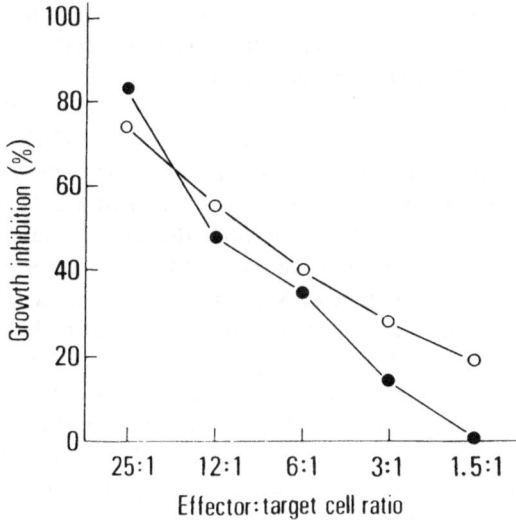

Figure 11. Effect of medium replenishment on the growth-inhibitory properties of Mc40A-derived macrophages. Targets were cultured Mc40A cells. Medium was unchanged throughout the duration (48 h) of the experiment (○−○); 50% of the medium was replenished with fresh medium after 18, 24, and 42 h (●−●).

V. DISCUSSION

If leukocyte infiltration is a manifestation of immunological recognition, as cumulative evidence appears to suggest, it might be expected that where a tumor is not composed of cells selected for immunoresistance, the various components would possess the characteristics of immunologically active cells and some of these (e.g., T cells) would express specific functions directed against the corresponding tumor targets. Although Mc40A possesses rejection antigen(s), no specific CTL were unequivocally detected at the tumor site. This deficit was either (1) intrinsic, the tumor providing insufficient stimulus for the attraction of intratumor CTL; (2) operational, in the sense that the expression of specific CTL might have been compromised by suppressive factors of a humoral or cellular nature; or (3) relative, their activity being obscured by NK cells which were the most pervasive cytotoxic effectors in this system. Although the proportion of committed cells entering even an allograft is small, a total absence of CTL is unlikely in view of the anamnestic and specific nature of Mc40A rejection *in vivo*. Failure to detect specific CTL at the tumor site is thus probably a reflection of (2) and/or (3). The strongest indication of specific CTL at a systemic level was obtained from tumor-bearer spleens 11–28 days after implantation. Even here, however, the evidence was not unequivocal in that specific CTL could not be distinguished from enhanced NK reactivity, although augmentation of the latter was inapparent in concomitant tests against the K562 cell line. In lymph nodes displaying minimal NK activity, specific CTL also could not be detected, a finding possibly related to the balance of inhibitory and stimulatory subpopulations known to exist in these lymphoid tissues (Brooks *et al.*, 1976).

To date there have been few reports of *in situ* CTL in experimental neoplasms. Specific CTL have been isolated from both regressing and progressing MSV-induced sarcomas, but from the latter only during the early phase of tumor growth. Although cytotoxicity data were not obtainable before day 11 of Mc40A growth, our system parallels that of MSV insofar as specific CTL could not be detected in TIL isolated from progressive tumors. In murine MC-induced tumors, the detection of *in situ* CTL is presently confined to a single report (DeLustro and Haskill, 1978) wherein T-cell-enriched tumor-derived fractions and spleen cells from mice bearing progressive MCA-2 tumors were shown to be cytotoxic *in vitro* for cultured MCA-2 cells in an assay of 18-h duration. The specificity of the reactions was established by resistance of SAD2 fibrosarcoma cells and T1699 which were susceptible to specific killing by effectors from the respective tumor-bearing hosts. This study, which takes no account of the possible participation of NK cells in the *in situ* cytotoxic reaction against MCA-2, contrasts with the present findings attributing most *in situ* cytotoxicity to NK cells. However, further comparison is limited by the fact that MC tumors vary considerably in the degree of immunogenicity and in the pattern of host-cell infiltration. Specific CTL has also been reported in ultraviolet light-induced murine tumors undergoing regression, but not in progressive neoplasms (Lill and Fortner, 1978). Ultraviolet tumors differ from MC-induced murine and rat tumors in that they will grow progressively only in immunosuppressed mice (Kripke and Fisher, 1976). The highly antigenic character and biological behavior of these tumors is thus reminiscent of MSV-induced sarcomas wherein a distinction in the cytotoxic status of T lymphocytes is apparent between progressors and regressors (Gillespie *et al.*, 1977).

The presence of NK cells *in situ* has likewise been reported. Lymphocytes cytotoxic for YAC (MLV-induced lymphoma) and RBL-5 (Rauscher-leukemia-virus-induced tumor) could be isolated from MSV tumors in high NK-reactive CBA mice but not in low NK-reactive A strain mice, in spite of the regularly occurring regression in the latter strain (Becker and Klein, 1976). There are several uncertainties about the basis of NK selectivity for different tumor targets *in vitro* and their biological relevance *in vivo*. Modulation of tumor susceptibility to NK cells occurs on explantation (Becker *et al.*, 1978) and in only a few instances has the extent to which the tumors are sensitive to NK cells *in vivo* been evaluated (Haller *et al.*, 1977b). Recently, this has extended to the use of isotopically prelabeled tumor cells to monitor *in vivo* cell death attributable to NK cells in lethally irradiated mice, from which the contribution of immune T cells was eliminated (Riccardi *et al.*, 1979). Presently, NK cells are widely attributed with a role in the immunosurveillance of neoplasia, an hypothesis which draws support from the stimulatory effects on NK cells of a diversity of agents with antitumor properties (Wolfe *et al.*, 1976; Tracey *et al.*, 1977; Oehler *et al.*, 1978*b*; Potter and M. Moore, 1980).

Preliminary information on the capacity of TIL derived from another methylcholanthrene-induced rat sarcoma (Mc7) to inhibit tumor growth in Winn assays has recently been presented (Robins *et al.*, 1979, and personal communication). These tests disclosed differences between spleen cells and TIL (the latter comprising about 50% T cells as determined by reactivity with the W 3/13 monoclonal antibody) which could not have been predicted on the basis of *in vitro* cytotoxicity tests. Spleen cells were inactive under conditions where the TIL population was highly active, even at low effector to target cell ratios, regardless of whether the transfers were performed with *in vivo*-derived cells or cultured target cells. Further studies of this type should help to identify the most cytotoxic lymphocyte subpopulations, their mode and specificity of action, and eventually provide greater insight into the requirements for more effective tumor restraint.

By contrast with NK cells which display very rapid cytolytic effects and represent the main natural effector cells in short-term assays, the cytotoxic effects of monocytes and macrophages—alternative natural effector cells—only became evident after 48-h incubation with target cells. In common with other studies, the expression of this cytotoxic reactivity was essentially nonspecific. These findings differed from those of Haskill and colleagues (Haskill and Fett, 1976) in respect to the T1699 mammary adenocarcinoma, where monocyte-mediated cytotoxicity was antibody-dependent, immunologically specific, and apparently closely associated with tumor regression. Despite the preliminary nature of our data, they are not incompatible with the circumstantial evidence (Section I) implicating macrophages in the local and systemic control of tumor growth. However, the properties of macrophages are so diverse that on presently available information the question of whether their intratumor role is primarily that of cytotoxic effector cells must remain open (cf. Section II.G). Macrophages are involved at all stages of the immune response and have the capacity to produce and respond to many different stimuli, including the elaboration of a wide range of biologically active substances which influence or condition the tumor environment. Currently much attention is focused on macrophages from tumor bearers which interfere with antitumor immunity (Herberman *et al.*, 1980). A predominant activity of suppressor macrophages is inhibition not only of lymphoproliferative responses to tumor antigens, but of proliferation-independent immune responses as well (Klimpel and Henney, 1978; Varesio *et al.*, 1979). In addition, macrophages are involved in *in vivo* regulation of NK activity (Oehler and Herberman, 1978). Although, as has been implied, *in vitro* cytotoxicity reactions studied with cultured tumor targets and isolated components of the immune response may have only limited relevance to antitumor reactivity *in vivo*, data from many sources now point to the existence of multifaceted anti-tumor reactions of potential importance in *in vivo* host defenses (Herberman, 1979). Elucidation of the interplay of these components *in situ* should eventually provide a more rational approach to the manipulation of the immune response in cancer.

ACKNOWLEDGMENTS

This study was supported by grants from the Medical Research Council and Cancer Research Campaign of Great Britain.

We are grateful to the following publishers for permission to reproduce material from our earlier articles: International Union Against Cancer (Figs. 1-4); Organisers and Editors of the European Reticuloendothelial Society "Macrophage and Cancer" Symposium, University of Edinburgh, Scotland (Fig. 5); H. K. Lewis and Co., Ltd. (Fig. 8 and Tables III, IV, VI, and VII).

VI. REFERENCES

Alexander, P., and Evans, R., 1971, Endotoxin and double stranded RNA render macrophages cytotoxic, *Nature (London) New Biol.* **232:**76.

Baldwin, R. W., Embleton, M. J., and Pimm, M. V., 1979, Host responses to spontaneous rat tumours, in: *Antiviral Mechanisms in the Control of Neoplasia* (P. Chandra, ed.), p. 333, Plenum Press, New York.

Becker, S., and Klein, E., 1976, Decreased "natural killer" effect in tumour-bearing mice and its relation to the immunity against oncornavirus-determined cell surface antigens, *Eur. J. Immunol.* **6:**892.

Becker, S., Kiessling, R., Lee, N., and Klein, G., 1978, Modulation of sensitivity to natural killer cell lysis after *in vitro* explantation of a mouse lymphoma, *J. Natl. Cancer Inst.* **61:**1495.

Blazar, B. A., and Heppner, G. H., 1978, *In situ* lymphoid cells of mouse mammary tumours. II. The characterisation of lymphoid cells separated from mouse mammary tumours, *J. Immunol.* **120:**1881.

Brooks, C. G., Rees, R. C., and Baldwin, R. W., 1976, Studies on the micro-cytotoxicity test. I. Evidence that the effect of normal lymphoid cells on tumour cell growth in microtest plates may be caused by non-immunological modifications of the culture medium, *Int. J. Cancer* **18:**778.

Brooks, C. G., Rees, R. C., and Robins, R. A., 1978, Studies on the micro-cytotoxicity test. II. The uptake of amino acids ([^{3}H]leucine or [^{75}Se]methionine) but not nucleosides ([^{3}H]thymidine or [^{125}I]IUdR) or ^{51}CrO$_4^{2-}$ provides a direct and quantitative measure of target cell survival in the presence of lymphoid cells, *J. Immunol. Meth.* **21:**111.

Brozna, J. P., and Ward, R. A., 1975, Antileukotactic properties of tumour cells, *J. Clin. Invest.* **56:**616.

Cerottini, J.-C., and Brunner, K. T., 1974, Cell mediated cytotoxicity, allograft rejection, and tumour immunity, *Adv. Immunol.* **18:**67.

Currie, G. A., 1978, Activated macrophages kill tumour cells by releasing arginase, *Nature (London)* **273:**758.

DeLustro, F., and Haskill, J. S., 1978, *In situ* cytotoxic T cells in a methylcholanthrene-induced tumour, *J. Immunol.* **121**:1007.

Eccles, S., and Alexander, P., 1974*a*, Macrophage content of tumours in relation to metastatic spread and host immune reaction, *Nature (London)* **250**:667.

Eccles, S. A., and Alexander, P., 1974*b*, Sequestration of macrophages in growing tumours and its effect on the immunological capacity of the host, *Br. J. Cancer* **30**:42.

Eccles, S. A., Bandlow, G., and Alexander, P., 1976, Monocytosis associated with the growth of transplanted syngeneic rat sarcomata differing in immunogenicity, *Br. J. Cancer* **34**:20.

Evans, R., 1972, Macrophages in syngeneic animal tumours, *Transplantation* **14**:468.

Evans, R., 1973, Preparation of pure cultures of tumour macrophages, *J. Natl. Cancer Inst.* **50**:271.

Evans, R., 1976, Tumor macrophages in host immunity to malignancies, in: *The Macrophage in Neoplasia* (M. A. Fink, ed.), p. 27, Academic Press, New York.

Evans, R., 1977, Macrophages in solid tumours, in: *The Macrophage and Cancer* (K. James, B. McBridge, A. E. Stuart, ed.), p. 321, Econoprint, Edinburgh, Scotland.

Evans, R., and Alexander, P., 1972, Role of macrophages in tumour immunity. II. Involvement of a macrophage cytophilic factor during syngeneic tumour growth inhibition, *Immunology* **23**:627.

Evans, R., and Alexander, P., 1976, Mechanisms of extracellular killing of nucleated mammalian cells by macrophages, in: *Immunobiology of the Macrophage* (D. S. Nelson, ed.), p. 536, Academic Press, New York.

Fauve, R. M., Hevin, B., Jacob, H., Gaillard, J. A., and Jacob, F., 1974, Antinflammatory effect of murine malignant cells, *Proc. Natl. Acad. Sci. USA,* **71**:4052.

Gillespie, G. Y., Hansen, C. B., Hoskins, R. G., and Russell, S. W., 1977, Inflammatory cells in solid murine neoplasms. IV. Cytolytic T lymphocytes isolated from regressing and progressing Moloney sarcomas, *J. Immunol.* **119**:564.

Hall, J. M., and Hallett, C., 1975, A simple precise method for measuring rodent paw volume, *J. Pharm. Pharmacol.* **27**:623.

Haller, O., Kiessling, R., Orn, A., Kärre, K., Nilsson, K., and Wigzell, H., 1977*a*, Natural cytotoxicity to human leukaemia mediated by mouse non-T cells, *Int. J. Cancer* **20**:93.

Haller, O., Hansson, M., Kiessling, R., and Wigzell, H., 1977*b*, Role of nonconventional natural killer cells in resistance against syngeneic tumour cells *in vivo, Nature (London)* **270**:609.

Hansen, C. B., Gillespie, G. Y., and Russell, S. W., 1977, Isolation of T lymphocytes from disaggregated tumours, with high purity and good percentage recovery, *J. Natl. Cancer Inst.* **59**:273.

Haskill, J. S., and Fett, J. W., 1976, Possible evidence for antibody-dependent macrophage-mediated cytotoxicity directed against murine adenocarcinoma cells *in vivo, J. Immunol.* **117**:1992.

Haskill, J. S., Proctor, J. W., and Yamamura, Y., 1975*a*, Host response within solid tumours. I. Monocyte effector cells within rat sarcomas, *J. Natl. Cancer Inst.* **54**:387.

Haskill, J. S., Yamamura, Y., and Radov, L., 1975*b*, Host responses within solid tumours: Non-thymus-derived specific cytotoxic cells within a murine mammary adenocarcinoma, *Int. J. Cancer* **16**:798.

Haskill, S., and Parthenais, E., 1978, Immunologic factors influencing the intratumour localization of ADCC effector cells, *J. Immunol.* **120**:1813.

Herberman, R. B., 1974, Cell-mediated immunity to tumour cells, *Adv. Cancer Res.* **19**:207.

Herberman, R. B., 1979, Host immune responses in experimental tumour systems, in: *Proceedings XIIth International Cancer Congress*, Vol. 6, *Basis for Cancer Therapy* (M. Moore, ed.), Buenos Aires, Argentina, p. 13, Pergamon Press, Oxford, United Kingdom.

Herberman, R. B., and Holden, H. T., 1978, Natural cell-mediated immunity, *Adv. Cancer Res.* **27**:305.

Herberman, R. B., Holden, H. T., Djeu, J. Y., Jerrells, T. R., Varesio, L., Tagliabue, A., White, S. L., Oehler, J. R., and Dean, J. H., 1980, Macrophages as regulators of immune responses against tumors, in: *Macrophages and Lymphocytes: Nature, Functions, and Interaction* (M. R. Escobar and H. Friedman eds.), Part B, p. 361, Plenum Press, New York.

Hibbs, J. B., 1976, The macrophage as a tumourididal effector cell: A review of *in vivo* and *in vitro* studies on the mechanisms of the activated macrophage non-specific cytotoxic reaction, in: *The Macrophage and Neoplasia* (M. Fink, ed.), p. 83, Academic Press, New York.

Holden, H. T., Haskill, J. S., Kirchner, H., and Herberman, R. B., 1976, Two functionally distinct anti-tumour effector cells isolated from primary murine sarcoma virus-induced tumours, *J. Immunol.* **117**:440.

Holm, G., 1972, Lysis of antibody-treated human erythrocytes by human leucocytes and macrophages in tissue culture, *Int. Arch. Allergy* **43**:671.

James, K., 1977, The influence of tumour cell products on macrophage function *in vitro* and *in vivo:* A review, in: *The Macrophage and Cancer* (K. James, B. McBride, and A. Stuart, eds.), p. 225, University of Edinburgh, Scotland.

Keller, R., 1977, Mononuclear phagocytes and antitumour resistance: A discussion, in: *The Macrophage and Cancer* (K. James, B. McBride, and A. Stuart, eds.), p. 31, University of Edinburgh, Scotland.

Keller, R., 1978, Macrophage-mediated natural cytotoxicity against various target cells *in vitro*. I. Macrophages from diverse anatomical sites and different strains of rats and mice, *Br. J. Cancer* **37**:732.

Kerbel, R. S., and Davies, A. J. S., 1974, The possible biological significance of Fc receptors in mammalian lymphocytes and tumor cells, *Cell* **3**:105.

Kerbel, R. S., and Pross, H. F., 1976, Fc receptor-bearing cells as a reliable marker for quantitation of host lymphoreticular infiltration of progressively growing solid tumours, *Int. J. Cancer* **18**:432.

Kerbel, R. S., Pross, H. F., and Elliot, E. V., 1975, Origin and partial characterisation of Fc receptor bearing cells found within experimental carcinomas and sarcomas, *Int. J. Cancer* **15**:918.

Klimpel, G. R., and Henney, C. S., 1978, A comparison of the effects of T and macrophage-like suppressor cells on memory cell differentiation *in vitro, J. Immunol.* **121**:749.

Kripke, M. L., and Fisher, M. S., 1976, Immunologic parameters of ultraviolet carcinogenesis, *J. Natl. Cancer Inst.* **57**:211.

Kung, J. T., Brooks, S. B., Jakway, J. P., Leonard, L. J., and Talmage, D. W., 1977, Suppression of *in vitro* cytotoxic response by macrophages due to induced arginase, *J. Exp. Med.* **146**:665.

Lay, W. H., and Nussenzweig, V., 1968, Receptors for complement on leucocytes, *J. Exp. Med.* **139**:991.

Levy, J. P., and Leclerc, J. C., 1977, The murine sarcoma virus-induced tumour—Exception or general model in tumour immunology? *Adv. Cancer Res.* **24**:1.

Lill, P. H., and Fortner, G. W., 1978, Identification and cytotoxic reactivity of inflammatory cells recovered from progressing or regressing syngeneic UV-induced murine tumours, *J. Immunol.* **121**:1854.

Ly, I. A., and Mishell, R. I., 1974, Separation of mouse spleen cells by passage through columns of Sephadex G-10, *J. Immunol. Meth.* **5**:239.

Mantovani, A., Evans, R., and Alexander, P., 1977, Non-specific cytotoxicity of spleen cells in mice bearing trasplanted chemically-induced fibrosarcomas, *Br. J. Cancer* **36**:35.

Meltzer, M. J., Stevenson, M. M., and Leonard, E. J., 1977, Characterisation of macrophage chemotaxis in tumour cell cultures and comparison with lymphocyte-derived chemotactic factors, *Cancer Res.* **37**:721.

Moore, K., and Moore, M., 1977a, Intra-tumour host cells of transplanted rat neoplasms of different immunogenicity, *Int. J. Cancer* **19**:803.

Moore, M., and Moore, K., 1977b, Kinetics of macrophage infiltration of experimental rat neoplasms, in: *The Macrophage and Cancer* (K. James, B. McBride, and A. Stuart, eds.), p. 330, University of Edinburgh, Scotland.

Moore, K., and Moore, M., 1979, Systemic and *in situ* natural killer activity in tumour-bearing rats, *Br. J. Cancer* **39**:636.

Nathan, C. F., Hill, V. M., and Terry, W. D., 1976, Isolation of a subpopulation of adherent peritoneal cells with anti-tumour activity, *Nature (London)* **260**:146.

Nelson, D. S., 1976, Non-specific immunoregulation by macrophages and their products, in: *Immunobiology of the Macrophage* (D. S. Nelson, ed.), p. 235, Academic Press, New York.

Oehler, J. R., and Herberman, R. B., 1978, Natural cell-mediated cytotoxicity in rats. III. Effects of immunopharmacologic treatments on natural reactivity and on reactivity augmented by polyinosinic-polycytidylic acid, *Int. J. Cancer* **21**:221.

Oehler, J. R., Lindsay, L. R., Nunn, M. E., and Herberman, R. B., 1978a, Natural cell-mediated cytotoxicity in rats. I. Tissue and strain distribution, and demonstration of a membrane receptor for the Fc portion of IgG, *Int. J. Cancer* **21**:204.

Oehler, J. R., Lindsay, L. R., Nunn, M. E., Holden, H. T., and Herberman, R. B., 1978b, Natural cell-mediated cytotoxicity in rats. II. *In vivo* augmentation of NK-cell activity, *Int. J. Cancer* **21**:210.

Plata, F., McDonald, H. R., and Sordat, B., 1976, Studies on the distribution and origin of cytolytic T lymphocytes present in mice bearing Moloney murine sarcoma virus (MSV)-induced tumours, in: *Comparative Leukaemia Research 1975, Bibliotheca Haematologica*, No. 43 (J. Clemmensen and D. S. Yohn, eds.), p. 274, Karger, Basel.

Pollack, S. B., Nelson, K., and Gransz, J. D., 1976, Separation of effector cells mediating antibody-dependent cellular cytotoxicity (ADC) to erythrocyte targets from those mediating ADC to tumour targets, *J. Immunol.* **116**:944.

Potter, M. R., and Moore, M., 1978, Organ distribution of natural cytotoxicity in the rat, *Clin. Exp. Immunol.* **34**:78.

Potter, M. R., and Moore, M., 1980, The effect of BCG stimulation on natural cytotoxicity in the rat, *Immunology* **39**:427.

Pross, H. F., and Kerbel, R. S., 1976, An assessment of intra-tumour phagocytic and surface marker bearing cells in a series of autochthonous and early passaged chemically-induced murine sarcomas, *J. Natl. Cancer Inst.* **57**:1157.

Riccardi, C., Puccetti, P., Santoni, A., and Herberman, R. B., 1979, Rapid *in vivo* assay of mouse NK cell activity, *J. Natl. Cancer Inst.* **63**:1041.

Robins, R. A., Flannery, G. R., and Baldwin, R. W., 1979, Tumour-derived lymphoid cells are able to prevent tumour growth *in vivo*, *Br. J. Cancer* **40**:946.

Rubin, B., and Hertel-Wulff, B., 1975, Biological significance of Fc receptor-bearing cells among activated T lymphocytes, *Scand. J. Immunol.* **4**:451.

Russell, S. W., and McIntosh, A. J., 1977, Macrophages isolated from regressing Moloney sarcomas are more cytotoxic than those recovered from progressing sarcomas, *Nature (London)* **268**:69.

Russell, S. W., Doe, W. F., Hoskins, R. G., and Cochrane, C. G., 1976a, Inflammatory cells in solid murine neoplasms. I. Tumour disaggregation and identification of constituent inflammatory cells, *Int. J. Cancer* **18**:322.

Russell, S. W., Gillespie, G. Y., Hansen, C. B., and Cochrane, C. G., 1976b, Inflammatory cells in solid murine neoplasms. II. Cell types found throughout the course of Moloney sarcoma regression or progression, *Int. J. Cancer* 18:331.

Russell, S. W., Doe, W. F., and McIntosh, A. T., 1977, Functional characterisation of a stable, non-cytolytic stage of macrophage activation in tumors, *J. Exp. Med.* 146:1511.

Shellam, G. R., 1977, Gross virus-induced lymphoma in the rat. V. Natural cytotoxic cells are non-T cells, *Int. J. Cancer* 19:225.

Snyderman, R., and Mergenhagen, S. E., 1976, Chemotaxis of macrophages, in: *Immunobiology of the Macrophage* (D. S. Nelson, ed.), p. 323, Academic Press, New York.

Snyderman, R., and Pike, M. C., 1976, An inhibitor of macrophage chemotaxis produced by neoplasms, *Science* 192:370.

Snyderman, R., Pike, M. C., Blaylock, B. L., and Weinstein, P., 1976, Effects of neoplasms on inflammation: Depression of macrophage accumulation after tumor implantation, *J. Immunol.* 116:585.

Szymaniec, S., and James, K., 1976, Studies on the Fc receptor bearing cells in a transplanted methylcholanthrene mouse fibrosarcoma, *Br. J. Cancer* 33:36.

Thomson, D. M. P., Steele, K., and Alexander, P., 1973, The presence of tumour-specific membrane antigen in the serum of rats with chemically induced sarcomata, *Br. J. Cancer* 27:27.

Tilney, N. L., Strom, T. B., Macpherson, S. G., and Carpenter, C. B., 1975, Surface properties of functional characteristics of infiltrating cells harvested from acutely rejecting cardiac allografts in inbred rats, *Transplantation* 20:323.

Tilney, N. L., Notis-McConarty, J., and Strom, T. B., 1978, Specificity of cellular migration into cardiac allografts in rats, *Transplantation* 26:181.

Tracey, D. E., Wolfe, S. A., Durdick, J. M., and Henney, C. S., 1977, BCG-induced murine effector cells. I. Cytolytic activity in peritoneal exudates: An early response to BCG, *J. Immunol.* 119:1145.

Van Loveren, H., and Den Otter, W., 1974, Macrophages in solid tumours. I. Immunologically specific effector cells, *J. Natl. Cancer Inst.* 53:1057.

Varesio, L., Herberman, R. B., Gerson, J. M., and Holden, H. T., 1979, Suppression of lymphokine production by macrophages infiltrating murine virus-induced tumors, *Int. J. Cancer* 24:97–102.

Walker, W. S., 1976, Functional heterogeneity of macrophages in the induction and expression of acquired immunity, *J. Reticuloendothel. Soc.* 20:57.

Werb, Z., 1975, Macrophage membrane synthesis, in: *Mononuclear Phagocytes in Immunity, Infection and Pathology* (R. van Furth, ed.), p. 331, Blackwell Scientific Publications, Oxford and London.

West, W. H., Cannon, G. B., Kay, D., Bonnard, G. D., and Herberman, R. B., 1977, Natural cytotoxic reactivity of human lymphocytes against a myeloid cell line: Characterisation of effector cells, *J. Immunol.* 118:355.

Winter, C. A., Risley, E. A., and Nuss, G. W., 1962, Carrageenin-induced edema in hind paw of the rat as an assay for antiinflammatory drugs, *Proc. Soc. Exp. Biol. Med.* 111:544.

Wolfe, S. A., Tracey, D. E., and Henney, C. S., 1976, Induction of "natural killer" cells by BCG, *Nature (London)* 262:584.

Wood, G. L., and Gillespie, Y., 1975, Studies on the role of macrophages in regulation of tumour growth and metastasis of murine chemically-induced tumours, *Int. J. Cancer* 16:1022.

Wood, G. W., Gillespie, G. Y., and Barth, R. F., 1975, Receptor sites for antigen-antibody complexes on cells derived from solid tumours: Detection by means of antibody-sensitised sheep erythrocytes labelled with Technetium-99m, *J. Immunol.* 114:950.

Chapter 6

Evidence for Mononuclear Phagocytes in Solid Neoplasms and Appraisal of Their Nonspecific Cytotoxic Capabilities

Stephen W. Russell, G. Yancey Gillespie, and Judith L. Pace

Department of Pathology and The Cancer Research Center
University of North Carolina School of Medicine
Chapel Hill, North Carolina 27514

I. INTRODUCTION

After years of being viewed as little more than scavengers, mononuclear phagocytes are now more properly regarded as cells with a multiplicity of functions. One of these, tumor cell killing, recently has attracted particular interest. Both antigenically specific and nonspecific effects have been reported (for reviews, see Evans and Alexander, 1976; Hibbs, 1976; and Keller, 1976). Of the two, nonspecific killing has been the most extensively studied, with a number of candidates for the cytolytic mechanism(s) now under consideration (Hibbs, 1974a; Bucana, et al., 1976; Ferluga, et al., 1978; Schorlemmer, et al., 1978; Currie, 1978; Adams, 1978). The process is nonphagocytic in its nature, either contact or extremely close juxtaposition of the target and effector cells is required, and only tumor cells appear to be susceptible to killing.

Macrophages that have become nonspecifically cytotoxic for tumor cells are commonly referred to as "activated." This operational definition is extended by some to include inflammatory macrophages that are stimulated but nontumoricidal. We will retain the more restricted use of the term, however, because we feel that expression of nonspecific cytotoxic activity denotes a functional state distinct and separable from other levels of macrophage stimulation.

The purpose of this presentation is to review comprehensively the evidence that tumors contain mononuclear phagocytes, that these cells may or may not

143

be nonspecifically cytotoxic for tumor cells *in vitro*, and that some tumors appear to be capable of subverting the process of macrophage activation. In addition, we will consider some of the more important technical problems that influence the assay of macrophage-mediated cytotoxic activity.

II. MACROPHAGES IN SOLID NEOPLASMS

Most of the evidence for macrophages in tumors has been obtained in one of three different ways: morphological studies, immune hemadsorption onto tumor tissue sections, and analysis of cell suspensions derived from mechanically or enzymatically disaggregated tumors. Each of these approaches has shortcomings; however, the composite of results obtained leads, inevitably, to the conclusion that many tumors contain substantial numbers of macrophages.

A. Morphological Studies

It is extremely difficult to differentiate members of the mononuclear phagocyte series from other mononuclear inflammatory cells by bright-field light-microscopic examination of tissues stained with hematoxylin and eosin. For this reason, cellular infiltrates associated with tumors usually have been described as containing mononuclear cells, lymphoreticular cells or, simply, lymphocytes. There have been exceptions. For example, Rosenau and Moon (1966) described macrophagelike cells as the principal constituent of inflammatory infiltrates seen 3–9 days after tissue or cells from primary, methylcholanthrene-induced sarcomas had been injected into syngeneic mice.

Histochemical staining of tumor tissue sections has been used in an attempt to decrease the subjectivity associated with light-microscopic recognition of macrophages. Judgmental decisions are required here too, however, because no single enzyme activity yet described can be used to unequivocally identify mononuclear phagocytes. Monis and Weinberg (1961) described cells containing large amounts of esterase activity evenly distributed in the stroma of human tumors. Woods and Papadimitriou (1977) examined methylcholanthrene-induced fibrosarcomas in rats for evidence of peroxidase, catalase, acid phosphatase, and nonspecific esterase activities. Of these, they felt that peroxidase staining was the most useful in demonstrating the distribution of mononuclear phagocytes. No differences were found between tumors and the subcutaneous connective tissues of age-matched controls. Lysosomal acid phosphatase activity has been selected by other groups as the histochemical marker of choice for macrophages. By this approach, Abraham and Barbolt (1978) identified large numbers of macrophages in the stroma of colonic adenomas induced in rats by the oral administration of dimethylhydrazine. Stromal macrophages in adenocarcinomas were, by contrast, fewer in number and contained less enzyme activity, especially if the tumors were poorly differentiated and invasive. As will be seen, the increased association of macrophages in this study with benign, compared to malignant, neoplasms is an uncommon finding. Lauder and colleagues (1977), also using acid phosphatase histochemistry, noted differences in the distribution of mononuclear phagocytes in infiltrative human breast carcinomas. These cells were confined to the peripheries of some of the neoplasms, while in others infiltration resulted in close juxtaposition of macrophages and neoplastic cells. No morphologic evidence of a cytotoxic effect was found, but extensive intercellular infiltration of tumors by lymphoreticular cells was associated with a reduced incidence of metastasis.

Ultrastructural studies, while limited in number, have confirmed the presence of macrophages in untreated solid neoplasms (for review, see Carr and Underwood, 1974). Within lymphomas of the hamster, Birbeck and Carter (1972) have identified mononuclear phagocytes of various appearances. In a nonmetastasizing lymphoma they found large, active-looking macrophages that contained numerous primary and secondary lysosomes. By contrast, macrophages in a type of lymphoma that characteristically metastasizes gave little evidence of stimulation, i.e., they were small and contained few phagolysosomes. Macrophages occurred with approximately the same frequency in each of the two types of lymphoma, and no evidence for specialized forms of contact between macrophages and tumor cells was found in either of the two tumors. Macrophages had gone unrecognized in the metastasizing tumor until it was examined ultrastructurally. This fact attests to the previously mentioned difficulty that attends the differentiation of macrophages from other mononuclear cell types at the light-microscopic level. Ultrastructural studies of human neoplasms (Underwood and Carr, 1972) and rat brain tumors (Lantos, 1975) also showed infiltrating mononuclear phagocytes of both mature and immature types, but no evidence that these cells were mediating injury to tumor cells could be found.

B. Immune Hemadsorption to Frozen Sections of Tumor Tissue

Adsorption of erythrocytes sensitized with antibody (EA) or complement (EAC) to cryostat-prepared sections has been a useful way of demonstrating the distribution of various receptor-bearing cell types in lymphoid tissues (Shevach et al., 1973). This same technique has been applied to the analysis of tumor tissue sections, with the result that Fc-receptor-bearing cells have unequivocally been associated with neoplasms. There has been controversy, however, as to whether such reactivity in nonlymphoreticular neoplasms is a property of the tumor cells or of host inflammatory cells that have infiltrated the neoplasm. As will be seen in this section, the bulk of accumulated evidence suggests that host inflammatory cells are the principal source of binding.

Immune hemadsorption of EA to frozen sections of a nonlymphoreticular murine tumor was described initially by Humphrey *et al.* (1967). Subsequently, Milgrom *et al.* (1968) presented four lines of evidence that the reaction was the result of interaction of the Fc portion of IgG antibody with cells in the tumor tissue sections: (1) enzymatic removal of the Fc fragment from sensitizing antibody abolished binding of EA without affecting hemagglutinating activity of the same preparation; (2) treatment of F(ab')$_2$-coated erythrocytes with intact antibody against Fab restored the reaction; (3) horse complement, used to "cover" the Fc portion of sensitizing antibody, blocked immune hemadsorption; and (4) preincubation of tissue sections with Cohn fraction II immunoglobulins, which undoubtedly contained immunoglobulin aggregates, blocked immune hemadsorption, while Cohn fraction V preparations (principally albumin) did not. Later work showed that preincubation of tissues with either Fc fragments (Matre, 1976) or various kinds of immune complexes (Wood *et al.*, 1975; Targowski *et al.*, 1977a,b) inhibited binding, while neither F(ab')$_2$, Fab, or Facb fragments, nor intact IgM or IgA blocked adherence (Matre, 1976; Turner *et al.*, 1978). Milgrom *et al.* (1968) demonstrated that extensive absorption of their antierythrocyte serum with a variety of malignant tissues failed to affect binding, thereby showing that adherence was not due to simple interaction of sensitizing antibody with cross-reacting antigens found both on erythrocytes and in tumor tissues. Further investigations established that the Fc receptors in malignant tissue are similar to those in spleen and liver with respect to binding characteristics and susceptibility to chemical degradation (Tønder *et al.*, 1974; Matre, 1976; Matre *et al.*, 1976). Animal studies were extended to show that neoplasms of man also contain Fc-receptor-positive cells (Tønder and Thunold, 1973; Tønder *et al.*, 1974, 1975, 1976; Matre, 1976; Matre *et al.*, 1976; Wood and Gollahon, 1977; Turner *et al.*, 1978; Morantz *et al.*, 1979b), while benign lesions of the human breast (Tønder *et al.*, 1975; Turner *et al.*, 1978) and prostate (Tønder *et al.*, 1975) were found not to bind antibody-sensitized erythrocytes.

In several reports (Edelson *et al.*, 1973, 1975), investigators have routinely failed to detect EA binding to frozen sections of several different primary human neoplasms. These particular primary tumors may have contained very few Fc-receptor-positive cells. However, in view of other studies (Tønder *et al.*, 1975; Wood and Gollahon, 1977) wherein 100% of tumors similar in type to those studied by Edelson *et al.* (1973, 1975) bound EA, another explanation seems likely. For example, Edelson *et al.* washed their sections in order to remove nonadherent erythrocytes and, by so doing, may have removed weakly bound EA inadvertently. The closed-chamber method of Tønder *et al.* (1964), as modified by Milgrom *et al.* (1968), avoids this problem, thereby giving a marked improvement in sensitivity (Tønder *et al.*, 1974, 1975). Briefly, the concavity of a microculture (depression) slide is filled with a suspension of indicator erythrocytes. A cover slip with test tissue affixed is inverted over the depression, after which the slide is inverted to allow erythrocytes to settle onto the tissue.

To read, the slide is righted, permitting unbound erythrocytes to fall away. No washing is required, allowing the detection of even the weakest erythrocyte binding. Using the closed-chamber method, 85–100% of the neoplasms in several different series (Tønder et al., 1975; Wood and Gollahon, 1977; Turner et al., 1978) have bound EA, whether or not they had histologic evidence of lymphoreticular infiltrates.

As techniques improved, observations were made with greater precision. For example, individual cells in sections were seen to bind different numbers of EA (Tønder et al., 1974, 1975). More importantly, it was discovered that tumors displayed different patterns of immune hemadsorption, ranging from focal to diffuse (Tønder et al., 1974, 1975; Wood and Gollahon, 1977, 1978; Turner et al., 1978; Morantz et al., 1979b). In some instances (Wood and Gollahon, 1977; Turner et al., 1978) it could be shown that erythrocytes were attached to stromal elements rather than tumor cells. Disaggregation studies (Tønder et al., 1975; Morantz et al., 1979b) revealed that neoplasms that yielded the highest percentage of Fc-receptor-positive cells in suspensions also exhibited the greatest degree of EA binding to tumor tissue sections. Not all cells in these suspensions rosetted and, significantly, many of those identifiable as tumor cells were without bound erythrocytes. Continued technical advances have shown that Fc-receptor binding by tumor tissue corresponds to the distribution of nonspecific esterase-positive cells (Wood and Gollahon, 1977) and, presumably the same thing, macrophages (Wood and Gollahon, 1978). The latter were identified by fluorescence microscopy using antimacrophage serum.

Thus it can be seen how questions raised by the natural evolution of immune hemadsorption studies fostered the belief that host rather than tumor cells were being detected by EA-binding assays. Data obtained by other approaches were required to confirm this hypothesis, however.

C. Cell Suspensions Derived from Disaggregated Neoplasms

Perhaps the most compelling evidence that tumors contain substantial numbers of normal host cells, especially macrophages, stems from the analysis of cell suspensions derived from mechanically or enzymatically disaggregated neoplasms. The first such examination was made by Cohen et al. (1971). These investigators disaggregated transmissible venereal tumors of the dog, as well as a methylcholanthrene-induced and a spontaneously occurring fibrosarcoma of the rat. They showed that 20–30% of the cells in resultant suspensions rosetted with antibody-sensitized erythrocytes, indicating the presence of Fc receptors. In contrast, fewer than 1% of the cells in a suspension culture, derived many passages before from a hamster fibrosarcoma, bound the indicator erythrocytes. Cytologic examination did not allow conclusive identification of the rosetting cells in primary explants, and carbonyl iron treatment followed by exposure of the cell suspensions to a magnet was equally uninstructive. The authors suggested that they could be detecting macrophages; however, they considered it unlikely that a tumor could contain 20–30% Fc-receptor-positive host cells. Cohen and his colleagues therefore concluded that tumor cells were the ones forming rosettes. Retrospectively we know that such percentages are not unrealistic for intratumoral inflammatory cells.

Because of controversy that had arisen from immune hemadsorption studies (see Section II.B), considerable effort was expended to show that the Fc-receptor-positive cells in suspensions were of host, and not of tumor, origin. Adherent, Fc-receptor-bearing cells derived from tumors did not produce neoplasms when injected into mice (Wood and Gillespie, 1975). Neoplastic cells isolated from the tumors of experimental animals (Kerbel *et al.*, 1975, 1977; Wood *et al.*, 1975) and human beings (Kerbel *et al.*, 1977) were negative for Fc and C3b receptors unless they were derived from a cell type that would be expected to express them. Reinjection of receptor-negative, cultured tumor cells gave rise to neoplasms that again contained cells subject to killing by antimacrophage serum/complement treatment (Evans, 1972) or that expressed Fc receptors (Kerbel *et al.*, 1975; Wood *et al.*, 1975; Pross and Kerbel, 1976; Szymaniec and James, 1976). In each of these cases, the percentage of macrophages or Fc-receptor-positive cells found in suspensions derived from the newly induced tumors was approximately the same as the percentage that had characterized the original suspension from which the cultured tumor cells had come. The percentage found appeared to be independent of the route of inoculation (Evans, 1972; Szymaniec and James, 1976). The most direct evidence that the intratumoral, Fc-receptor-positive population is of host origin has come from studies in which F_1 hybrid mice were inoculated with tumor cells obtained from one of the parental strains. Treatment of cell suspensions derived from resultant tumors with alloantisera (directed against H-2 specificities of the other parental strain) and complement killed the Fc-receptor-positive population (Kerbel *et al.*, 1975; Pross and Kerbel, 1976). In similar studies, using fluorescence microscopy and rat alloantisera (K. Moore and Moore, 1977*a*), it was shown that, after passage into F_1 hybrids, parental strain tumors contained cells that expressed the histocompatibility antigens of both parents. The percentage of such cells approximated the combined percentages of Fc-receptor-positive cells and T lymphocytes found in the same tumors.

Assays for Fc receptors could theoretically detect any of the many inflammatory and noninflammatory cell types that express them (Kerbel and Davies, 1974; Kerbel *et al.*, 1977). Operationally, however, the majority of Fc-receptor-positive cells in suspensions derived from disaggregated tumors has been composed of mononuclear phagocytes (Kerbel *et al.*, 1975; Wood and Gillespie, 1975; Szymaniec and James, 1976; Wood and Gollahon, 1977, 1978; Korn *et al.*, 1978*a*). Multiple criteria have usually been used to identify the macrophages in these cell suspensions, including morphologic appearance, capacity to adhere to surfaces and resist detachment by trypsin, ability to phagocytose particles, content of nonspecific esterase activity, expression of Fc and/or C3b receptors, and expression of macrophage-specific antigens detectable by antimacrophage serum (either complement-mediated cytolysis or fluorescence). Values reported in the literature for the percentage of total cells recovered from tumors that are macrophages have ranged from 0 to 65%, with the majority falling between 15 and 45%. These figures have been derived from the examination of naturally occurring and experimentally induced tumors of mice and rats, as well as a variety of human neoplasms (Table I). When it has been sought, correlation has been good between the percentage of macrophages in cell suspensions and the extent to which the parent tumors have been infiltrated by macrophages, as estimated by histologic (Stutman, 1975; Pross and Kerbel, 1976), immune hemadsorption (Wood and

Table I. Relative Macrophage Content of Cell Suspensions Derived from Disaggregated Neoplasms

Species	Neoplasms[a]	Macro-phages[b] (%)	References
Mouse	Sarcomas and carcinomas, mostly chemically induced and transplanted in syngeneic hosts	0–60	Evans (1972), Owen and Seeger (1973), van Loveren and Den Otter (1974), Kerbel et al. (1975), Stutman (1975), Wood and Gillespie (1975), Holden et al. (1976), Pross and Kerbel (1976), Russell et al. (1976a,c), Szymaniec and James (1976), Mendiondo et al. (1978), Normann and Cornelius (1978), Stewart and Beetham (1978), Wood and Gollahon (1978)
Rat	Sarcomas and carcinomas, chemically induced and transplanted in syngeneic hosts	2–65	Evans (1972), Eccles and Alexander (1974a,b), van Loveren and Den Otter (1974), Currie and Eccles (1976), Gauci (1976), K. Moore and Moore (1977a), M. Moore and Moore (1977b), Normann and Cornelius (1978)
Human	Breast carcinoma, melanoma, squamous cell carcinoma, adenocarcinoma of the gastrointestinal tract, thyroid carcinoma, bronchial carcinoma, giant cell tumor of bone, renal cell carcinoma, meningioma, neurofibroma	0–56	Alexander et al. (1976), Wood and Gollahon (1977), Wood et al. (1978)

[a]The vast majority in the murine systems was sarcomas, usually fibrosarcomas. Virus-induced tumors were mouse Moloney rhabdomyosarcomas.
[b]Ranges of values reported. The majority of percentages fell in midrange. The criteria used to identify macrophages were one or more (usually more) of the following: morphologic appearance, adherence, resistance to detachment by trypsin, phagocytic, cell surface antigen(s) detectable by antimacrophage serum, Fc receptor positive, nonspecific esterase positive.

Gollahon, 1977; Wood *et al.*, 1978), and immunofluorescence (Wood and Gollahon, 1978) analyses.

A given inoculum of tumor cells from an established cell line will usually induce tumors that have a highly predictable content of macrophages and other inflammatory cell types. In some instances the pattern of host response is so distinctive that the tumor can actually be identified on this basis (Pross and Kerbel, 1976). Implicit in this latter statement is recognition that the inflammatory cell response engendered by each neoplasm is different qualitatively and quantitatively from that of others (Haskill *et al.*, 1976; Pross and Kerbel, 1976; Wood and Gollahon, 1978). Appreciating this fact, it is understandable why reports in the literature may appear to be in conflict. For example, the percentage of macrophages in primary neoplasms may either fall (Pross and Kerbel, 1976) or rise (Wood and Gillespie, 1975) with successive transplantation. Depending on the study, there is a higher percentage of macrophages in larger tumors (Wood and Gollahon, 1978) or in smaller tumors (Haskill *et al.*, 1975*a*; Szymaniec and James, 1976; M. Moore and Moore, 1977*b*; Normann and Cornelius, 1978; Stewart and Beetham, 1978), or tumor size has no bearing on intratumoral macrophage content (Evans, 1972; Gauci, 1976). A few generalizations can be made, however. Regressing tumors usually have had a higher content of macrophages than progressing tumors, whether rejection was spontaneous (Haskill *et al.*, 1975*b*; Stutman, 1975; Russell *et al.*, 1976*a,c*) or induced (Snodgrass and Hanna, 1973; Mendiondo *et al.*, 1978). Locally recurrent and metastatic tumors contain macrophages (Gauci, 1976; Currie and Eccles, 1976), although metastases may contain relatively fewer mononuclear phagocytes than primary neoplasms of the same type (Alexander *et al.*, 1976). The extent of intratumoral necrosis has little effect on the percentage of macrophages in a neoplasm (Evans, 1972) and likewise does not affect their distribution (Elston, 1968). Finally, the macrophage content of a tumor neither affects its growth rate (Pross and Kerbel, 1976) nor predicts whether a neoplasm will regress or progress (Evans, 1973*a*; Mendiondo *et al.*, 1978).

A direct relationship between the macrophage content of a tumor and its immunogenicity has been suggested (Evans, 1972; Eccles and Alexander, 1974*a*; K. Moore and Moore, 1977*a*; M. Moore and Moore, 1977*b*; Morantz *et al.*, 1979*a*). Accumulating evidence supports this contention by implicating the host's immunologic response in mobilizing macrophages in tumors. S. Haskill and Parthenais (1978) showed that neither delayed hypersensitivity nor antibody responsiveness was solely responsible for recruiting mononuclear phagocytes into transplantable mouse mammary carcinomas, but that one or the other had to be operative before a cellular infiltrate would develop. A number of other reports indicate that whole-body irradiation, alone or in conjunction with thymectomy, will eliminate or markedly reduce the intratumoral content of macrophages (Eccles and Alexander, 1974*b*; Haskill *et al.*, 1975*b*; Currie and Eccles, 1976; Evans, 1977; Mendiondo *et al.*, 1978). On the other hand, Szymaniec and James (1976) showed that thymectomized, lethally irradiated mice reconstituted with anti-Thy-1/complement-treated bone marrow cells had as many Fc-receptor-positive cells in their tumors as did sham thymectomized, irradiated, reconstituted mice. Both of these populations had higher levels of intratumoral Fc-receptor-positive cells than did untreated controls. These same workers also found that immunosuppressive doses of cyclophosphamide increased, rather than decreased, the percentage of phagocytic, Fc-receptor-positive cells in neoplasms. The significance of this latter finding is difficult to assess, however, because the drug concomitantly diminished tumor size. Evans (1979) determined that cyclophosphamide-induced remission of FS6 murine fibrosarcoma was characterized by parallel decreases in numbers of both neoplastic cells and host inflammatory cells, most of which were macrophages. In transplanted mouse mammary carcinomas controlled for tumor size, cyclophosphamide therapy had no influence on the relative content of Fc-receptor-positive cells (Gebhardt and Fisher, 1979). Evidence specifically suggesting that T-lymphocyte responsiveness is needed to mobilize macrophages in tumors has come from studies of unirradiated, T-cell-deficient animals. Nude mice had fewer macrophages, especially on an absolute basis, in virus-induced Moloney sarcomas than did heterozygotic controls (Stutman, 1975). Similarly, thoracic duct drainage decreased the macrophage content of rat sarcomata (Eccles and Alexander, 1974b), as did neonatal thymectomy (Gauci, 1976). Thymectomy did not affect mobilization of the few macrophages found in a nonimmunogenic sarcoma (Guaci, 1976).

D. Indirect Means of Associating Macrophages with Tumors

A novel roentgenographic technique employing a brominated fluorocarbon (perfluorocytlbromide) emulsion has been used to show the presence of macrophages in a variety of primary, as well as transplanted, neoplasms of experimental animals. Long and his co-workers (1978) injected the contrast agent intravenously and demonstrated subsequent long-term (days to weeks) radiopacification of seven of eight neoplasms, as well as the spleens and livers of recipient mice, rats and hamsters. By electron-microscopic examination they demonstrated that the principal cause of radiopacification was inclusion of the fluorocarbon emulsion in macrophages present in these tissues. Distribution of the contrast agent in tumors was irregular, but allowed visualization of neoplasms as small as 3–4 mm in diameter.

Indirect evidence of macrophages in neoplasms also has been obtained by documenting elevated serum lysozyme levels in tumor-bearing animals. Gordon et al., (1974) showed that macrophages secrete large amounts of lysozyme at a rate that is relatively independent of their level of stimulation. These workers further suggested that production of this enzyme could be a useful measure of macrophage numbers. Given this background and a growing appreciation that many tumors contain macrophages, it was a natural extension of research in this area that serum lysozyme levels be examined in tumor-bearing animals.

The potential importance of lysozyme as a means of indirectly quantifying mononuclear phagocyte activity in host–tumor relationships was suggested over 15 years ago by Perri et al. (1963). Currie and Eccles (1976) were the first, however, to provide evidence for a direct relationship between macrophage content of tumors and levels of serum lysozyme. Irradiation, which decreased the percentage of macrophages in tumors, also decreased serum levels of lysozyme (Currie and Eccles, 1976; Mendiondo *et al.*, 1978). Similarly, amputation of tumors reversed the elevation of activity in serum. Isolating enriched populations from disaggregated neoplasms demonstrated conclusively that intratumoral macrophages, and not tumor cells, were the secretors of lysozyme (Bordin and Young, 1976; Currie and Eccles, 1976).

III. NONSPECIFIC KILLING OF TUMOR CELLS BY MACROPHAGES ISOLATED FROM SOLID NEOPLASMS

Based on the above data, the conclusion that many neoplasms contain macrophages is inescapable. The question now is, what functions, if any, do intratumoral mononuclear phagocytes have? Consideration of all possibilities, given the range of macrophage functions, is beyond the scope of this presentation. The following section, therefore, will focus on nonspecific cytolytic activity mediated by macrophages recovered from neoplasms, and how the genesis of this function, i.e., activation, may be subverted by progressively growing tumors.

A. Assay of Macrophage-Mediated Cytotoxicity

It is important to recognize that the term "cytotoxicity," as Evans (1975) has so clearly stated, can refer to either cytostasis, cytolysis, or a combination of these two effects. Assays based on the release of radioisotope from prelabeled tumor target cells primarily, if not exclusively, measure cytolysis. It is unfortunately not possible to make such a statement about assays that are purported to detect cytostasis. All of these are based on demonstrating, either directly or indirectly, that fewer target cells are present in experimental, compared to control, cultures. Such a difference may, indeed, be the result of cytostasis; however, decreased cell number caused by the lysis of target cells must be rigorously excluded in order to reach this conclusion. The finding that, during the assay period, target cell numbers remain above the number initially seeded does *not* exclude cytolysis. Lysis balanced, to a greater or lesser degree, by proliferation continuing in the same culture is just as capable of producing a "static" result as is simple failure of the target cells to either replicate or die. That such balancing is a real, rather than hypothetical, phenomenon has been shown directly by Stewart and Beetham (1978). Using time-lapse cinemicrography these investigators showed that tumor cells not in contact with effector macrophages continued to divide alongside target cells that lysed as a consequence of contact with macrophages.

Another major artifact in measuring cytostasis has stemmed from reliance on assays of incorporation of radiolabeled DNA precursors (principally [^{3}H] thymidine or [^{125}I] iododeoxyuridine) by target cells. Decreased incorporation has been equated with decreased DNA synthesis and, by extrapolation, to interference by macrophages with target cell division. However, macrophages secrete large amounts of a compound, most likely thymidine or a very similar molecule, that interferes with uptake of these radiolabeled precursors (Opitz et al., 1975; Evans and Booth, 1976; Russell et al., 1977b; Stadecker et al., 1977). The decreased incorporation that has been interpreted as cytostasis could, therefore, in many instances have been due to competitive inhibition of uptake of radiolabel.

In spite of these technical difficulties, there are enough data from well-controlled experiments that little doubt is left that tumor macrophages can mediate cytostatic, as well as cytolytic, effects. Whether or not these represent different mechanisms or are simply quantitative differences in expression of the same mediation pathway remains to be determined.

B. Evidence for the Mediation of Nonspecific Cytotoxic Effects by Macrophages Isolated from Solid Neoplasms

Using assays based on cell counting, Evans (1973a) was the first to show that intratumoral macrophages can mediate nonspecific cytotoxic effects in vitro. Macrophages isolated from transplantable, syngeneic tumors of both the rat and mouse were held under serum-free-culture conditions for 24–48 h before being challenged with tumor target cells. Further investigations (Evans, 1975, 1976) in these same systems were performed using an assay based on pulse labeling of cultures with [^{125}I]-IUdR. Careful visual analysis and testing of culture supernates confirmed that the effects obtained did not result from competitive inhibition of radioisotope uptake by secreted products of the macrophages (Robert Evans, personal communication). Macrophages from some of the tumors tested after 24–48 h in vitro were very efficient at arresting the growth of target cells and later killing them. Macrophages from other tumors were, by contrast, only weakly cytotoxic or were completely lacking in their capacity to affect the growth or survival of target cells. As pointed out by Evans (1976), failure to detect killing under these conditions may have been wholly or in part attributable to the time spent in culture by macrophages before they were challenged with tumor target cells (see Section IV.B).

Two different groups have investigated macrophages isolated from spontaneously regressing Moloney sarcomas. Russell et al. (1977a,b) measured only cytolytic activity, assayed as release of chromium-51 (^{51}Cr) from prelabeled target cells. In these studies, neoplasms induced by the injection of cultured sarcoma cells were disaggregated enzymatically and the macrophages in resultant suspensions plated to form confluent monolayers. These cells were capable of lysing a variety of tumor target cells; however, the rate at which ^{51}Cr was released differed for each target cell type, suggesting either differences in susceptibility to macrophage-mediated killing or in the way the radioisotope leaked from injured cells. Release of ^{51}Cr from most cell types tested was detectable as early as 4–8 h. These points are illustrated in the left panel of Fig. 1.

The investigations of Holden *et al.* (1976), Korn *et al.* (1978*b*), and Puccetti and Holden (1979) also have been of macrophages isolated from regressing Moloney sarcomas, but these were virus, rather than cell, induced. The principal contribution of these workers has been to show that the population of nonspecifically cytotoxic macrophages obtained from regressing sarcomas is separable by velocity sedimentation at unit gravity into two, and sometimes three, peaks of activity. These findings suggest that cytotoxic macrophages, at least in this system, are heterogeneous with regard to size. The two subpopulations observed routinely had peak sedimentation velocities of 4–5 mm/h and 5–6 mm/h, with the

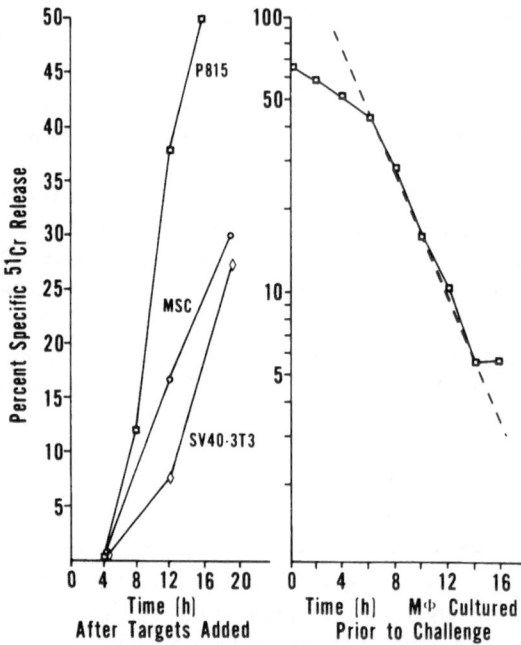

Figure 1. Macrophages (MΦ) from enzyme-disaggregated, regressing Moloney sarcomas were plated at a population density of $6 \times 10^3/\text{mm}^2$ in 16-mm-diameter, flat-bottomed wells (Russell *et al.*, 1976*b*, 1977*a,b*). The left panel depicts the rate at which ^{51}Cr was released from prelabeled cells of three different antigenically unrelated tumor cell lines (P815 mastocytoma; MSC, the Moloney sarcoma cell line that had been used to induce the tumors from which macrophages were recovered; and a BALB 3T3 cell transformed by SV40 virus). The target cells were introduced into assay cultures shortly after the macrophages were explanted from tumors. The right panel illustrates how rapidly macrophages from regressing Moloney sarcomas lost their capacity to kill *in vitro*. In this experiment, macrophages were held *in vitro* for various times before P815 mastocytoma cells were added. The amount of ^{51}Cr release from these targets was then measured, for each point shown, 16 h later.

irregularly observed third peak falling at 7 mm/h. When they were detected, the latter, largest macrophages contributed least to the total cytotoxic activity observed. Both cytolytic and cytostatic activities have been claimed by these workers for Moloney macrophages. There is no doubt that cytolysis was detected, since ^{51}Cr release was obtained; however, the assays (separate use of [^{3}H] thymidine incorporation or electronic cell-counting) employed to measure cytostasis leave open to question whether or not macrophages from the tumors mediated this cytotoxic effect. Peritoneal macrophages from tumor-bearing mice were, on the other hand, examined *concurrently* by ^{51}Cr release and cell-counting assays, allowing a judgment regarding cytostatic effects to be made. Results here showed that peritoneal macrophages reduced target cell numbers markedly, compared to controls, at effector-to-target-cell ratios that did not result in detectable cytolysis. The finding that resident and inflammatory peritoneal macrophages were cytolytic is in direct contrast to the negative findings of Russell et al. (1977a). This apparent discrepancy is probably explainable on the basis of differences in the tumor (virus-induced vs. cell-induced) and/or assay systems.

Analysis by time-lapse cinemicrography showed that macrophages isolated from progressively growing EMT6 tumors could either be cytostatic (target cells neither divided nor lysed) or cytolytic (Stewart and Beetham, 1978). The target cell had to be in prolonged contact with one or more macrophages in order for either effect to be seen. Targets not contacted by macrophages, or contacted infrequently, continued to divide. On the rare occasion when tumor cells divided after they had been in prolonged contact with macrophages, both of the daughter cells died synchronously within one hour of the time of division.

C. Evidence That Activation of Macrophages is Subverted in Some Progressively Growing Tumors

While some progressively growing neoplasms contain nonspecifically cytotoxic, i.e., activated, macrophages (Evans, 1973a, 1975, 1976; Stewart and Beetham, 1978), others do not (Evans, 1973a, 1975, 1976; Russell et al., 1977a). A similar, but more intriguing, difference is found within the Moloney sarcoma system: regressing tumors contain activated, cytolytic macrophages (Russell et al., 1977b; Puccetti and Holden, 1979), while progressively growing sarcomas of this same type contain macrophages that either do not kill, or that kill with greatly reduced efficiency (Russell and McIntosh, 1977; Taniyama and Holden, 1979). These observations raise several questions. Are macrophages in some progressively growing neoplasms unable to mediate cytotoxicity because they have been entirely without the stimuli needed to effect activation, or have they been activated only partially? Alternatively, have they been fully activated at one time, but for some reason have lost their cytotoxic capability *in vivo*, much as activated tumor macrophages do when they are explanted and held as a purified population *in vitro* (Evans, 1976; Russell *et al.*, 1977*a,b*; Fig. 1, right panel)? The answers to these questions are not yet fully known; however, some insight has been obtained through the use of bacterial lipopolysaccaride (LPS) as a probe of macrophage activation (Russell *et al.*, 1977*a*). Noncytolytic macrophages from two different kinds of progressively growing mouse tumors responded to concentrations of LPS in the pg-to-ng/ml range by developing high levels of nonspecific cytolytic activity within hours. Similar treatment had no detectable effect on thioglycollate-elicited peritoneal macrophages. Thioglycollate-elicited (Table II) and other types of inflammatory peritoneal macrophages (Hibbs *et al.*, 1977; Ruco and Meltzer, 1978) will respond cytolytically to such minute amounts of LPS, however, if they have first been exposed to nonactivating concentrations of lymphokine.

Whether or not such exquisite sensitivity to stimulation by LPS characterizes the noncytotoxic macrophages recovered from the neoplasms of other species is not yet known. Weakly cytotoxic macrophages isolated from rat sarcomas became cytolytic when exposed *in vitro* to LPS (Evans, 1973*a*). However, the concentration of LPS and time of *in vitro* exposure used in these studies (50 μg/

Table II. LPS-Mediated Activation of Thioglycollate-Elicited Macrophages (TG-MΦ) Primed *in Vitro* by Exposure to Lymphokine-Rich Supernates[a]

Treatment of TG-MΦ monolayers	Counts per minute of released [51]Cr[b]	Specific ^{51}Cr release (%)[c]
Untreated	1328 ± 57	0
Lymphokine (1:5)	1370 ± 26	1
LPS (125 ng/ml)	1371 ± 54	1
Lymphokine plus LPS	4093 ± 69	62

[a]Macrophages, elicited by the intraperitoneal injection of 3 ml of thioglycollate given 4 days previously, were plated in 16-mm-diameter, flat-bottomed wells (CoStar #3524) at an approximate population density of $5 \times 10^3/mm^2$. After washing to remove nonadherent cells, the monolayers were incubated (4 h, 37°C) in minimum essential tissue culture medium supplemented to 10% with fetal bovine serum alone or in combination with lymphokine (1:5), LPS (125 ng/ml), or both lymphokine and LPS. Lymphokine-rich supernates were from cultures of concanavalin-A-stimulated (2 μg/ml, 72 h) spleen cells of BALB/c mice.
[b]Radioactivity released in 16 h from P815 mastocytoma cells (10^5/well) prelabeled with [51]Cr. The mean for three wells, ± standard deviation, is given. Rate of spontaneous release was 1.4 %/h. Total counts released by osmotic lysis were 5771 ± 127/min.
[c]Specific release was calculated as previously described (Russell *et al.*, 1977*a,b*).

ml, 48 h) were in the range that will cause activation of macrophages *de novo* (Alexander and Evans, 1971; Doe and Henson, 1978).

Based on results obtained with the LPS probe, it has been proposed (Russell *et al.*, 1977*a*) that noncytolytic macrophages in some progressively growing tumors are partially activated, or "primed." The latter term is meant to convey that these macrophages have been readied to express cytotoxic activity, but that they cannot do so without a final stimulus or combination of stimuli.

It remains to be determined how widely found the phenomenon of partial activation will be, and whether or not stimulation of macrophages will be totally lacking in some progressively growing neoplasms. Where these "deficient" states are found, it will be important to identify the mechanisms responsible for causing them. Inherent in such an undertaking are the technical difficulties to which we have previously alluded in this review. These are of sufficient importance in the conduct and interpretation of experiments to warrant a brief description of them in the final section.

IV. TECHNICAL CONSIDERATIONS IN ASSAYING CYTOTOXICITY MEDIATED BY MACROPHAGES RECOVERED FROM TUMORS

Most of the items to be considered here have a negative influence on results, i.e., they have the potential to interfere with either the expression or detection of macrophage-mediated cytotoxic activity. As will be seen, however, several can produce falsely positive results.

A. Population Density of Macrophage Monolayers

Low population density of macrophage monolayers is, in our opinion, the single most important cause of falsely negative findings in cytolytic assays. The degree to which differences in population density can affect the expression of cytolytic activity has been demonstrated conclusively by Stewart *et al.* (1977) and Doe and Henson (1978). The former group investigated peritoneal macrophages activated *in vivo* by the injection of viable bacilli Calmette–Guérin (BCG). It was shown by time-lapse cinemicrography that cytolytic events decreased in frequency as population density was reduced. Macrophage-to-target-cell ratios were held constant. The need for contact between effector and target cells was invoked as the most likely explanation for the observed population-density-dependent effects. Doe and Henson (1978) used inflammatory (thioglycollate-elicited) peritoneal macrophages activated *in vitro* by LPS. Here, target cell numbers were held constant while the number of macrophages in assay cultures was reduced concomitantly. A population density was reached at which killing declined precipitously. To show that the effect was not due solely to changes in the effector-to-target-cell ratio, the converse experiment was performed. At a macrophage population density that was optimal for killing, the number of target cells per well could be varied over a 100-fold range without greatly affecting the percentage of ^{51}Cr release obtained.

The observations of Stewart *et al.* (1977) and Doe and Henson (1978) not only point out the important role of population density in assaying macrophage-mediated cytolysis, but also indicate the relative unimportance of effector-to-target-cell ratios, given adequate population density.

Cytotoxicity mediated by macrophages recovered from tumors is similarly population density dependent. In the time-lapse studies of Stewart and Beetham (1978), target cells continued to proliferate normally when monolayers were sparse, and as a consequence, contact between target cells and macrophages was reduced. As macrophage population density, and therefore the opportunity for contact with target cells, was increased, both cytostatic and cytolytic effects were observed with increasing frequency. Table III shows that the full cytolytic potential of LPS-stimulated tumor macrophages would not have been reflected had the assay been conducted at the lowest population density. Similar results (not shown) have been obtained when macrophages activated *in vivo* were explanted from regressing Moloney sarcomas and challenged immediately with target cells.

In the Moloney system it has been our experience that 5×10^3–7.5×10^3 macrophages/mm^2 are needed to obtain maximum rates of ^{51}Cr release. How-

Table III. Effect of Monolayer Population Density on Killing Mediated by LPS-Stimulated Macrophages (MΦ) Isolated from Moloney Sarcomas[a]

Macrophages[b] per monolayer $(\times 10^{-5})$	Macrophage[b] population density $(\times 10^{-3}/mm^2)$	Counts per minute[c] released by:		Specific ^{51}Cr release[d] (%)
		Unstimulated macrophages	MΦ + LPS (100 ng/ml)	
6.7	3.4	733 ± 15	933 ± 96	12
15	7.5	793 ± 36	1628 ± 37	41
29	14.4	863 ± 35	1712 ± 100	44

[a]Macrophages recovered from tumors disaggregated with a combination of trypsin, collagenase, and DNase and plated in 16-mm-diameter, flat-bottomed wells (Russell *et al.*, 1977a,b). After overnight culture, supernatant media in wells were replaced with fresh, minimum essential tissue culture medium containing 30% fetal bovine serum, with or without 100 ng/ml LPS.
[b]Cells were washed from the bottoms of wells after overnight culture (during which time macrophages from these tumors became loosely adherent) and directly counted in a hemacytometer. Population density was obtained by dividing the total number of cells recovered by the surface area of the well (201 mm^2).
[c]Radioisotope released in 16 h from P815 mastocytoma cells (10^5/well) prelabeled with ^{51}Cr. The mean for three wells, ± standard deviation, is given. Rate of spontaneous release was 1.6–1.9 %/h.
[d]Specific release was calculated as previously described (Russell *et al.*, 1977a,b).

ever, cytotoxic efficiency can vary with the source and treatment of macrophages, as well as with the assay used. The influence that population density has on results should therefore be determined for each tumor and assay system.

B. Loss of Cytolytic Activity *in Vitro*

Macrophages isolated from regressing Moloney sarcomas are cytolytic when explanted and challenged immediately with tumor target cells, but are incapable of killing after spending 12-24 h in culture (Russell *et al.*, 1977*a,b*; Puccetti and Holden, 1979). As shown in Fig. 1 (left panel), when freshly explanted from regressing Moloney sarcomas, macrophages killed target cells from three different antigenically unrelated cell lines. However, after only 14 h in culture, macrophages from the same source had lost almost all of their cytolytic activity (Fig. 1, right panel). A completely erroneous impression of the cytolytic capabilities of these macrophages would have been obtained if they had, for example, been held overnight before target cells were introduced. Similar findings have been made using macrophages recovered from rat and other mouse sarcomas (Evans, 1976).

The rate at which cytolytic activity is lost *in vitro* appears to vary with the source of macrophages. Some of the tumors studied by Evans (1976), for example, yielded macrophages capable of mediating cytotoxic activity only if they were exposed to tumor target cells immediately upon explantation. By contrast, it took 3-5 days for macrophages from other neoplasms to lose their cytotoxic potential completely. In view of this variability, the safest course, and the one that ensures that full cytotoxic activity will be detected, is to introduce target cells into assay cultures as soon after tumor macrophages are explanted as is practicable.

C. Contamination of Macrophage Monolayers with Other Cell Types

While vigorously washing monolayers of peritoneal macrophages makes it possible to remove all but a few contaminating cell types, levels of contamination of monolayers established from tumors are invariably higher. A number of manipulations have been suggested that will reduce contamination to a minimum, however. Evans (1973*a,b*) has proposed culturing for 24-48 h in serum-free medium, as stimulated macrophages survive well under these conditions, while other cell types do not. Inherent in this approach, however, is the danger of partial or complete loss of macrophage-mediated cytolytic activity (see Section IV.B). Another procedure that can be tried is plating of the macrophages in the enzyme solution used to disaggregate the neoplasm (Evans, 1973*b*). Under these conditions it has been reported that few tumor cells will adhere. Alternatively, monolayers can be exposed to a dilute (0.02-0.1%) solution of trypsin after they have become established (Evans, 1972, 1973*b*). Such treatment enhanced the spreading of macrophages and removed adherent tumor cells. The efficacy of these enzyme-based approaches may vary with the tumor system, however. In our hands, neither plating in an enzyme solution nor exposure of monolayers to a solution of trypsin removed a significant proportion of the cell types that contaminated monolayers established from MSC cell-induced Moloney sarcomas. Our greatest success in reducing contamination in this, and other, tumor systems has come from relying on the capacity tumor macrophages have to adhere rapidly and tightly to surfaces. Advantage can be taken of this property by repetitively (usually two to three times) exposing the bottoms of 16-mm-diameter, flat-bottomed wells to tumor-derived cell suspensions for short periods of time (5-10 min). When the desired population density has been reached by this means, resultant monolayers are washed to remove any remaining nonadherent cells. With this approach, adherent cell populations that are 90–95% macrophages can be obtained routinely. The principal contaminants usually are tumor cells, polymorphonuclear leukocytes (when they are a component of the intact tumor), and T lymphocytes.

Granted that some contamination of tumor-derived monolayers by cells other than macrophages is unavoidable, the nature and extent of contamination should be known and controlled for adequately. For example, the kinds of cells present can be documented by washing, or otherwise removing, adherent cells from wells for differential analysis in stained cytocentrifuge preparations or by fluorescence-microscopic examination. Alternatively, monolayers can be fixed and examined directly by these techniques.

Contaminating cell types can potentially cause either falsely negative or positive results in assays of macrophage-mediated cytotoxicity. As an example of the former, tumor cells that contaminate monolayers may competitively inhibit the killing of added neoplastic target cells. Falsely positive results might originate through stimulation of macrophages by lymphokines (e.g., macrophage-activating factor) produced by adherent lymphocytes. This latter consideration is an especially important one if LPS is being used to probe the level of activation of tumor-derived macrophages, as several groups of investigators (Hibbs *et al.*, 1977; Ruco and Meltzer, 1978; Weinberg *et al.*, 1978) have shown that minute amounts of lymphokine-rich material can act synergistically with LPS to induce cytolytic activity in otherwise noncytotoxic macrophages. This phenomenon is reflected by the data in Table 2.

D. Contamination of Tissue Culture Reagents with LPS

Noncytolytic macrophages in some tumors are exquisitely sensitive to stimulation by LPS (Russell *et al.*, 1977a). Weinberg *et al.* (1978) and Martin *et al.* (1978) have shown that reagents commonly employed in tissue culture may contain detectable amounts of endotoxinlike contaminants. If the final concentrations of such contaminants in assay media are sufficient to trigger the onset of cytolytic activity in primed macrophages, it is a foregone conclusion that falsely positive data will result.

V. CONCLUDING REMARKS

Work completed in the last five years has called attention to the fact that many tumors contain macrophages. This "descriptive" era is now concluding, with investigators in the field beginning to characterize the functions that intratumoral macrophages may have. It is unlikely that all of these will prove to be of benefit to the tumor-bearing animal; indeed, there is increasing evidence for activities that may be detrimental. For example, in some instances mononuclear phagocytes may sustain, rather than inhibit, the proliferation of neoplastic cells *in vivo* (Evans, 1976, 1977, and this volume; Mantovani, 1978), or may interfere with the production of cytotoxic T lymphocytes in tumors (Gillespie *et al.*, 1978; Gillespie and Russell, 1978). Such potentially negative influences need to be considered in any therapeutic regimen directed toward stimulating intratumoral mononuclear phagocytes. A comprehensive understanding of the functions expressed by these cells should make it possible to manipulate them selectively, thereby augmenting activities of benefit to the tumor-bearing host while at the same time suppressing those of a detrimental nature. Thus, the "functional" phase of research being entered most assuredly has clinically relevant, as well as purely academic, meaning.

ACKNOWLEDGMENTS

This work was supported by National Cancer Institute Research Grant CA23686 and Contract CB84271, as well as by American Cancer Society Institutional Grants IN-15S and IN-15T. S.W.R. is the recipient of Research Career Development Award CA00497 from the National Cancer Institute. The authors extend their thanks to Mrs. Patricia Coke for typing the manuscript.

VI. REFERENCES

Abraham, R., and Barbolt, T. A., 1978, Lysosomal enzymes in macrophages of colonic tumors induced in rats by 1,2-dimethylhydrazine dihydrochloride, *Cancer Res.* 38:2763–2767.

Adams, D. O., 1978, Culture supernatants of activated macrophages (AM) selectively lyse neoplastic cells, *J. Reticuloendothel. Soc.* 24:21a.

Alexander, P., and Evans, R., 1971, Endotoxin and double stranded RNA render macrophages cytotoxic, *Nature (London) New Biol.* 232:76–78.

Alexander, P., Eccles, S. A., and Gauci, C. L. L., 1976, The significance of macrophages in human and experimental tumours, *Ann. N.Y. Acad. Sci.* 276:124–133.

Birbeck, M. S. C., and Carter, R. L., 1972, Observations on the ultrastructure of two hamster lymphomas with particular reference to infiltrating macrophages, *Int. J. Cancer* 9:249–257.

Bordin, S., and Young, E. T., 1976, Tumor-associated macrophages as the primary source of lysozyme in the urine of mice bearing GPC-11, a transplantable reticulum cell sarcoma, *J. Natl. Cancer Inst.* 57:827–835.

Bucana, C., Hoyer, L. C., Hobbs, B., Breesman, S., McDaniel, M., and Hanna, M. G., 1976, Morphological evidence for the translocation of lysosomal organelles from cytotoxic macrophages into the cytoplasm of tumor target cells, *Cancer Res.* 36:4444–4458.

Carr, I., and Underwood, J. C. E., 1974, The ultrastructure of the local cellular reaction to neoplasia, *Int. Rev. Cytol.* 37:329–347.

Cohen, D., Gurner, B. W., and Coombs, R. R. A., 1971, A phenomenon resembling opsonic adherence shown by disaggregated cells of the transmissible venereal tumour of the dog, *Br. J. Exp. Pathol.* 52:447–451.

Currie, G. A., 1978, Activated macrophages kill tumour cells by releasing arginase, *Nature (London)* 273:758–759.

Currie, G. A., and Basham, C., 1975, Activated macrophages release a factor which lyses malignant cells but not normal cells, *J. Exp. Med.* 142:1600–1605.

Currie, G. A., and Eccles, S. A., 1976, Serum lysozyme as a marker of host resistance. I. Production by macrophages resident in rat sarcomata, *Br. J. Cancer* 33:51–59.

Doe, W. F., and Henson, P. M., 1978, Macrophage stimulation by bacterial lipopolysaccharides. I. Cytolytic effect on tumor target cells, *J. Exp. Med.* 148:544–556.

Eccles, S. A., and Alexander, P., 1974a, Macrophage content of tumours in relation to metastatic spread and host immune reaction, *Nature (London)* 250:667–669.

Eccles, S. A., and Alexander, P., 1974b, Sequestration of macrophages in growing tumours and its effect on the immunological capacity of the host, *Br. J. Cancer* 30:42–49.

Edelson, R. L., Smith, R. W., Frank, M. M., and Green, I., 1973, Identification of subpopulations of mononuclear cells in cutaneous infiltrates. I. Differentiation between B cells, T cells and histiocytes. *J. Invest. Dermatol.* 61:82–89.

Edelson, R. L., Hearing, V. J., Dellon, A. L., Frank, M., Edelson, E. K., and Green, I., 1975, Differentiation between B cells, T cells and histiocytes in melanocytic lesions: Primary and metastic melanoma and halo and giant pigmented nevi, *Clin. Immunol. Immunopathol.* 4:557–568.

Elston, C. W., 1968, Cellular reaction to choriocarcinoma, *J. Pathol.* 97:261–268.

Evans, R., 1972, Macrophages in syngeneic animal tumours, *Transplantation* 14:468–473.

Evans, R., 1973a, Macrophages and the tumour bearing host, *Br. J. Cancer* 28 (Suppl. I):19–25.

Evans, R., 1973b, Preparation of pure cultures of tumor macrophages, *J. Natl. Cancer Inst.* 50:271–273.

Evans, R., 1975, Macrophage-mediated cytotoxicity: Its possible role in rheumatoid arthritis, *Ann. N.Y. Acad. Sci.* 256:275–287.

Evans, R., 1976, Tumor macrophages in host immunity to malignancies, in: *The Macrophages in Neoplasia* (M. Fink, ed.), pp. 27–42, Academic Press, New York.

Evans, R., 1977, Effect of X-irradiation on host-cell infiltration and growth of a murine fibrosarcoma, *Br. J. Cancer* 35:557–566.

Evans, R., 1979, Host cells in transplanted murine tumors and their possible relevance to tumor growth, *J. Reticuloendothel. Soc.* 26:427–437.

Evans, R., and Alexander, P., 1976, Mechanisms of extracellular killing of nucleated mammalian cells by macrophages, in: *Immunobiology of the Macrophage* (D. S. Nelson, ed.), pp. 535–576, Academic Press, New York.

Evans, R., and Booth, C. G., 1976, Inhibition of [125]IUdR incorporation by supernatants from macrophages and lymphocyte cultures: A cautionary note, Cell. Immunol. 26:120–126.

Ferluga, J., Schorlemmer, H. U., Baptista, L. C., and Allison, A. C., 1978, Production of the complement cleavage product, C3a, by activated macrophages and its tumorolytic effects, Clin. Exp. Immunol. 31:512–517.

Gauci, C. L., 1976, The significance of the macrophage content of human tumours, in: Recent Results in Cancer Research, Vol. 56 (G. Mathé, I. Florentin, and M. -C. Simmler, eds.), pp. 122–130, Springer-Verlag, New York.

Gebhardt, M. C., and Fisher, B., 1979, Further observations on the inhibition of tumor growth by Corynebacterium parvum with cyclophosphamide. IX. Macrophage content of tumors in mice, J. Natl. Cancer Inst. 62:1035–1041.

Gillespie, G. Y., and Russell, S. W., 1978, Development and persistence of cytolytic T lymphocytes in regressing or progressing Moloney sarcomas, Int. J. Cancer 21:94–99.

Gillespie, G. Y., Hansen, C. B., and Russell, S. W., 1978, Resurgence of killing and in vivo protection mediated by lymphocytes cultured from lymph nodes draining Moloney sarcomas, Br. J. Cancer 38:365–374.

Gordon, S., Todd, J., and Cohn, Z. A., 1974, In vitro synthesis and secretion of lysozyme by mononuclear phagocytes, J. Exp. Med. 139:1228–1248.

Haskill, J. S., Proctor, J. W., and Yamamura, Y., 1975a, Host responses within solid tumors. I. Monocytic effector cells within rat sarcomas, J. Natl. Cancer Inst. 54:387–393.

Haskill, J. S., Yamamura, Y., and Radov, L., 1975b, Host responses within solid tumors: Nonthymus-derived specific cytotoxic cells within a murine mammary adenocarcinoma, Int. J. Cancer 16:798–809.

Haskill, J. S., Radov, L. A., Yamamura, Y., Parthenais, E., Korn, J. H., and Ritter, F. L., 1976, Isolation and identification of specific and non-specific effector cells in experimental solid tumors, J. Reticuloendothel. Soc. 20:233–241.

Haskill, S., and Parthenais, E., 1978, Immunologic factors influencing the intratumor localization of ADCC effector cells, J. Immunol. 120:1813–1817.

Hibbs, J. B., 1974, Heterocytolysis by macrophage activated by bacillus Calmette–Guérin: Lysosome exocytosis into tumor cells, Science 184:468–471.

Hibbs, J. B., 1976, The macrophage as a tumoricidal effector cell: A review of in vivo and in vitro studies on the mechanism of the activated macrophage nonspecific cytotoxic reaction, in: The Macrophage in Neoplasia (M. Fink, ed.), pp. 83–111, Academic Press, New York.

Hibbs, J. B., Taintor, R. R., Chapman, H. A., and Weinberg, J. B., 1977, Macrophage tumor killing: Influence of the local environment, Science 197:279–282.

Holden, H. T., Haskill, J. S., Kirchner, H., and Herberman, R. B., 1976, Two functionally distinct anti-tumor effector cells isolated from primary murine sarcoma virus-induced tumors, J. Immunol. 117:440–446.

Humphrey, L. J., Milgrom, F., Tønder, O., and Witebsky, E., 1967, Hemadsorption by murine tumors, Fed. Proc. 26:702.

Keller, R., 1976, Cytostatic and cytocidal effects of activated macrophages, in: Immunobiology of the Macrophage (D. S. Nelson, ed.), pp. 487–508, Academic Press, New York.

Kerbel, R. S., and Davies, A. J. S., 1974, The possible biological significance of Fc receptors on mammalian lymphocytes and tumor cells, Cell 3:105–112.

Kerbel, R. S., Pross, H. F., and Elliott, E. V., 1975, Origin and partial characterization of Fc receptor-bearing cells found within experimental carcinomas and sarcomas, Int. J. Cancer 15:918–932.

Kerbel, R. S., Pross, H. F., and Leibovitz, A., 1977, Analysis of established human carcinoma cell lines for lymphoreticular-associated membrane receptors, Int. J. Cancer 20:673–679.

Korn, J. H., Haskill, J. S., Holden, H. T., Radov, L. A., and Ritter, F. L., 1978a, In situ Fc receptor-bearing cells in two murine tumors. I. Isolation and identification, *J. Natl. Cancer Inst.* 60:1387-1390.

Korn, J. H., Haskill, J. S., Holden, H. T., Rodov, L. A., and Ritter, F. L., 1978*b*, In situ Fc receptor-bearing cells in two murine tumors. II. Role in tumor immunity, *J. Natl. Cancer Inst.* 60:1391-1397.

Lantos, P. L., 1975, Macrophages in brain tumours induced transplacentally by N-ethyl-N-nitrosourcea in rats: An electron-microscope study, *J. Pathol.* 116:107-115.

Lauder, I., Aherne, W., Stewart, J., and Sainsbury, R., 1977, Macrophage infiltration of breast tumours: A prospective study, *J. Clin. Pathol.* 30:563-568.

Long, D. M., Multer, F. K., Greenburg, A. G., Peskin, G. W., Lasser, E. C., Wickham, W. G., and Sharts, C. M., 1978, Tumor imaging with x-rays using macrophage uptake of radiopaque fluorocarbon emulsions, *Surgery* 84:104-112.

Mantovani, A., 1978, Effects on *in vitro* tumor growth of murine macrophages isolated from sarcoma lines differing in immunogenicity and metastasizing capacity, *Int. J. Cancer* 22:741-746.

Martin, F., Martin, M., Jeannin, J. -F., and Lagneau, A., 1978, Rat macrophage-mediated toxicity to cancer cells: Effect of endotoxins and endotoxin inhibitors contained in culture media, *Eur. J. Immunol.* 8:607-611.

Matre, R., 1976, Specificity of Fc_γ receptors in human malignant tissue and normal lymphoreticular tissue, *Scand. J. Immunol.* 5:963-968.

Matre, R., Tønder, O., Thunold, S., and Solhaug, J. H., 1976, Properties of Fc_γ receptors in normal and malignant human tissues, *Scand. J. Immunol.* 5:361-368.

Mendiondo, O., Suit, H., and Fixler, H., 1978, Lysozyme levels and macrophage content of tumor tissue in CH_3 mice bearing fibrosarcoma transplants treated by radiation and *Corynebacterium parvum*, *Int. J. Radiat. Biol.* 4:829-834.

Milgrom, F., Humphrey, L. J., Tønder, O., Yasuda, J., and Witebsky, E., 1968, Antibody-mediated hemadsorption by tumor tissues, *Int. Arch. Allergy Appl. Immunol.* 33:478-492.

Monis, B., and Weinberg, T., 1961, Cytochemical study of esterase activity of human neoplasms and stromal macrophages, *Cancer* 14:369-377.

Moore, K., and Moore, M., 1977*a*, Intra-tumour host cells of transplanted rat neoplasms of different immunogenicity, *Int. J. Cancer* 19:803-813.

Moore, M., and Moore, K., 1977*b*, Kinetics of macrophage infiltration of experimental rat neoplasms, in: *The Macrophage and Cancer* (K. James, B. McBride, and A. Stuart, eds.), pp. 330-339, Department of Surgery, University of Edinburgh Medical School, Scotland.

Morantz, R. A., Wood, G. W., Foster, M., Clark, M., and Gollahon, K., 1979*a*, Macrophages in experimental and human brain tumors. Part 1: Studies of the macrophage content of experimental rat brain tumors of varying immunogenicity, *J. Neurosurg.* 50:298-304.

Morantz, R. A., Wood, G. W., Foster, M., Clark, M., and Gollahon, K., 1979*b*, Macrophages in experimental and human brain tumors. Part 2: Studies of the macrophage content of human brain tumors, *J. Neurosurg.* 50:305-311.

Normann, S. J., and Cornelius, J., 1978, Concurrent depression of tumor macrophage infiltration and systemic inflammation by progressive cancer growth, *Cancer Res.* 38:3453-3459.

Opitz, H. -G., Niethammer, D., Jackson, R. C., Lemke, H., Huget, R., and Flad, H. -D., 1975, Biochemical characterization of a factor released by macrophages, *Cell. Immunol.* 18:70-75.

Owen, J. J. T., and Seeger, R. C., 1973, Immunity to tumours of the murine leukaemia-sarcoma virus complex, *Br. J. Cancer* 28 (Suppl. I):26-34.

Perri, G. C., Cappuccino, J. G., Faulk, M., Mellors, J., and Stock, C. C., 1963, Variations of the content of lysozyme in normal rats and in rats bearing Jensen sarcoma following surgery, *Cancer Res.* 23:431–435.

Pross, H. F., and Kerbel, R. S., 1976, An assessment of intratumor phagocytic and surface marker-bearing cells in a series of autochthonous and early passaged chemically induced murine sarcomas, *J. Natl. Cancer Inst.* 57:1157–1167.

Puccetti, P., and Holden, H. T., 1979, Cytolytic and cytostatic anti-tumor activities of macrophages from mice injected with murine sarcoma virus, *Int. J. Cancer* 23:123–133.

Rosenau, W., and Moon, H. D., 1966, Cellular reactions to methylcholanthrene-induced sarcomas transplanted to isogenic mice, *Lab. Invest.* 15:1212–1224.

Ruco, L. P., and Meltzer, M. S., 1978, Macrophage activation for tumor cytotoxicity: Development of macrophage cytotoxic activity requires completion of a sequence of short-lived intermediary reactions. *J. Immunol.* 121:2035–2042.

Russell, S. W., and McIntosh, A. T., 1977, Macrophages isolated from regressing Moloney sarcomas are more cytotoxic than those recovered from progressing sarcomas, *Nature (London)* 268:69–71.

Russell, S. W., Doe, W. F., and Cochrane, C. G., 1976a, Number of macrophages and distribution of mitotic activity in regressing and progressing Moloney sarcomas, *J. Immunol.* 116:164–166.

Russell, S. W., Doe, W. F., Hoskins, R. G., and Cochrane, C. G., 1976b, Inflammatory cells in solid murine neoplasms. I. Tumor disaggregation and identification of constituent inflammatory cells, *Int. J. Cancer* 18:322–330.

Russell, S. W., Gillespie, G. Y., Hansen, C. B., and Cochrane, C. G., 1976c, Inflammatory cells in solid murine neoplasms. II. Cell types found throughout the course of Moloney sarcoma regression or progression, *Int. J. Cancer* 18:331–338.

Russell, S. W., Doe, W. F., and McIntosh, A. T., 1977a, Functional characterization of a stable, noncytolytic stage of macrophage activation in tumors, *J. Exp. Med.* 146:1511–1520.

Russell, S. W., Gillespie, G. Y., and McIntosh, A. T., 1977b, Inflammatory cells in solid murine neoplasms. III. Cytotoxicity mediated *in vitro* by macrophages recovered from disaggregated regressing Moloney sarcomas, *J. Immunol.* 118:1574–1579.

Schorlemmer, H. U., Hadding, U., Bitter-Suerman, D., and Allison, A. C., 1978, The role of complement cleavage products in killing of tumour cells by macrophages, in: *The Macrophage and Cancer* (K. James, B. McBride, and A. Stuart, eds.), pp. 68–77, Department of Surgery, University of Edinburgh Medical School, Scotland.

Shevach, E. M., Jaffe, E. S., and Green, I., 1973, Receptors for complement and immunoglobulin on human and animal lymphoid cells, *Transplant. Rev.* 16:3–28.

Snodgrass, M. J., and Hanna, M. G., Jr., 1973, Ultrastructural studies of histiocyte-tumor cell interactions during tumor regression after intralesional injection of *Mycobacterium bovis, Cancer Res.* 33:701–716.

Stadecker, M. J., Calderon, J., Karnovsky, M. L., and Unanue, E. R., 1977, Synthesis and release of thymidine by macrophages, *J. Immunol.* 119:1738–1743.

Stewart, C. C., and Beetham, K. L., 1978, Cytocidal activity and proliferative ability of macrophages infiltrating the EMT6 tumor, *Int. J. Cancer* 22:152–159.

Stewart, C. C., Adles, C., and Hibbs, J. B., 1977, Interaction of macrophages with tumor cells, in: *The Reticuloendothelial System in Health and Disease* (H. Friedman and M. R. Escobar, eds.), pp. 423–433, Plenum Press, New York.

Stutman, O., 1975, Delayed tumour appearance and absence of regression in nude mice infected with murine sarcoma virus, *Nature (London)* 253:142–144.

Szymaniec, S., and James, K., 1976, Studies on the Fc receptor bearing cells in a transplanted methylcholanthrene induced mouse fibrosarcoma, *Br. J. Cancer* 33:36–49.

Taniyama, T., and Holden, H. T., 1979, Cytolytic activity of macrophages isolated from primary murine sarcoma virus (MSV)-induced tumors, *Int. J. Cancer* 24:151–160.

Targowski, S. P., Abeyounis, C. J., and Milgrom, F., 1977*a*, Studies on adsorption by tumor tissue of erythrocytes sensitized by IgG antibodies, *Int. Arch. Allergy Appl. Immunol.* 54:262–268.

Targowski, S. P., Abeyounis, C. J., and Milgrom, F., 1977*b*, Effect of murine tumor sera on adsorption of IgG-sensitized erythrocytes by murine sarcoma tissue, *Proc. Soc. Exp. Biol. Med.* 154:365–367.

Tønder, O., and Thunold, S., 1973, Receptors for immunoglobulin Fc in human malignant tissues, *Scand. J. Immunol.* 2:207–215.

Tønder, O., Milgrom, F., and Witebsky, E., 1964, Mixed agglutination with tissue sections, *J. Exp. Med.* 119:265–274.

Tønder, O., Morse, P. A., and Humphrey, L. J., 1974, Similarities of Fc receptors in human malignant and normal lymphoid tissue, *J. Immunol.* 113:1162–1169.

Tønder, O., Humphrey, L. J., and Morse, P. A., 1975, Further observations on Fc receptors in human malignant tissue and normal lymphoid tissue, *Cancer* 35:580–587.

Tønder, O., Krishnan, E. C., Jewell, W. R., Morse, P. A., and Humphrey, L. J., 1976, Tumor Fc receptors and tumor-associated immunoglobulin, *Acta Pathol. Microbiol. Scand.* 84C:105–111.

Turner, D. T. L., Connolly, C. E., Isaacson, P., and Turnbull, A. R., 1978, Receptors for Fc and complement in human breast carcinoma, *Clin. Oncology* 4:87–92.

Underwood, J. C. E., and Carr, I., 1972, The ultrastructure of the lymphoreticular cells in non-lymphoid human neoplasms, *Virchows Arch. B.* 12:39–50.

van Loveren, H., and Den Otter, W., 1974, Macrophages in solid tumors. I. Immunologically specific effector cells, *J. Natl. Cancer Inst.* 53:1057–1060.

Weinberg, J. B., Chapman, H. A., Jr., and Hibbs, J. B., Jr., 1978, Characterization of the effects of endotoxin on macrophage tumor cell killing, *J. Immunol.* 121:72–80.

Wood, G. W., and Gillespie, G. Y., 1975, Studies on the role of macrophages in regulation of growth and metastasis of murine chemically induced fibrosarcomas, *Int. J. Cancer* 16:1022–1029.

Wood, G. W., and Gollahon, K. A., 1977, Detection and quantitation of macrophage infiltration into primary human tumors with the use of cell-surface markers, *J. Natl. Cancer Inst.* 59:1081–1087.

Wood, G. W., and Gollahon, K. A., 1978, T-lymphocytes and macrophages in primary murine fibrosarcomas at different stages in their progression, *Cancer Res.* 38:1857–1865.

Wood, G. W., and Morantz, R. A., 1979, Immunohistologic evaluation of the lymphoreticular infiltrate of human central nervous system tumors, *J. Natl. Cancer Inst.* 62:485–491.

Wood, G. W., Gillespie, G. Y., and Barth, R. F., 1975, Receptor sites for antigen-antibody complexes on cells derived from solid tumors: Detection by means of antibody sensitized sheep erythrocytes labeled with technetium-99m, *J. Immunol.* 114:950–957.

Wood, G. W., Neff, J. R., Gollahon, K. A., and Gourley, W. K., 1978, Macrophages in giant cell tumours of bone, *J. Pathol.* 125:53–58.

Woods, A. E., and Papadimitriou, J. M., 1977, The effect of inflammatory stimuli on the stroma of neoplasms: The involvement of mononuclear phagocytes, *J. Pathol.* 123:163–174.

Woodward, J. G., and Daynes, R. A., 1978, Cell-mediated immune response to syngeneic UV induced tumors. I. The presence of tumor associated macrophages and their possible role in the *in vitro* generation of cytotoxic lymphocytes, *Cell. Immunol.* 41:304–319.

Chapter 7

Mononuclear Cells and IgG Associated with Human Malignant Tissue

O. Tønder, R. Matre, and F. Wesenberg

*Broegelmann Research Laboratory for Microbiology
and Department of Microbiology
The Gade Institute
University of Bergen
Bergen, Norway*

I. INTRODUCTION

Surface receptors have become important as markers for the characterization and classification of mononuclear cells. Most attention has been focused on the receptors for sheep erythrocytes (E receptors), complement (C receptors), and the Fc region of the immunoglobulin molecule (Fc receptors). Rosette techniques are convenient for the detection of these receptors on cells in suspension. By applying the technique of hemadsorption to tissue sections, it is also possible to use the receptors as markers in studies of the topographic distribution of mononuclear cells in normal lymphoid organs, as well as in the characterization of neoplastic and inflammatory mononuclear cell infiltrates (Shevach *et al.*, 1973; Jaffe *et al.*, 1975; Stingl *et al.*, 1977; Berard *et al.*, 1978; Bjerke *et al.*, 1978).

Human nonlymphoid malignant tissues of various histopathological types (Tønder *et al.*, 1974) and carcinomas and sarcomas in animals (Milgrom *et al.*, 1968; Cohen *et al.*, 1971; Kerbel *et al.*, 1975) possess Fc_γ receptors (FcR). The FcR has been demonstrated using IgG-sensitized erythrocytes (EA), soluble antigen-antibody complexes, or aggregated IgG.

It is well established that malignant tissues contain varying amounts of infiltrating host cells known to have Fc receptors (Underwood, 1974; Kerbel *et al.*, 1975; Roubin *et al.*, 1975; Evans, 1976; Wood and Gollahon, 1977). These host cells could account for all the FcR activity. But since the malignant

167

tissues show very high activity, even exceeding that in normal lymphoid tissues, it is natural to speculate whether some of the malignant cells may possess FcR (Tφnder and Thunold, 1973; Kerbel and Pross, 1976). We are therefore continuously faced with the problem of identifying the FcR-positive cells in malignant tissues, irrespective of whether cell suspensions or tissue sections are used. Isolation and characterization of the tumor-associated immunoglobulins represent another challenge (Witz, 1977). The biological significance of these immunoglobulins is unclear. They can be bound to tumor cells or to infiltrating host cells, but the mechanisms of binding have not been clarified (Witz, 1977).

We have studied approximately 500 human malignant tumors of various histopathological types. In this communication we will report some of the results obtained on the relation of FcR to host or tumor cells and to tumor-associated IgG.

II. MONONUCLEAR CELL MARKERS IN SOLID TUMORS

The main techniques of studying mononuclear cells in tumor tissues have been based on liberating the cells by mechanical disintegration and/or enzymatic treatment (Russell *et al.*, 1976), followed by characterization using surface markers and functional tests. These techniques have certain disadvantages: it is difficult to liberate cells from fibrous tissues, the various enzymes used can affect the receptors, and no information on the topographic distribution is obtained. Much effort has therefore been put into developing techniques that allow the use of unfixed, frozen tissue sections as the substrate for studying cells *in situ*.

A. Detection Using Tissue Sections

Two substantially different procedures have been developed; we have called one an "open" technique and the other a "closed chamber" technique. Using the open technique, the indicator cells are layered on the sections, which are washed after incubation to remove the unbound indicator cells (Silveira *et al.*, 1972; Brubaker and Whiteside, 1977). Using the closed-chamber technique, the indicator cells are applied to the sections in small closed chambers, and unattached cells detach by gravity (Tφnder *et al.*, 1974; Christensen *et al.*, 1978). The last procedure can also be used to study weak bonds, e.g., the attachment of sheep erythrocytes to human T lymphocytes or the attachment of EA to B lymphocytes. Until recently, many authors have claimed that these interactions could not be demonstrated using tissue sections. Since the procedure is essential in our studies, a brief outline of the technique is given in Fig. 1.

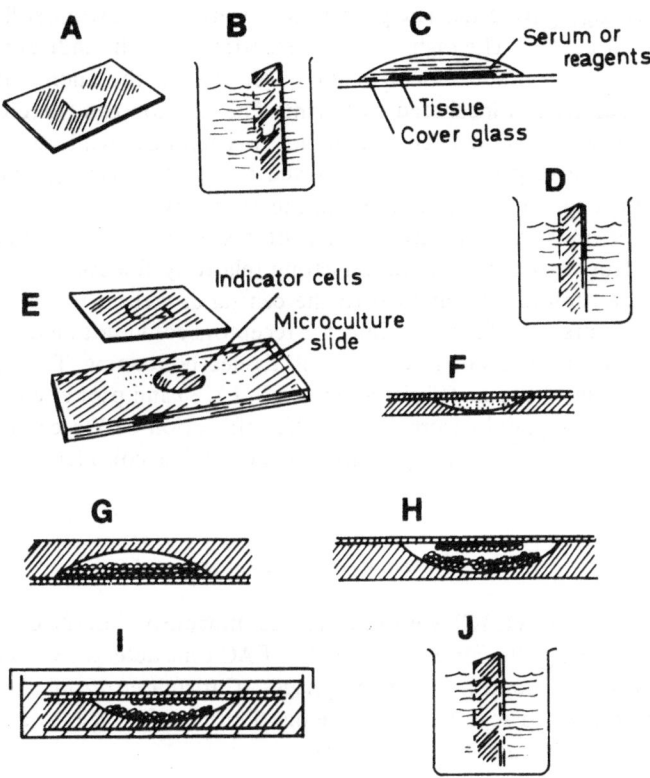

Figure 1. Illustration of the procedure of hemadsorption to tissue sections. Cryosections 6–8 μm thick are placed on cover glasses (A). The sections can be washed or treated with fixatives (B), incubated with various reagents (C), and washed (D) before testing. The concavity in microculture slides (hanging drop slides) is filled with a 1% suspension of the indicator cells (E). The cover glass with the tissue section is pressed into place on to the slide with the section in the center of the concavity (F). The slide is then inverted to allow the indicator cells to settle on to the tissue section (G). The slides are incubated at a suitable temperature and for a suitable length of time, dependent on the membrane markers being studied. The slides are then turned over and left at a suitable temperature so that the indicator cells detach from the cover glass and from nonreactive tissue and settle into the concavity of the microculture slide (H). The degree of hemadsorption is recorded microscopically. The sections can be fixed (I) and stained for histological studies (J). (From Tønder and Krogh, 1980.)

1. Presence of E Receptors

Sheep erythrocytes were treated with the sulfhydryl reagent 2-aminoethyl-isothiouronium bromide (AET) according to a procedure described by Kaplan and Clark (1974). The tissue sections were incubated at 4°C overnight with E_{AET} suspended in phosphate-buffered saline (PBS) containing 25% heat-inactivated fetal calf serum. The slides were then turned over and left at 4°C to allow the unattached E_{AET} to settle. The preparations were studied while still cold, and they were fixed at $4°C$. The high serum concentration in the indicator cell suspension can cause firm attachment of the cover glass to the microculture slide when the preparation is incubated overnight. The fixation can therefore be inadequate because of a slow exchange of fluids. Therefore, while submerged in the fixative, the cover glass if carefully moved to one side, leaving a small opening between the edge of the cover glass and the concavity.

Sections of most tumors, irrespective of histological type, showed only scanty and diffuse adsorption of E, indicating relatively few E-receptor-positive cells within the tumors. This applied to the central as well as to the peripheral parts of the tumors. The failure to detect E receptors could not be due to inadequate technique, since sections of control tissues containing T lymphocytes [T areas in lymphoid organs (Christensen et al., 1978) and psoriatic skin lesions (Bjerke et al., 1978)], did adsorb E_{AET}. The infiltration of E-receptor-positive cells around the tumors in nonlymphoid tissues varied considerably, but was mostly low.

2. Presence of C Receptors

The indicator cells (EAC) were prepared as previously described (Matre and Tønder, 1976). Using the control tissues, the EAC cells detected C receptors on B lymphocytes, monocytes, and macrophages (Christensen et al., 1978). The tumor tissues showed a scanty and diffuse distribution of C receptors, very similar to the patterns obtained for E receptors.

3. Presence of Fc Receptors

The indicator cells (EA) were prepared by sensitizing E with rabbit IgG antibodies (A) in various amounts, expressed as agglutinating units. One agglutinating unit is defined as the amount of the highest dilution of antiserum that agglutinates an equal amount of a 1% suspension of E. The sections were incubated with EA for 30 min at room temperature. The hemadsorption was graded as earlier (Tønder et al., 1974). Approximately 95% of the tumors adsorbed EA, on an average equal to the adsorption observed using normal human liver and spleen. The occurrence of Fc receptors in malignant tissues was marked compared to the E and C receptors.

B. Detection Using Cell Suspensions

Surgically removed tumors were carefully cleared of necrotic tissue, fat, and blood. The tissue was then minced with iris scissors, suspended in PBS, and treated with collagenase and DNase (Russell et al., 1976). Some types of tumors,

Table I. E, Fc, and C Receptors in Malignant Human Tissues. Relation between Receptor Activities on Cells in Suspension and in Tissue Sections, Detected Using E, EA, and EAC Indicator Cells

Tissue		Percent rosetting cells in 3 cell suspensions			Reactivity in 3 tissue sections		
No.	Type	E	EA	EAC	E	EA	EAC
	Normal spleen	36	37	45	++	++	+++
	Carcinoma of						
1	Kidney	2	25	10	–	++	+
2	Stomach	17	31	12	+	+	+
3	Thyroid	7	38	3	–	+	+
4	Ovary	2	12	7	–	+++	+
5	Stomach	7	14	7	+	+++	+

especially breast carcinomas, were impossible to disintegrate into single cells. The cell suspensions were adjusted to 4×10^6 cells/ml and were tested as previously described (Matre *et al.*, 1977) for rosette-forming cells, using the indicator cells described for the tissue section technique. Mononuclear cells from the peripheral blood of the same patient were also usually tested.

The amount of rosette-forming cells varied considerably from tumor to tumor (Table I). Generally, cell suspensions of tumor tissue contained few cells carrying E or C receptors, as expected from the results obtained with tissue sections.

However, there was no relation between the amount of FcR-bearing cells in the suspensions and the strength of FcR reaction in tissue sections. Three patterns emerged: (1) tumor tissue behaved much as normal spleen tissue (No. 1), (2) the content of FcR-positive single cells was higher than expected from the reaction with tissue sections (Nos. 2 and 3), and (3) the content of FcR-positive single cells was lower than expected (Nos. 4 and 5). This variation could be due to the difficulties present in liberating cells from the various tissues.

III. LOCALIZATION OF Fc RECEPTORS IN SOLID TUMORS

The low amounts of FcR-positive cells in suspensions of some of the tumors were unexpected. One explanation might be that the amount of intracellular FcR is high, which agrees with previous findings (Tønder *et al.*, 1978). This localization would result in stronger FcR activity when tissue sections were used. However, an intercellular FcR would give similar results. Investigations on the localization of the FcR have therefore been extended.

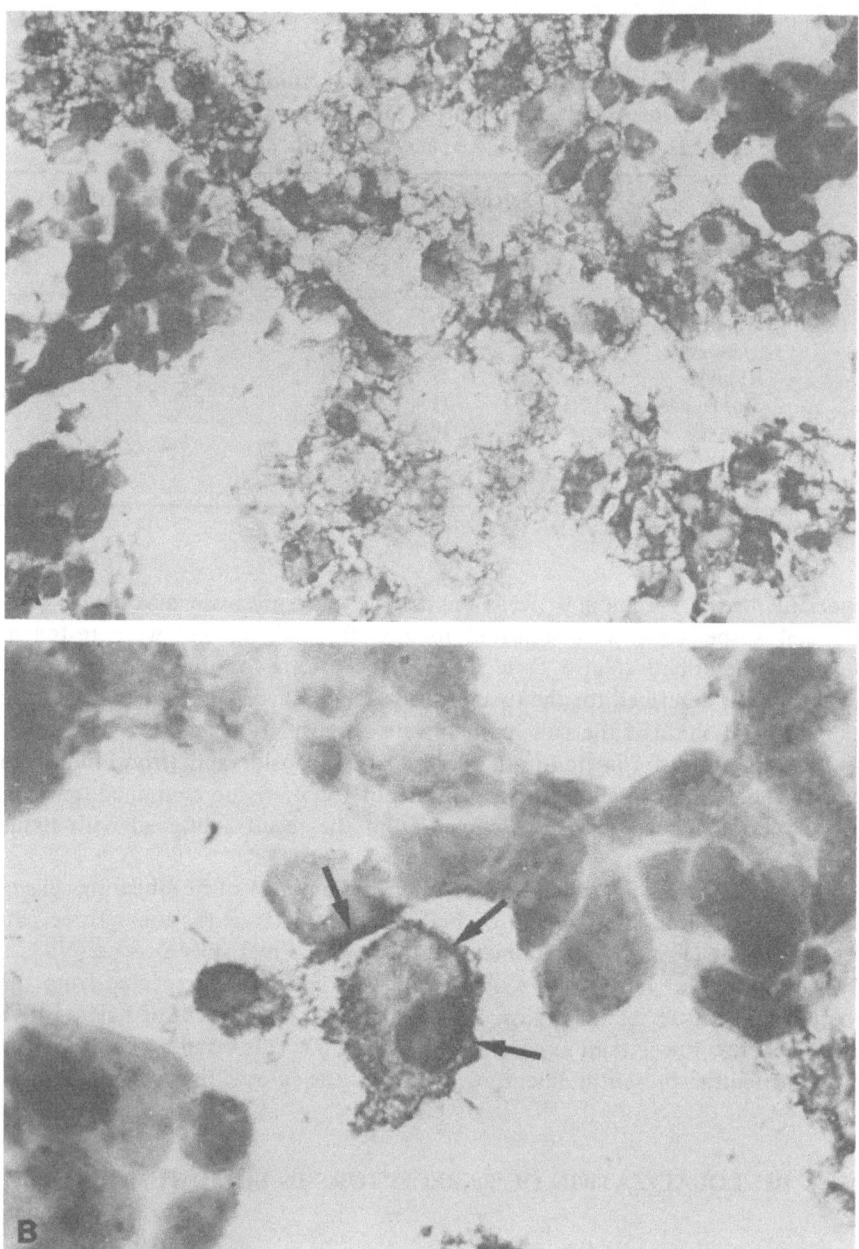

Figure 2. Sections of carcinoma of the ovary tested for Fc receptors using complexes of horseradish peroxidase (HRP)–anti-HRP. (A) Receptor activity revealed in most of the central area, with nonreactive clusters of cells to the left and upper right (×448). (B) Receptor activity on a probable tumor cell (one arrow) and on a probable macrophage (two arrows) (×1120).

Immune complexes of horseradish peroxidase (HRP)–anti-HRP were prepared at various ratios of antigen to antibody (Matre and Haugen, 1978). Sections were incubated with the complexes in a moist chamber at room temperature for 30 min and washed in PBS. After the peroxidase activity had occurred, the sections were counterstained. Control sections were incubated with HRP solution only, or with immune complexes prepared of HRP and $F(ab')_2$ fragments of IgG anti-HRP. The dark-brown reaction products were easily traced with a light microscope.

So far, 10 tumors have been tested using this technique. Characteristic patterns obtained with a carcinoma of the ovary are shown in Fig. 2. Apparently the complexes were localized intercellularly to the membranes of the mononuclear cells and possibly also to some of the malignant cells. Immune complexes prepared at equivalence or slight antigen excess blocked the reaction with the labeled complexes.

The intercellular localization raised the possibility that FcR in malignant tissue might be free or bound to IgG complexes.

IV. IMMUNOGLOBULINS IN SOLID TUMORS

Extract and eluates of tissues were prepared as described previously (Wesenberg and Tønder, 1978). In brief, the tissue was gently minced with scissors and homogenized. The homogenate was centrifuged, and the supernatant beneath the lipid layer was collected (extract). The sediment was resuspended, placed between glass fiber filters and glass wool in a short glass column, and washed at 4°C in a continuous upward flow of PBS. The procedure was monitored by the optical density of the effluent. Elution was performed by submerging the column in a water bath at 37, 45, and 56°C successively. Immunoglobulins in the eluates were quantified. Agglutinins to rabbit erythrocytes served as "marker" antibodies for nonspecifically bound IgG.

Eluates of the tumors contained higher amounts of IgG than eluates of normal tissue. This is consistent with other reports (for review, see Witz, 1977). IgA was present in small quantities in eluates from some of the tumors, while IgM and IgD were not detected in any.

The marker antibodies were detected in eluates of some of the tumors (Wesenberg and Tønder, 1978), indicating that at least part of the IgG is nonspecifically bound. Since most of the IgG eluted at 56°C, the binding is probably strong.

It has not been possible to determine to which cells the IgG is bound. It is more likely bound to the tumor cells than to the infiltrating host cells. The finding that eluates from normal human liver and spleen contained no detectable IgG is of special interest in this regard.

V. RELATION BETWEEN Fc RECEPTORS AND IgG

A series of experiments have been performed to study the relationship between FcR and IgG in tissue. Since homogenized tissue is the most utilized material for studies of bound Ig, the effect of homogenization on FcR activity was studied. Homogenization of the tissue for more than 2 min partly abolished the FcR activity, irrespective of temperature. Tissues were therefore homogenized for 1 min only, and then eluted at 37, 45, and 56°C. The FcR activity was not altered after washing and elution of the tissue at 37 and 45°C, but was abolished after 56°C.

So far, FcR activity has not been traced in the eluates, indicating that the FcR were probably destroyed at 56°C.

In one series of experiments, we found an inverse relationship between the amount of IgG on cells in suspension (RIA technique) and the FcR activity in the corresponding tissue sections in 7 out of 10 tumors (Tφnder *et al.*, 1976). In another series using heat elution, 3 out of 13 tumors showed such a relationship (Wesenberg, 1978). These results indicate that part of the IgG may be bound to FcR in the tumors.

VI. CONCLUDING REMARKS

The results discussed indicate that (1) the infiltration by mononuclear cells within tumors is generally low, (2) the infiltrating mononuclear cells have lost some of their membrane receptors, or (3) the receptors on the infiltrating mononuclear cells are blocked. Additional results support the first possibility, e.g., cells with phagocytic, peroxidase, and esterase activity were few in both tissue sections and cell suspensions (<10%).

The regularity with which FcR are detected in tumor tissue is noteworthy. We have indications that FcR can be found intracellularly, on cell membranes and in the intercellular space. As a consequence, soluble antigen–antibody complexes may be bound in at least three different locations in tumors. Such bindings can account for the nonspecifically bound IgG, and even for the specifically bound IgG if complexes are shedded from the tumor cells.

There is still a lot of uncertainty concerning the origin of FcR in solid human tumors. Mononuclear cells may be the only source, but malignant cells cannot be overlooked. FcR may be produced by the malignant cell itself, or it may be adsorbed from the shedded FcR of infiltrating host cells (Lee and Paraskevas, 1978). In the clarification of these questions, we are faced with the technical problems in liberating, identifying, and enumerating the cells in solid tumors. The topographic distribution of all types of cells is also a central question.

ACKNOWLEDGMENTS

The experimental work described has been supported in part by a grant to R. M. from the Norwegian Cancer Society. F. W. is a fellow of the Norwegian Research Council for Science and the Humanities (C. 01.04-4).

VII. REFERENCES

Berard, C. W., Jaffe, E. S., Braylan, R. C., Mann, R. B., and Nanba, K., 1978, Immunologic aspects and pathology of the malignant lymphomas, *Cancer* 42:911.

Bjerke, J. R., Krogh, H.-K., and Matre, R., 1978, Characterization of mononuclear cell infiltrates in psoriatic lesions, *J. Invest. Dermatol.* 71:340.

Brubaker, D. B., and Whiteside, T. L., 1977, Localization of human T lymphocytes in tissue sections by a rosetting technique, *Am. J. Pathol.* 88:323.

Christensen, B. E., Jønsson, V., Matre, R., and Tønder, O., 1978, Traffic of T and B lymphocytes in the normal spleen, *Scand. J. Haematol.* 20:246.

Cohen, D., Gurner, B. W., and Coombs, R. R. A., 1971, A phenomenon resembling opsonic adherence shown by disaggregated cells of the transmissible venereal tumour of the dog, *Br. J. Exp. Pathol.* 52:447.

Evans, R., 1976, Tumor macrophages in host immunity to malignancies, in: *The Macrophage in Neoplasia* (M. Fink, ed.), pp. 27–42, Academic Press, New York.

Jaffe, E. S., Shevach, E. M., Sussman, E. H., Frank, M., Green, I., and Berard, C. W., 1975, Membrane receptor sites for the identification of lymphoreticular cells in benign and malignant conditions, *Br. J. Cancer* 31:107.

Kaplan, M. E., and Clark, C., 1974, An improved rosetting assay for detection of human T lymphocytes, *J. Immunol. Methods* 5:131.

Kerbel, R. S., and Pross, H. F., 1976, Fc receptor-bearing cells as a reliable marker for quantitation of host lymphoreticular infiltration of progressively growing solid tumors, *Int. J. Cancer* 18:432.

Kerbel, R. S., Pross, H. F., and Elliot, E. V., 1975, Origin and partial characterization of Fc receptor-bearing cells found within experimental carcinomas and sarcomas, *Int. J. Cancer* 15:918.

Lee, S.-T., and Paraskevas, F., 1978, Macrophage–T cell interactions. I. The uptake by T cells of Fc receptors released from macrophages, *Cell. Immunol.* 40:141.

Matre, R., and Haugen, Aa., 1978, The placental Fc_γ receptors studied using immune complexes of peroxidase, *Scand. J. Immunol.* 8:187.

Matre, R., and Tønder, O., 1976, Complement receptors in human renal glomeruli, *Scand. J. Immunol.* 5:917.

Matre, R., Talstad, I., and Haugen, Aa., 1977, Surface markers in non-phagocytic hairy cell leukemia, *Acta Pathol. Microbiol. Scand. Sect. C* 85:406.

Milgrom, F., Humphrey, L. J., Tønder, O., Yasuda, J., and Witebsky, E., 1968, Antibody-mediated hemadsorption by tumor tissues, *Int. Arch. Allergy Appl. Immunol.* 33:478.

Roubin, R., Césarini, J.-P., Fridman, W. H., Pavie-Fischer, J., and Peter, H. H., 1975, Characterization of the mononuclear cell infiltrate in human malignant melanoma, *Int. J. Cancer* 16:61.

Russell, S. W., Doe, W. F., Hoskins, R. G., and Cochrane, C. G., 1976, Inflammatory cells in solid murine neoplasms. I. Tumor disaggregation and identification of constituent inflammatory cells, *Int. J. Cancer* **18**:322.

Shevach, E. M., Jaffe, E. S., and Green, I., 1973, Receptors for complement and immunoglobulin on human animal lymphoid cells, *Transplant. Rev.* **16**:3.

Silveira, N. P. A., Mendes, N. F., and Tolnai, M. E. A., 1972, Tissue localization of two populations of human lymphocytes distinguished by membrane receptors, *J. Immunol.* **108**:1456.

Stingl, G., Wolff, K., Diem, E., Baumgartner, G., and Knapp, W., 1977, *In situ* identification of lymphoreticular cells in benign and malignant infiltrates by membrane receptor sites, *J. Invest. Dermatol.* **69**:231.

Tønder, O., and Krogh, H. K., 1980, Hemadsorption techniques for the *in situ* characterization of mononuclear cells in tissue, in: *Autoimmunity in Psoriasis,* (E. H. Beutner, S. Jablonska, and T. P. Chorzelski, eds.), Yearbook Medical Publishers, Chicago, in press.

Tønder, O., and Thunold, S., 1973, Receptors for immunoglobulin Fc in human malignant tissues, *Scand. J. Immunol.* **2**:207.

Tønder, O., Morse, P. A., Jr., and Humphrey, L. J., 1974, Similarities of Fc receptors in human malignant tissue and normal lymphoid tissue, *J. Immunol.* **113**:1162.

Tønder, O., Krishnan, E. C., Jewell, W. R., Morse, P. A., Jr., and Humphrey, L. J., 1976, Tumor Fc receptors and tumor-associated immunoglobulins, *Acta Pathol. Microbiol. Scand. Sect. C* **84**:105.

Tønder, O., Krishnan, E. C., Morse, P. A., Jr., Jewell, W. R., and Humphrey, L. J., 1978, Localization of Fc receptors in human and rat malignant tissues, *Acta Pathol. Microbiol. Scand. Sect. C* **86**:173.

Underwood, J. C. E., 1974, Lymphoreticular infiltration in human tumours: Prognostic and biological implications: A review, *Br. J. Cancer* **30**:538.

Wesenberg, F., 1978, Fc_γ receptors and IgG associated with human malignant tumours, *Acta Pathol. Microbiol. Scand. Sect. C* **86**:259.

Wesenberg, F., and Tønder, O., 1978, Evidence for nonspecifically bound IgG in human tumours, *Acta Pathol. Microbiol. Scand. Sect. C* **86**:251.

Witz, I. P., 1977, Tumor-bound immunoglobulins: *In situ* expressions of humoral immunity, *Adv. Cancer Res.* **25**:95.

Wood, G., and Gollahon, K. A., 1977, Detection and quantitation of macrophage infiltration into primary human tumors with the use of cell-surface markers, *J. Natl. Cancer Inst.* **59**:1081.

Chapter 8

Evidence for Membrane-Bound Antibodies Directed against Antigens Expressed on Tumors

S. von Kleist

Institute of Tumor Immunology
University of Freiburg
Freiburg im Breisgau, Germany

M. King and C. Huet

Institut de Recherches Scientifiques sur le Cancer
Villejuif, France.

I. ANTIGENS ASSOCIATED WITH HUMAN CANCER TISSUE

The possible existence in the cancer patient of an effective defense mechanism against his malignancy is of high clinical interest and has prompted numerous investigations yielding both positive and negative results (for reviews, see Baldwin *et al.*, 1973; Sjögren, 1976; Prehn, 1976; Witz, 1977).

The importance of cellular immunity has been stressed in a positive sense—mostly in experimental animal systems—for the rejection of allografts and tumor transplants (Kahan, 1967; Churchill *et al.*, 1968; Thomson and Alexander, 1973; Haskill *et al.*, 1976; Saksela *et al.*, 1975; Lamon *et al.*, 1975; Cohen *et al.*, 1973; Haskill and Fett, 1976). Delayed hypersensitivity reactions have provided evidence that similar mechanisms may prevail in humans (Herberman and Oren, 1969; J. Hellström *et al.*, 1970, 1971a; Oren and Herberman, 1971; Hollinshead *et al.*, 1972; Mavligit *et al.*, 1973; Bull *et al.*, 1973; Herberman, 1974; Baldwin and Price, 1976; Bernstein *et al.*, 1976).

Humoral tumor immunity, usually considered of lesser importance, or sometimes even affecting adversely the tumor-bearing host, has been investigated less extensively in man, and reports are still scarce on the implicated antigens. The antigens in question have not been isolated; hence their physicochemical nature is unknown, and in most cases their presence was shown only by indirect methods such as immunfluorescence or *in vitro* cytotoxicity or migration-inhibition tests (J. B. Graham and Graham, 1955; Itoh and Southam, 1964; Hodkinson and Taylor, 1969; Muna *et al.*, 1969; Eilber and Morton, 1970; Edynak *et al.*, 1970; Fossati *et al.*, 1971; K. E. Hellström and Hellström, 1974; Schultz *et al.*, 1975).

However, those antigens that have been isolated and characterized from human tumors have either been found to be not autoantigenic or their autoantigenicity is still a matter of controversy (Gold, 1967; Collatz *et al.*, 1971; Lo Gerfo *et al.*, 1972; Gold *et al.*, 1972; Sorokin *et al.*, 1973).

Practically all the antigens isolated so far from human tumors fall into the category of carcinofetal antigens (Table I). These are substances present in high quantities in both carcinomas and homologous fetal tissues and virtually absent from normal tissues or present only in trace amounts.

Among these antigens the carcinoembryonic antigen (CEA) of Gold and Freedmann (1965) has been thoroughly investigated concerning its molecular composition, immunological role, and clinical role. This is the main of three antigens that we have previously isolated from human colonic tumors.

The other antigens are the nonspecific crossreacting antigen (NCA) (von Kleist *et al.*, 1972), also known as normal-glycoprotein (NGP) (Mach *et al.*, 1972) and by several other synonyms, and the membrane-associated tissular autoantigen (MTA) (von Kleist *et al.*, 1974).

NCA is the principal of several different antigens giving a strong cross-reaction with CEA (von Kleist and Burtin, 1979) (Table II). It is present not only in colonic tumors but also in appreciable amounts in several normal tissues. Hence it is neither cancer- nor organ-specific, which explains its name. NCA is a tenacious contaminant during CEA purification because the physicochemical properties of both molecules are strikingly similar.

However, CEA and NCA have, in addition to a cross-reacting moiety, differ-

Table I. Carcinofetal Antigens in Man[a]

Abbreviation	Full name
AFP	α-Fetoprotein
CEA	Carcinoembryonic antigen
FSA	Fetal sulfoglycoprotein antigen
α2H-Fe	α-2-Hepatic ferro globulin
MTA	Membrane-associated tissular autoantigen
BOFA	β-Oncofetal antigen

[a]From von Kleist and Burtin, 1977.

Table II. Antigens Cross-Reacting with CEA[a]

Name	Abbreviation
Nonspecific cross-reacting antigen	NCA
Normal glycoprotein	NGP
Fetal sulfoglycoprotein antigen	FSA
CEA-associated protein	CEX
Colonic carcinoembryonic antigen 2	CCEA-2
Colonic carcinoma antigen III	CCA-III
Breast cancer glycoprotein	BCGP
Beta external protein	βE
Second nonspecific cross-reacting antigen	NCA-2
Biliary glycoprotein II	BGPII
Gastric CEA-like antigen	–

[a]From von Kleist and Burtin, 1977.

ent specific antigenic determinants on their molecules. This was proven by absorption experiments using radioimmunoassays. Like CEA, NCA circulates also in the sera of cancer patients; however, the extent of its elevation in the serum of cancer patients is only moderate and not significantly different from the circulating levels of this antigen in nonmalignant diseases (von Kleist et al., 1977).

MTA, the third antigen, which like the two preceding ones is also perchlorosoluble, has no immunological relationship with CEA or NCA. It is of α-globulin electrophoretic mobility, compared to the β-globulin mobility of CEA and NCA. It is present in appreciable amounts in fetal and in normal adult colonic mucosa and in colonic and many other solid tumors. By immunofluorescence we showed that MTA, CEA, and NCA are membrane-associated antigens. (von Kleist et al., 1975).

Circulating antibodies directed against only MTA and CEA have been described so far (Gold et al., 1972; Constanza et al., 1973; von Kleist et al., 1974). Recently we have identified in patients' sera antibodies directed also against NCA (von Kleist et al., 1978), and we have evidence that these antibodies have the ability to fix specifically onto the tumor cell membrane, as shall be outlined in the present paper.

II. EXPERIMENTAL

Two hundred and ten human sera were collected from three main groups of patients: (1) cancer patients who all had histologically confirmed solid carcinomas of different tissue origin, including the colon, the lung, and various other organ sites; (2) patients with nonmalignant diseases, all hospitalized for known illnesses;

and (3) professional blood donors–apparently healthy, but clinically uncontrolled, subjects, who tested negative for the Australia antigen. The latter two groups comprised the controls. All sera were screened for the presence of antibodies by the passive hemagglutination technique, as previously described in detail (Collatz *et al.*, 1971).

In order to investigate whether the antibodies detectable by passive hemagglutination were able to fix to the membrane of tumor cells, the indirect immunofluorescence technique was employed (Coons *et al.*, 1955). Cultured HT29 cells, derived from a human colonic tumor and graciously furnished by Dr. J. Føgh (Sloan-Kettering Institute), were used as targets for antibodies present in artificially prepared antisera directed against the purified colonic tumor antigens and in the patients' sera.

Both the antisera and the purified antigens were prepared according to known and repeatedly published procedures (von Kleist *et al.*, 1972). The unfixed living HT29 cells were first incubated with antisera directed against CEA, NCA, and MTA in order to establish that these main antigens are still expressed on the tumor cell membrane. The cell line was also tested for its blood group antigens and for the expression of Fc receptors. The technical details of this study and the results have been described elsewhere (von Kleist *et al.*, 1975).

All the antisera tested gave strong, reproducible fluorescence, indicating the presence of CEA, MTA, and NCA on the HT29 tumor cell surface. Among the sera against the principal ABO blood group substances, only the antiblood group A serum gave a positive reaction, confirming the tumor donor's known blood group.

Incubation of the HT29 cells with heat-aggregated human γ-globulins did not yield fluorescence, indicating the absence of Fc receptors on these cells. A bright fluorescence was observed when the same solution of aggregates was applied to a preparation of peripheral white blood cells.

In order to test the ability of the antibodies to fix onto the tumor cell membrane *in vivo*, membrane-rich fractions of surgically removed tumors were prepared by ultracentrifugation steps. The 105,000g pellets, considered as membrane-enriched fractions, were subjected to elution by an acid buffer (HCl-glycine, pH 2.8), and the eluates were tested for their antibody content by the passive hemagglutination technique, following the technique of Avrameas *et al.* (1969), and by the Ouchterlony double diffusion method. The eluted antibodies were tested for their ability to attach to the tumor cell membrane by the indirect immunofluorescence technique.

Both tumor cell membranes and membranes from the adjacent tissue of comparative wet weights and obtained by the same technique were eluted in parallel, and the eluates were tested for antibody activity as described above.

The incubated HT29 cells were examined by both light and electronmicroscopy, and photomicroscopy was carried out with a Leitz–Orthostat fluorescence microscope equipped with an automatic camera Orthomat (Leitz, Wetzlar,

Germany); colored slides were taken on Fuji films. A Siemens EM 102 electron microscope was used for micrographs.

The specificity of the reaction was controlled for by using patients' sera negative in passive hemagglutination assays and by utilizing antisera absorbed with tissue extracts as well as with purified antigens.

A. Passive Hemagglutination

When the patients' sera were tested in the passive hemagglutination technique, positive titers were observed in all groups. However, the frequency and the titers varied with the sensitizing extracts employed: Erythrocytes coated with perchloricacid (PCA) extracts agglutinated less frequently and at lower titers than erythrocytes coated with saline extracts; i.e., the purer the extract, the less frequent were high antibody titers. When purified CEA was employed as sensitizing antigen, titers became naught. When NCA was used as the sensitizing antigen in the passive hemagglutination technique, positive titers were observed in all groups of patients tested. However, in the two control groups the titers were always below 1/64. High titers were observed exclusively in sera from patients suffering from malignant diseases. In the cancer group the titers spread from negative to over 1/64 (Fig. 1).

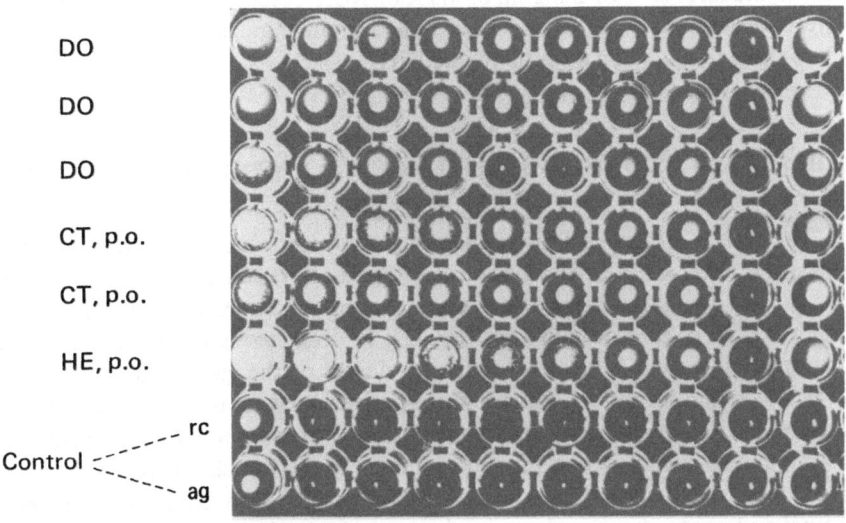

Figure 1. Passive hemagglutination (HA) titers of three blood donors (DO), two colonic cancer patients (CT), and one hepatoma patient (HE) being tested postoperatively (p.o.). The first dilution of the sera was 1/2. Titers were (from top to bottom) neg., neg., 1/2, 1/16, 1/8, 1/128. (rc) Red cells, (ag) antigen.

B. Immunofluorescence

The wide range of circulating antibody titers in the cancer patients suggested that the tumor stage or the tumor mass might influence the expression of systemic humoral antitumor immunity by absorbing antibodies onto the tumor cell membrane, hence rendering them no longer demonstrable in the circulation. In order to test this possibility we incubated the HT 29 cells with positive patients' sera of blood group A, (because, as mentioned above, we found that the HT 29 cells expressed blood group A substance on their surface). Of the 23 sera thus tested in the immunofluorescence technique, 11 (48%) gave concordant results, being positive in both the passive hemagglutination and in the immunofluorescence assays or negative in both techniques. In 52%, the results were discordant insofar as all of these sera had positive titers in the hemagglutination technique (though none greater than 1/64), while no fluorescence was seen when tested on the target cells. These antibodies, although able to agglutinate antigen-coated erythrocytes, were unable to attach specifically to the tumor cell membranes of the HT 29 cell line.

Absorption experiments done on eight positive sera showed that these antibodies were apparently directed against an antigen present in normal colon mucosa. The serological reactivity assayed by the two techniques, hemmagglutination as well as fluorescence, could be abolished by absorbing the sera with either 5 mg of PCA extract of colonic tumors, 4 mg of PCA extract of normal colonic mucosa, or 1 or 2 mg/ml of MTA or NCA, respectively. These quantities were excess amounts. We did not seek to determine minimal quantities necessary for complete absorption of antibody activity.

III. ANALYSIS OF SURGICAL TUMOR CELL MEMBRANE ELUATES

The results presented above indicated that sera of cancer patients apparently contained antibodies directed against antigens expressed at the membrane of colonic tumor cells and that the antibodies were able to bind specifically to the membrane of cultured tumor cells (Fig. 2). In order to show whether the same phenomenon occurs *in vivo* we analyzed eluates of the membrane fractions of surgically removed tumors. Eluates were first analyzed for their immunoglobulin content by the Ouchterlony technique. In all eluates we found large quantities of IgG, and to a lesser extent immunoglobulins of the IgA class (Fig. 3).

The antibody activity of the eluate immunoglobulins obtained from both normal and cancerous tissues was demonstrated by both the immunofluorescence and hemmagglutination techniques. About half of the tested eluates had hemagglutination titers against sheep red blood cells coated with purified NCA, and stained HT 29 cells in immunofluorescence (Table III).

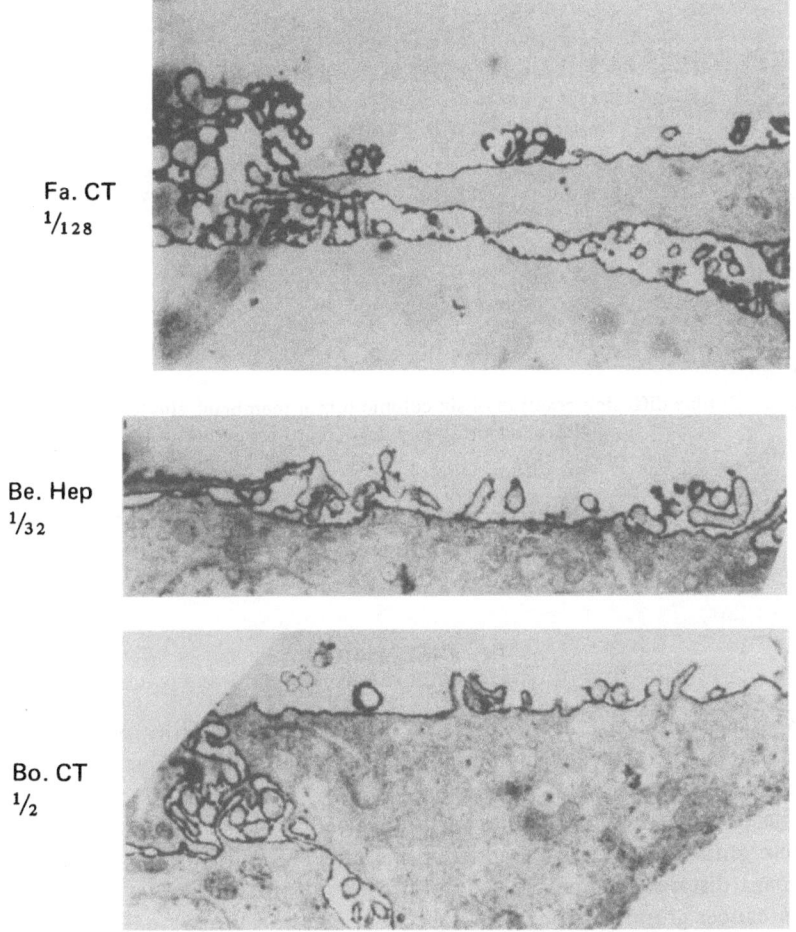

Fa. CT
1/128

Be. Hep
1/32

Bo. CT
1/2

Figure 2. Electron micrograph of HT 29 cells incubated with HA-positive patients' sera and stained by the immune peroxydase method. CT, colonic tumor; Hep, hepatoma.

In order to exclude the possibility that other antigenic systems, such as the HL-A system, were involved in these reactivities, we tested the serum and the tumor cell eluate of the patient on his own frozen tumor sections. We also obtained fluorescence patterns in this autologous system (Fig. 4). Moreover, when the immunoglobulins eluted off surgical tumor membrane fractions were tested in the passive hemagglutination assay, many, but not all, gave positive results.

The fact that the eluted immunoglobulins were able to agglutinate NCA-conjugated sheep red blood cells indicated to us their antibody nature. This

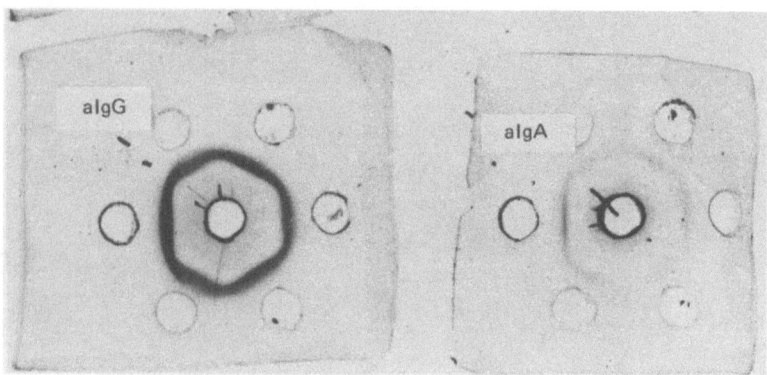

Figure 3. Double diffusion reaction of six colonic tumor membrane eluates with antihuman
IgG (left) and antihuman IgA (right) antiserum.

is reinforced by their ability to fix to the tumor cell membranes of cultured
cells, which were shown to contain no Fc receptors.

IV. DISCUSSION

We have observed that in the sera of virtually all healthy or diseased individuals tested, there are circulating antibodies directed against antigens that
are expressed on tumor cell membranes.

The titers of these antibodies vary, however. A marked increase in the titers
of these antibodies occurs in sera from patients suffering from nonmalignant or
malignant diseases as compared with normal controls. The highest titers are seen
in the cancer group, provided that the tumor has been removed. Low titers in
cancer patients have been observed in the preoperative state. This might indicate
either of two mechanisms:

1. The antibodies have been bound by their corresponding antigen to form

**Table III. Passive Hemagglutination of NCA-Conjugated Sheep
Erythrocytes by Eluates from Human Tissues**

Number of eluates	Source of eluate	Reaction		Reciprocal titers[a]		
		Pos.	Neg.	2	4	8
24	Colonic tumors	15	9	5	4	6
19	Normal mucosa	6	13	2	4	–

[a]All eluates were concentrated to equal volume/weight.

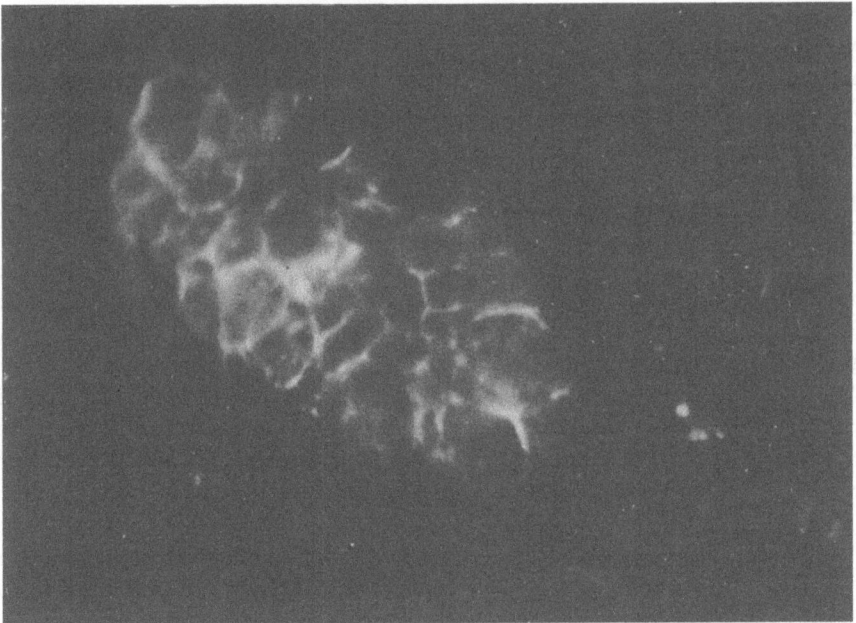

Figure 4. Immunofluorescence pattern of a frozen section of a colonic tumor incubated
with its autologous HA-positive serum.

soluble, circulating complexes. Evidence is accumulating that immune-
complex formation is a common phenomenon both in tumor bearing
animals and in cancer patients, though the role of these complexes is not
quite elucidated (Sjögren et al. 1971; Lewis et al., 1971; Baldwin et al.,
1973; Jose and Seshadri, 1974; Samayoa et al., 1977).

2. The second mechanism might be that the antibodies bind specifically to
the tumor cell membranes. This has been studied extensively in experimental animal systems and described repeatedly by many authors (Witz,
1973; Ran et al., 1974; Witz et al., 1974; Ran et al., 1976; Braslawsky
et al., 1976; see also the complete review by Witz, 1977). There are also
some reports of similar findings in cancer patients describing in vivo and
in vitro binding of specific antitumor antibodies to different human
tumors such as melanomas, ovarian, breast, and bladder carcinomas (Lewis
and Phillips, 1972; Thunold et al., 1973; Johannson and Ljunqvist,
1974; Dorsett et al., 1975; Gupta and Morton, 1975; Lewis et al., 1976;
Sulitzeanu et al., 1976).

Apparently the antibodies we demonstrated in this study are also able to ab-
sorb onto the tumor cell membrane in a specific way. Elution experiments using
surgically removed tumors showed that immunoglobulins with antibody activity

could indeed be obtained. Such eluates agglutinated sheep red blood cells coated with purified tumor antigens such as NCA. Furthermore it was shown that the antibodies can fix onto the plasma membrane of colonic cultured tumor cells. We believe that Fc receptors were not involved, since we were unable to demonstrate them on the tumor cells.

The presence of these antibodies in the sera of supposedly healthy blood donors suggests that they are not directly linked with an attack upon the neoplasia that is, to begin with, hypothetical. The fact that the antibodies are found in all groups of patients seems to indicate that the antibody titers are apparently more related to the antigen release than to the malignant character of the disease. Furthermore, the fact that the antibodies are found on the cell membranes of growing tumors may indicate that they belong to the category of antibodies called "enhancing or facilitating" antibodies rather than to those that have a cytotoxic effect on the tumor cell, and hence are beneficial for the tumor patient. The existence of this kind of antibodies has been previously shown by J. Hellström *et al.* (1971*b*), Sjögren *et al.* (1971, 1972), and K. E. Hellström and Hellström (1974).

However, whether the antibodies we demonstrated on the tumor cells belong to the so-called blocking antibodies or whether they play any role at all in the defense mechanism of the cancer patient has still to be shown.

V. REFERENCES

Avrameas, S., Taudou, B., and Chuilon, S., 1969, Glutaraldehyde, cyanuric chloride and tetrazotized *O*-dianizide as coupling reagents in the passive hemagglutination test, *Immunochemistry* 6:67–76.

Baldwin, R. W., and Price, M.R., 1976, Nature and expression of tumour antigens associated with experimental animal and human tumours, *Ann. Clin. Biochem.* 13:488–94.

Baldwin, R. W., Bowen, J. G., and Price, M. R., 1973, Detection of circulating hepatoma D23 antigen and immune complexes in tumor bearer serum, *Br. J. Cancer* 28:16–24.

Baldwin, R. W., Embleton, M. J., Jones, J. S., *et al.*, 1973, Cell-mediated and humoral immune reactions to human tumours, *Int. J. Cancer* 12:73–83.

Bernstein, I., Hellström, K. E., and Wright, P. W., 1976, Immunity to tumor antigens: Potential implications in human neuroblastoma, *J. Natl. Cancer Inst.* 57:711–715.

Braslawsky, G., Ran, M., and Witz, I. P., 1976, Tumor-bound immunoglobulins: The relationship between the *in vivo* coating of tumor cells by potentially cytotoxic antitumor antibodies and the expression of immune complex receptors, *Int. J. Cancer* 18:116–121.

Bull, D. M., Leibach, J. R., Williams, M. A., *et al.*, 1973, Immunity to colon cancer assessed by antigen induced inhibition of mixed mononuclear cell migration, *Science* 181:957–959.

Churchill, W. H., Jr., Rapp, H. J., Kronman, B. S., *et al.*, 1968, Detection of antigens of a new diethyl-nitrosamine induced transplantable hepatoma by delayed hypersensitivity, *J. Natl. Cancer Inst.* 41:13–17.

Cohen, A. M., Ketcham, A. S., and Morton, D. L., 1973, Tumor specific cellular cytotoxicity to human sarcomas: Evidence for a cell mediated host immune response to a common sarcoma cell surface antigen, *J. Natl. Cancer Inst.* 50:585–589.

Collatz, E., von Kleist, S., and Burtin, P., 1971, Further investigations of circulating antibodies in colon cancer patients on the autoantigenicity of the carcino-embryonic antigen, *Int. J. Cancer* 8:298–303.

Constanza, M. E., Pim, V., Schwartz, R. S., *et al.*, 1973, Carcinoembryonic antigen–antibody complexes in a patient with colonic carcinoma and nephrotic syndrome, *N. Engl. J. Med.* 289:520–522.

Coons, A. H., Leduc, E. H., and Connolly, J. M., 1955, Studies on the antibody production, *J. Exp. Med.* 102:49–59.

Dorsett, B. H., Ioachim, H. L., Stollbach, L., *et al.*, 1975, Isolation of tumor-specific antibodies from effusions of ovarian carcinomas, *Int. J. Cancer* 16:779–786.

Edynak, E. M., Old, L. J., Vrana, M., *et al.*, 1970. A fetal antigen in human tumours: Detection by an antibody in the serum of cancer patients, *Proc. Am. Assoc. Cancer Res.* 11:22.

Eilber, F. R., and Morton, D. L., 1970, Sarcoma-specific antigens: Detection by complement fixation with serum from sarcoma patients, *J. Natl. Cancer Inst.* 44:651–656.

Fossati, G., Colnaghi, M. J., Porta, G. D., *et al.*, 1971, Cellular and humoral immunity against human malignant melanoma, *Int. J. Cancer* 8:344–350.

Gold, Ph., 1967, Circulating antibodies against carcinoembryonic antigens of the human digestive system, *Cancer* 20:1663–1664.

Gold, Ph., and Freedman, S. O., 1965, Specific carcinoembryonic antigens of the human digestive system, *J. Exp. Med.* 122:467–481.

Gold, J. M., Freedman, S. O., and Gold, Ph., 1972, Human anti-CEA antibodies detected by radioimmunoelectrophoresis, *Nature (London) New Biol.* 239:60–62.

Graham, J. B., and Graham, R. M., 1955, Antibodies elicited by cancer in patients, *Cancer* 8:406–419.

Gupta, K. R., and Morton, D. L., 1975, Suggestive evidence for *in vivo* binding of specific antitumor antibodies of human melanomas, *Cancer Res.* 35:58–62.

Haskill, J. S., and Fett, J. W., 1976, Possible evidence for antibody dependent macrophage-mediated cytotoxicity directed against murine adenocarcinoma cells *in vivo*, *J. Immunol.* 117:1992–1998.

Haskill, J. S., Radov, L. A., Yamamura, Y., *et al.*, 1976, Isolation and indentification of specific and non-specific effector cells in experimental solid tumors, *J. Reticuloendothel. Soc.* 20:233–243.

Hellström, K. E., and Hellström, J., 1974, Lymphocyte-mediated cytotoxicity and blocking serum activity to tumor antigens, *Adv. Immunol.* 18:209–277.

Hellström, J., Hellström, K., and Shepard, T., 1970, Cell mediated immunity against antigens common to human colonic carcinomas and fetal gut epithelium, *Int. J. Cancer* 6:346–351.

Hellström, J., Hellström, K. E., Sjögren, H. O., *et al.*, 1971a, Demonstration of cell-mediated immunity to human neoplasms of various histological types, *Int. J. Cancer* 7:1–16.

Hellström, J., Sjögren, H. O., Warner, G., *et al.*, 1971b, Blocking of cell-mediated tumor immunity by sera from patients with growing neoplasmas, *Int. J. Cancer* 7:226–237.

Herberman, R. B., 1974, Delayed hypersensitivity skin reactions to antigens on human tumors, *Cancer* 34(Suppl.):1469–1473.

Herberman, R. B., and Oren, M. E., 1969, Delayed cutaneous hypersensitivity reactions to membrane extracts of human tumor cells, *Clin. Res.* 17:403–405.

Hodkinson, M., and Taylor, G., 1969, Autoimmune responses to human tumour antigens, *Br. J. Cancer* 23:510–514.

Hollinshead, A. C., Macwright, C. G., and Glew, D. H., 1972, Separation of skin reactive intestinal cancer antigen from the carcinoembryonic antigen of Gold, *Science* 177:887–889.

Itoh, T., and Southam, C. M., 1964, Isoantibodies to human cancer cells in cancer patients following cancer homotransplants, *J. Immunol.* 93:916–936.

Johannson, B., and Ljunqvist, A., 1974, Localization of immunoglobulin in urinary bladder tumors, *Acta Pathol. Microbiol. Scand. Sect. A* 82:559-563.

Jose, D. G., and Seshadri, R., 1974, Circulating immune complexes in human neuroblastoma: Direct assay and role in blocking specific cellular immunity, *Int. J. Cancer* 13:824-838.

Kahan, B. D., 1967, Cutaneoushypersensitivity reactions of guinea pigs to proteinaceous transplantation antigen, *J. Immunol.* 99:1121-1127.

Lamon, E. W., Whitten, H. D., Skurzak, H. M., *et al.*, 1975, IgM antibody dependent cell mediated cytotoxicity in the moloney sarcoma virus system: The involvement of T and B lymphocytes as effector cells, *J. Immunol.* 115:1288-1297.

Lewis, M. G., and Phillips, T. M., 1972, The specificity of surface membrane immunofluorescence in human malignant melanoma, *Int. J. Cancer* 10:105-111.

Lewis, M. G., Loughridge, L. W., and Phillips, T. M., 1971, Immunologic studies in nephrotic syndrome associated with extravenal malignant disease, *Lancet* 2:134-135.

Lewis, M. G., Proctor, J. W., Thomson, D. M. P., *et al.*, 1976, Cellular localization of immunoglobulin within human malignant melanoma, *Br. J. Cancer* 33:260-266.

Lo Gerfo, P., Herter, F. P., and Bennett, S. J., 1972, Absence of circulating antibodies to carcinoembryonic antigen in patients with gastrointestinal malignancies, *Int. J. Cancer* 9:344-348.

Mach, J. P. and Pusztaszeri, G., 1972, CEA: Demonstration of a partial identity between CEA and a normal glycoprotein, *Immunochemistry* 9:1031-1034.

Mavligit, G. M., Ambus, U., Gutterman, J. U., *et al.*, 1973, Antigen solubilized from human solid tumours—Lymphocyte stimulation and cutaneous delayed-hypersensitivity, *Nature (London) New Biol.* 243:188-190.

Muna, N. M., Marcus, S., and Smart, C., 1969, Detection of immunofluorescence of antibodies specific for human malignant melanoma cells, *Cancer* 23:88-95.

Oren, M. E., and Herberman, R. B., 1971, Delayed cutaneus hypersensitivity reactions to membrane extracts of human tumour cells, *Clin. Exp. Immunol.* 9:45-56.

Prehn, R. T., 1976, Do tumors grow because of the immune response of the host? *Transplant. Rev.* 28:34-42.

Ran, M., Fish, F., Witz, I. P., *et al.*, 1974, Tumor-bound immunoglobulins: The *in vitro* disappearance of immunoglobulin from the surface of coated tumor cells, and some properties of released components, *Clin. Exp. Immunol.* 16:335-359.

Ran, M., Klein, G., and Witz, I. P., 1976, Tumor-bound immunoglobulins. Evidence for the *in vivo* coating of tumor cells by potentially cytotoxic anti-tumor antibodies, *Int. J. Cancer* 17:90-97.

Saksela, E., Imir, T., and Mäkelä, O., 1975, Specifically cytotoxic human and mouse lymphoid cells induced with antibody antigen or antibody complexes, *J. Immunol.* 115:1488-1492.

Samayoa, E. A., McDuffie, F. C., Nelson, A. M., *et al.*, 1977, Immunoglobulin complexes in sera of patients with malignancy, *Int. J. Cancer* 19:12-17.

Schultz, R. M., Woods, W. A., and Chirigos, M. A., 1975, Detection in colorectal carcinoma patients of antibody cytotoxic to established cell strains derived from carcinoma of the human colon and rectum, *Int. J. Cancer* 16:16-23.

Sjögren, H. O., 1976, Immunological aspects of colorectal cancer *Clin. Gastroenterol* 5:563-571.

Sjögren, H. O., Hellström I., Bansal, S. C., *et al.*, 1971, Suggestive evidence that the "blocking antibodies" of tumor bearing individuals may be antigen–antibody complexes, *Proc. Natl. Acad. Sci. USA* 68:1372-1375.

Sjögren, H. O., Hellström, I., Bansal, S. C., *et al.*, 1972, Elution of "blocking factors" from human tumors capable of abrogating tumor cell destruction by specifically immune lymphocytes, *Int. J. Cancer* 9:274-283.

Sorokin, J. J., Kupchick, H. Z., and Zamcheck, N., 1973, Carcinoembryonic antigen in colon cancer: Absence in perchloric acid precipitates of plasma, *J. Natl. Cancer Inst.* **51**:1081–1083.

Sulitzeanu, D., Gorsky, Y., and Morecky, S., 1976, Membrane bound immunoglobulin on cells of effusions from patients with malignant diseases, *Isr. J. Med. Sci.* **12**:1329–1331.

Thomson, D. M. B., and Alexander, P., 1973, A cross-reacting embryonic antigen in the membrane of rat sarcoma cells which is immunogenic in the syngeneic host, *Br. J. Cancer* **27**:35–47.

Thunold, S., Tönder, O., and Larsen, O., 1973, Immunoglobulins in eluate of malignant human tumors, *Acta Pathol. Microbiol. Scand. Suppl.* **236**:97–100.

von Kleist, S., and Burtin, P., 1977, The carcinoembryonic antigen (CEA) and other carcinofetal antigens in gastrointestinal cancers and benign diseases, *Prog. Gastroenterol.* **III**: 595–615.

von Kleist, S., and Burtin, P., 1979, Antigens crossreacting with CEA, in: *Immunodiagnosis of Cancer* (R. B. Herbermann and K. R. McIntire, eds.), pp. 322–342, Marcel Dekker, Inc., New York.

von Kleist, S., Chavanel, G., and Burtin, P., 1972, Identification of a normal antigen that cross reacts with the carcinoembryonic antigen. *Proc. Natl. Acad. Sci. USA* **69**:2492–94.

von Kleist, S., King, M., and Burtin, P., 1974, Charactization of a normal tissular antigen extracted from human colonic tumors, *Immunochemistry* **11**:249–253.

von Kleist, S., Chany, E., Burtin, P., *et al.*, 1975, Immunohistological study of the antigenic pattern of a continuous human colonic tumor cell line (HT 29), *J. Natl. Cancer Inst.* **55**:555–560.

von Kleist, S., Tronpel, S., King, M., *et al.*, 1977, A clinical comparison between non-specific crossreacting antigen (NCA) and CEA in patients' sera, *Br. J. Cancer* **35**:875–880.

von Kleist, S., King, M., and Haveysmann, K., 1978, Demonstration of antibodies in patients' sera directed against non specific cross-reacting antigen, *J. Natl. Cancer Inst.* **61**:1385–1391.

Witz, I. P., 1973, The biological significance of tumor-bound immunoglobulins, *Curr. Top. Microbiol. Immunol.* **61**:151–171.

Witz, I. P., 1977, Tumor-bound immunoglobulins: *In situ* expressions of humoral immunity, *Adv. Cancer Res.* **25**:95–148.

Witz, I. P., Kinnamon, S., and Ran, M., *et al.*, 1974, Tumor-bound immunoglobulins: The *in vitro* fixation of radioiodine labeled anti-immunoglobulin reagents by tumor cells, *Clin. Exp. Immunol.* **16**:321–334.

Chapter 9

Tumor-Localizing Lymphocytotoxic Antibodies

Maya Ran, Margalit Yaakubowicz, Ora Amitai, and Isaac P. Witz

Department of Microbiology
The George S. Wise Faculty of Life Sciences
Tel Aviv University
Tel Aviv, Israel

I. INTRODUCTION

A. Tumor-Associated Immunoglobulins

Humoral tumor immunity as expressed within the tumor tissue has been studied in several laboratories, including ours (Witz, 1977). There is little doubt that immunoglobulin molecules are associated with cells lodging in the tumors of humans and of animals. A preferential association between Ig and tumor tissues was indicated in some cases (Ran and Witz, 1970).

In view of this finding, which seems to be general for many types of tumors, several sets of questions emerge.

The first set of questions concerns the nature of the cells to which tumor-associated Ig is bound and the nature of binding. Tumor masses contain heterogeneous populations of cells: malignant cells proper, in addition to a variety of host cells such as stromal elements as well as infiltrating lymphocytes or macrophages. Conceivably each of these cell types or all of them could express membrane Ig.

Some cells, such as infiltrating B cells, could synthesize Ig *in situ*, whereas other cell types, notably Fc-receptor (FcR)-positive cells such as macrophages or certain types of lymphocytes, could possibly transfer Fc-bound Ig molecules into the tumor. Tumor cells *per se* could have Ig molecules on their membrane either as antibodies coating membrane antigens or bound onto Fc receptors expressed on some nonlymphoid tumor cells.

It seems that these possibilities are not mutually exclusive. Plasma cell infiltrates have been demonstrated in some tumor systems (Ioachim, 1976), raising the possibility of an *in situ* synthesis of Ig by host cells. On the other hand, Fc receptors have been demonstrated to be expressed in tumor cell areas and not in the areas of infiltrating lymphocytes both in human tumors (Tønder *et al.*, 1976) and in experimental tumors (Braslawsky *et al.*, 1976*a*). Some of those Fc receptors were saturated with Ig (Tønder *et al.*, 1976). A binding of Ig via Fc has been demonstrated in various types of human cancer (Tønder and Thunold, 1973; Tønder *et al.*, 1976) and in experimental animal tumors (Milgrom *et al.*, 1968; Kerbel and Davies, 1974; Kerbel *et al.*, 1975; Wood *et al.*, 1975; Braslawsky *et al.*, 1976*a*). In some systems it has been proven that at least some of the tumor-associated Ig molecules are in fact antitumor antibodies (Witz, 1977). We have demonstrated, for example, the *in vivo* localization of cytotoxic antitumor antibodies on SEYF-a tumor cells (a polyoma-virus-induced sarcoma) following the appearance of such antibodies in the serum of tumor bearers (Ran *et al.*, 1976). Collectively these results show that tumor-associated immunoglobulins are in many cases a heterogeneous population of molecules. In those cases in which Ig is associated with tumor cells through its binding site to an antigen, the opportunity presents itself to identify and isolate this antigen. It should be emphasized that such antibody-coated membrane antigens are of particular interest because they clearly are immunogenic in the tumor bearer and are also exposed and available for immune effectors.

The second set of questions concerns the biological functions, if any, of tumor-associated Ig molecules. Some of the proven and of the postulated roles such Ig molecules may play were raised in a review published two years ago (Witz, 1977). A study performed recently concerning this question warrants special attention. Jacquemin *et al.* (1978) obtained the interesting finding that specifically purified IgG molecules isolated from eluates derived from peripheral leukocytes of patients with chronic myelogenous leukemia (CML) at blastcrisis, neutralized *in vitro* the catalytic activity of reverse transcriptase from several retroviruses, most notably that of feline leukemia virus (FeLV). Based on these findings (which were confirmed by one of the authors—I.P.W.), Jacquemin *et al.* (1978) proposed that the response was directed either against FeLV-related reverse transcriptase, (or reverse-transcriptase precursor) present in the membrane of the leukemic cells or against a cell-surface protein crossreacting with such an enzyme.

When analyzing documented or postulated biological effects of tumor-associated Ig molecules, it is important to remember that such molecules could play a significant role in the immune relationship between the tumor bearer and his malignancy, even though they may not be antitumor antibodies and although the cell they consort with is a host, rather than a tumor, cell. For example, it is easily conceivable that immune complexes, although being serologically unrelated to tumor antigens, when saturating Fc receptors on host-derived immunocytes could interfere with the proper functions of such cells.

Another research area totally open at this time concerns the usefulness for the clinician of analyzing various aspects of Ig presence within tumors. It is tempting, for instance, to consider the possibility of developing assays that, by assessing the pattern of Ig molecules in the surgically operable primary local tumor, would provide reliable predictions concerning the prognosis of the patient, his chances to develop metastasis, and his response to various treatments.

Ig eluted from primary tumors could conceivably be used as a homing device for detectors of residual occult tumor foci or for therapeutic agents.

Even a thorough literature survey would indicate that no attempts to approach these problems were made as yet.

B. Methodology Used to Study Tumor-Associated Immunoglobulins

Tumor-associated immunoglobulins can be studied at the level of the Ig-expressing cell and in solution, after the molecules have been eluted from the cells.

The scope of studies on tumor-associated Ig molecules at the level of the cell is limited to showing whether or not Ig can be detected on cells, the class and subclass characterization of the Ig molecules, and the nature of the Ig-associated cells. Labeled reagents such as anti-Ig antisera or staphylococcal protein A are required in such assays. Studies aimed to elucidate the specificity pattern of tumor-associated Ig molecules or their biological functions require such molecules in solution. Some attention should, therefore, be paid to procedures aimed to dissociate Ig molecules including antibodies from sensitized, viable target cells.

An ideal dissociation procedure is one that offers maximal recovery of active antibody while not affecting its structure or function. A minimal damage to the coated cells is also desirable in order to reduce as far as possible the extraction of cellular components and thus the artificial formation of immune complexes.

In a recent study we (Ehrlich and Witz, 1979) compared, according to the criteria described above, various low-pH elution procedures described in the literature. We used two murine ascites tumor cells (EL4 and TA3/st) sensitized with radioiodinated allogeneic or xenogeneic antibodies.

The ability of several low-pH buffers to dissociate these antibodies from the sensitized living tumor cells was compared. Two buffers (glycine and citrate) were further tested for their dissociation abilities under different conditions of time and temperature, and for their influence on the eluted antibodies. The cytotoxicity mediated by these low-pH buffers was also determined by viability assays. Optimal results were obtained with 0.1 M citrate buffer at pH 3.5. This buffer eluted relatively high amounts of bound antibody, showed relatively little cytotoxicity towards the cells, and had essentially no denaturing effect on the eluted antibodies, and the antibodies eluted by this buffer exhibited increased specificity. The glycine buffer, on the other hand, although eluting quantitatively more antibodies than the citrate buffer, caused denaturation or degradation of a larger fraction of the eluted antibody than citrate buffer. This degradation may also explain the increased nonspecific binding of the antibody present in the glycine eluate compared with that in the citrate eluate. Furthermore, the glycine buffer exhibited a significantly higher cytoxicity towards the cells than the citrate buffer. Citrate buffer is therefore utilized in the studies described below.

C. Autoantibodies in Tumor Bearers

In studying the activity spectrum of antibodies eluted from SEYF-a tumors we discovered that tumor eluates mediated complement-dependent lysis (CdL) of normal lymphocytes. Such an activity was hardly detected in the serum of tumor bearers (Ran *et al.*, 1978).

Below we briefly review some of the evidence showing that various types of antiself-reactivities can be detected in tumor bearers.

Autoantibodies detected in cancer patients belong mainly to two categories:

1. Antibodies against the normal correlate of the tumor tissue. Among these are antirenal collecting duct antibodies present in patients with renal cell carcinoma (Forbes *et al.*, 1976).
2. Antibodies to seemingly unrelated antigens. Among these are anti-smooth-muscle antibodies in patients with breast carcinomas (Wasserman *et al.*, 1975) with various other carcinomas and with melanoma (Nelson, 1977). Also detected were antibodies directed against thymic antigens in naso-pharingeal cancer patients (Yasuda-Yasaki and Yoshida, 1975), auto-lymphocytotoxins in patients with cervical cancer (Müller and Koenig, 1977), and antilymphocyte antibodies in melanoma patients (Shiku *et al.*, 1977).

The stimulus to the production of autoantibodies in patients with cancer is not known. It has been suggested that these antibodies arise in response to either a direct stimulation by the abnormal cells or their products, or by passenger or oncogenic viruses present in tumor-bearing individuals (Nelson, 1977). In accordance with the suggestion of direct stimulation is the demonstration of auto-antibodies (Nelson, 1977) present in tumor-bearing animals whose tumors contain increased amounts of contractile protein (Toh and Müller, 1975). Similar results were reported for human malignancies (Gabbioni *et al.*, 1975). The second possibility is supported by the finding that viral infections are sometimes associated with abnormal autoantibody production (P. Andersen and Andersen, 1975).

A cross-reactivity between antibodies directed against tumor cells and those directed against normal tissue correlates could be easily explained if one accepts the possibility that malignant transformation is manifested by rearrangement of the membrane of normal cells (Garrido et al., 1976). This is supported by the findings that immunization with hapten-modified self-antigens (Galili et al., 1976) or treatment with adjuvant (Furnie et al., 1974) results in the formation of autoantibodies. A mechanism of abnormal T–B-cell cooperation has been suggested by Allison et al. (1971) as a model for autoantibody formation stimulated either by hapten-modified self-antigens or by viral infection of immunocytes. Profitt et al. have demonstrated autoreactive thymocytes following viral infection (1975). It is possible that the mechanism operating in autoreactivity following viral infection is different from the one operating in autoimmunity following hapten modification of self-antigens. Yet one or both of these mechanisms could possibly take place in mice bearing the SEYF-a tumor mentioned above where lymphocytotoxic antibodies of the IgG class appear following tumor inoculation (Ran et al., 1978).

Another type of autoimmunity in cancer patients is the appearance of antibodies directed against various parts of the IgG molecule. Antibodies directed against the Fc portion have been detected in the serum and in tumor-tissue elutes from various carcinomas and other types of tumors in humans (Thunold et al., 1970). Both anti-Fc and anti-Fab antibodies have recently been reported to occur in breast cancer patients (Humphrey et al., 1977).

It should be noted that both tumor-bound Fc receptors and tumor-bound anti-Fc antibodies may have very similar if not identical functions (Tønder and Thunold, 1973). Both types of molecules could play a role in regulation of the humoral immune response of cancer patients (Kerbel and Davies, 1974).

D. T-Cell-Related Abnormalities in Tumor Bearers

In autoimmune diseases, the appearance of autoantibodies is probably a result of the loss of effective suppressor T cells as proposed by several authors (Allison et al., 1971; Talal and Steinberg, 1974). Supporting this hypothesis are the findings that after the loss of suppressor T cells natural antithymocyte antibodies appear in NZB mice (Steinberg et al., 1975). Equally, antibodies against erythrocytes detectable in mice with experimental autoimmune hemolytic anemia appear only after suppressor T cells have disappeared (Cooke et al., 1978).

Although there is no direct proof that a T-cell-mediated regulation of antiself-reactivity is impaired in cancer patients, some T-cell-related abnormalities do occur in such patients, however. These could be divided into specific and nonspecific T-cell-related reactions. A specific suppressive effect mediated by T cells or by a T-cell factor was demonstrated with thymic cells of mice bearing methylcholanthrene-induced sarcomas (Fujimoto et al., 1976). Thymocytes or splenocytes from tumor-bearing mice infused into immune syngeneic mice receiving simultaneously a challenge of tumor cells, suppressed the rejection of the tumor by the immune mice. This immunosuppressive activity was specific to the tumor type and did not affect other tumors. A soluble factor with an identical suppressor activity was extracted from thymic cells (Fujimoto *et al.*, 1976). Evidence also suggests that the tumor-specific blocking factor purified from sera of mice bearing a chemically induced sarcoma is a T-cell factor (Nepom *et al.*, 1976).

Nonspecific abnormalities in cancer patients include a decreased percentage of peripheral T cells (determined by E rosettes) and impaired responses to phyto-hemagglutinin (Rand *et al.*, 1977) or to other mitogens (Quan and Burtin, 1978). Although most of these phenomena occur in patients with invasive cancer, a decrease in E-rosette-forming T cells was also reported to occur in preinvasive disease, raising the possibility that this T-cell suppression may be, at least partially, responsible for the spread of the disease (Rand *et al.*, 1977). There is still an argument about the types of cells involved in this suppression (Quan and Burtin, 1978).

In some malignant states a nonspecific but selective suppression of some T-cell activities occurs, among these a suppression of T helper cells (Haba *et al.*, 1976) and of alloreactive T cells (McMaster *et al.*, 1977; Brooks *et al.*, 1972; Succi-Foca *et al.*, 1973). There is some evidence that a soluble factor is involved in this sup-pression (McMaster *et al.*, 1977). The factor operative in these cases seems to be different from the specific T-cell factor mentioned above (Fujimoto *et al.*, 1976) both in function and in biochemical characteristics (Waksmann and Tada, 1977). It is possible that in tumor bearers T cells are stimulated for an increased release of such immunosuppressive factors.

In previous studies we demonstrated the occurance of antilymphocyte anti-bodies in mice bearing syngeneic sarcomas, (Ran *et al.*, 1978). The hypothesis underlying the present and further studies on the lymphocytotoxic autoanti-bodies in mice bearing nonlymphoid malignancies is that there is a causative relationship between some of the impaired T-cell functions discussed above and the formation of such antibodies.

II. EXPERIMENTAL RESULTS

A. Tumor-Bound Lymphocytotoxic Antibodies

SEYF-a is an ascites murine tumor originally induced by polyoma virus (Sjörgren, 1964*a,b*). It is at present at its 350th transplant generation in A.BY (H-2^b) mice. Studies on the immunogenicity of, and the transplantation resistance to, this and other polyoma-virus-induced tumors were performed by Sjörgren (1964*a,b*).

With the aid of an assay measuring complement-dependent cytotoxicity (CdL) we analyzed the antigenic specificities on the membrane of SEYF-a cells by antibodies present in artificially raised syngeneic or semisyngeneic antisera (Witz et al., 1976). The presence of several separate antigenic specificities on in vivo-propagated SEYF-a cells became apparent. The cells expressed a membrane antigen shared by other allogeneic polyoma-virus-induced murine sarcomas, but not by a considerable number of nonpolyma-virus-induced murine tumors (Klein et al., 1979).

A.BY mice bearing syngeneic SEYF-a tumors develop circulating antitumor antibodies mediating CdL of SEYF-a cells (Ran et al., 1976). It was thus of interest to compare the specificity pattern of the hyperimmune artificially produced anti-SEFY-a antibodies with that of the circulating antibodies present in tumor bearers (Ran et al., unpublished). It is evident that sera drawn from tumor bearers have a restricted specificity compared to the hyperimmune antisera. In particular, sera drawn from tumor-bearing mice shortly after inoculation (10–12 days) react with fewer antigenic specificities than sera drawn later on. Ran et al. (1976) supplied evidence that the circulating cytotoxic antitumor antibodies present in SEYF-a-bearing mice find their way to the tumor cells in vivo. Tumor-localized antibodies mediated CdL of tumor cells, either after addition of exogeneous complement to freshly harvested cells or after elution by low-pH buffers, when added with complement to indicator cells. The in vivo coating of different types of tumor cells by tumor antibodies was later also confirmed by other investigators (Witz, 1977). The SEYF-a-bound antibodies belong to the IgG2 a subclass (Moav and Witz, 1978), and their reactivity pattern was found to be more restricted (i.e., they reacted with fewer specificities) than the corresponding sera of tumor-bearing mice (Ran et al., unpublished). One may regard this restriction as evidence for a selective localization of circulating antibodies on tumor cells.

Selectivity of localization was also pronounced with the lymphocytotoxic antibodies mentioned above. These antibodies whereas hardly detectable in serum, are present in tumor eluates in titers similar to that of tumor antibodies, (Ran et al., 1978).

The induction and in vivo localization of lymphocytotoxic antibodies occurs also in tumor systems other than the SEYF-a tumor. These include SA-601, a solid, methylcholanthrene-induced sarcoma in NZW mice in its early transplant generations. Preliminary results indicate that lymphocytotoxic antibodies also localize within tumors of early passages of a spontaneous mammary carcinoma in R III mice (kindly given to us by Professor A. Frensdorff from our department).

B. Induction and Selective Tumor Localization
of Lymphocytotoxic Antibodies

We asked whether the in vivo localization of lymphocytotoxic antibodies on tumor-resident cells is a selective process, namely, would all types of antibodies present in a tumor bearer localize on tumor cells?

CdL by SEYF-a bearers against:

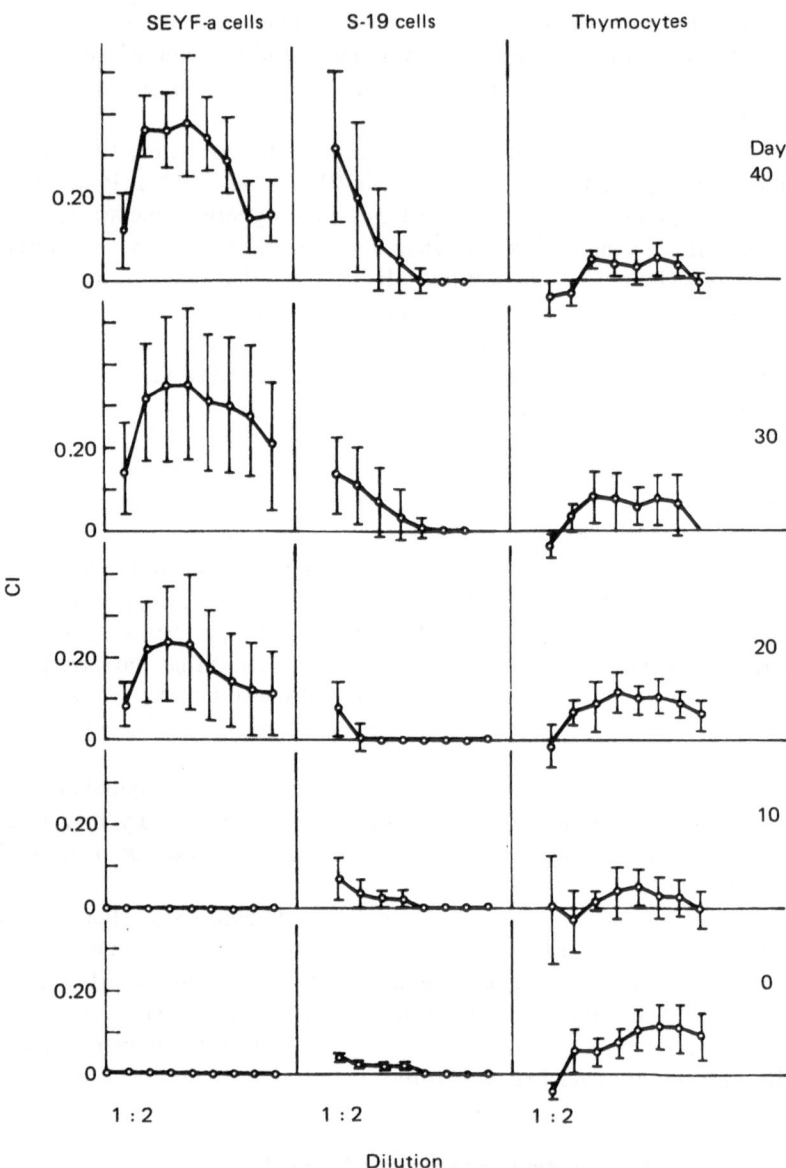

Figure 1. CdL mediated by sera of SEYF-a bearers towards SEYF-a cells, S-19 cells, and C57B1/6 thymocytes assayed by ^{51}Cr release. Cytotoxicity index (CI) values of sera drawn at the indicated day after tumor inoculation are shown. The values are mean ± standard deviation (SD) of six to eight serum samples.

To answer this question we compared the CdL reactivity pattern of serum and of eluates. The sera were not heat inactivated in order to enable the detection of both stable and heat-labile antibodies. As seen in Fig. 1, SEYF-a bearers formed circulating cytotoxic antibodies against the corresponding SEYF-a cells and against seemingly unrelated S-19, IgG2-synthesizing mouse plasmacytoma cells. The plasmacytoma cells were chosen as representatives of seemingly unrelated target cells against which reactivity is induced following tumor inoculation (Ran *et al.*, unpublished). The sera also contained low titers of thymocytotoxic antibodies. Eluates from SEYF-a and Sa-601 tumors were tested for CdL activity against these same target cells. As shown in Table I, the reactivity pattern of eluates was different from that of serum. A preferential tumor localization of thymocytotoxic antibodies (compared to anti-S-19 plasmacytoma) antibodies was evident (compare Fig. 1 with Table I). The results represented in Tables I and II suggest that the sera and eluates from the Sa-601 sarcoma is probably behaving in a similar fashion. In this tumor, there is also a preferential binding of thymocytotoxic antibodies onto cells within the tumor.

A similarity can be seen in the pattern of CdL mediated by eluates of SEYF-a and of Sa-601 towards various lymphoid lines (Table I). Both eluates react against L5178Y cells significantly higher than against EL4 or S-19 cells. Such a similarity, however, could not be demonstrated with sera of mice bearing the SEYF-a tumors (Table II). Serum for Sa-601 bearers, for example, reacted almost to the same degree with thymocytes, S-19 cells, and L5178Y cells and less with EL4 cells. sera of SEYF-a bearers, on the other hand, reacted equally well with EL4, L5178Y, and S-19 cells but essentially not with thymocytes. Sera from both SEYF-a bearers and Sa-601 bearers reacted with the lymphoid cells in a different pattern

Table I. Complement-Dependent Lymphocytotoxicity Mediated by Tumor Eluates

	SEYF-a eluates[a]			Sa-601 eluates[a]		
Target cells	Positive[b] per total	CI[c] mean ± SD[e]	$p <$[d]	Positive per total	CI[c] mean ± SD[e]	$p <$[d]
Thymocytes	12/12	0.35 ± 0.06		12/12	0.32 ± 0.12	
EL4	33/34	0.12 ± 0.03	0.001	3/7	0.07 ± 0.03	0.005
L5178Y	12/14	0.19 ± 0.07	0.025	4/6	0.24 ± 0.06	0.005
S-19	11/31	0.13 ± 0.05		9/9	0.08 ± 0.03	

[a] Low pH eluates of the indicated tumors were assayed.
[b] A positive reaction is defined as CI > 0.05. The indicated number of tumor eluates was assayed for CdL activity.
[c] CI, cytotoxicity index. Mean values were calculated for positive eluates only.
[d] Significance was evaluated using Student's *t* test.
[e] SD, standard deviation.

Table II. Complement-Dependent Lymphocytotoxicity Mediated by
Mouse Sera

Serum from	Serum dilution	Cytotoxicity index			
		Thymocytes	EL4	L5178Y	S-19
Normal 129 mice	1:2	0.29	0.05	0.00	NT
	1:4	0.37	0.03	0.00	NT
A.BY mice with SEYF-a[a]	1:2	0.00	0.41	0.53	0.32
	1:4	0.06	0.37	0.48	0.20
NZW mice with Sa-601[a]	1:2	0.26	0.10	0.22	0.27
	1:4	0.26	0.07	0.00	0.20

[a] Serum was drawn 20–40 days following tumor inoculation at the time when tumor cells were harvested for preparation of eluates.
[b] NT, not tested.

than the serum of normal 129 mice, which have high titers of natural thymocytotoxic antibodies (W. J. Martin and Martin, 1975).

C. Partial Identification of the Target Cell and the Target Antigen for the Tumor-Associated Antilymphocyte Antibody

We performed some experiments to identify the target lymphocytes for the cytotoxicity mediated by the antilymphocyte antibodies. CdL mediated by SEYF-a eluates was assayed using lymphocytes originating from various organs. Thymocytes and lymph node cells were found to be more sensitive than splenocytes, while bone marrow cells were much less sensitive (Ran *et al.*, 1978). For further identification of the sensitive target-cell population we used enrichment and elimination methods. As demonstrated in Fig. 2, treatment of mice with cortisone partially (using SEYF-a eluates) or completely (using Sa-601 eluates and eluates from other tumors) eliminated the sensitive population from the thymus. Using a percoll gradient separation of splenocytes, a minor subpopulation of cells having a density higher than that of the main population of splenocytes. The density of this subpopulation was similar to that of thymocytes. This subpopulation of cells was more sensitive to CdL mediated by eluates than the major population of splenocytes (Fig. 3). The minor subpopulation showed also a higher sensitivity than the major splenocyte subpopulation towards cytotoxicity mediated by an anti-Thy-1 antiserum.

In addition, it was found that thymocytes treated with an anti-Thy-1 antiserum and complement lost their sensitivity to the tumor-associated lymphocytotoxic antibodies (TALCA). Although more experiments are required to

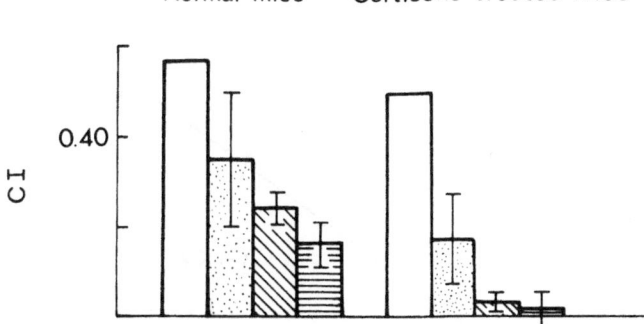

Figure 2. CdL mediated by eluates from SEYF-a ([▨▨▨]), Sa-601 ([◥◥◥]), and other tumors ([▤▤▤]) (see Section II) toward thymocytes from normal and from cortisone-treated C57B1/6 mice. For comparison, the cytotoxicity induced by an antiserum directed against Thy 1 is also shown. CI values (mean ± SD) of a ^{51}Cr release assay of 5–10 eluates is shown.

ascertain the exact nature of the lymphocyte subpopulation sensitive to the TALCA, the evidence obtained so far argues strongly for the possibility that these cells are T cells. The fact that thymocytes of the A.BY, C5 7B1/6 C3H, BALB/c, and AKR mouse strains (Ran *et al.*, 1978) and of NZW and 129 (results not shown) were all sensitive, indicated that neither Thy-1 nor G 1X serves as determinants for TALCA. These results also indicate that the sensitive subpopulation is probably present in most, if not in all, strains of mice.

We were intrigued by the possibility that the lymphocyte subpopulation sensitive to TALCA is a FcR bearing T cell. This possibility was supported by the results showing that L5178Y cells expressing FcR (Leclerc *et al.*, 1977) were significantly more sensitive to CdL mediated by tumor eluates than EL4 cells that are FcR-negative T cells (Table I). To test the hypothesis that TALCA are directed against FcR-expressing T cells, we treated L5178Y cells with tumor eluates and rabbit complement and then measured the ability of the treated cells to form rosettes with antibody-coated sheep erythrocytes (EA rosettes). Nontreated L5178Y cells served as controls. A 40–80% reduction of rosette formation was brought about by tumor eluates (Table III). Rosetting was not inhibited by eluates of normal spleen or of myeloma S-19 cells. These control eluates also did not mediate CdL of L5178Y cells. A correlation between anti-T-cell reactivity of tumor eluates and inhibition of rosetting was also demonstrated with activated T cells (ATC). As demonstrated in Table IV (experiment I), EA rosetting, between ATC and sRBC coated with either an unseparated mouse antiserum directed against sRBC or with a 7 S preparation of a rabbit antiserum against

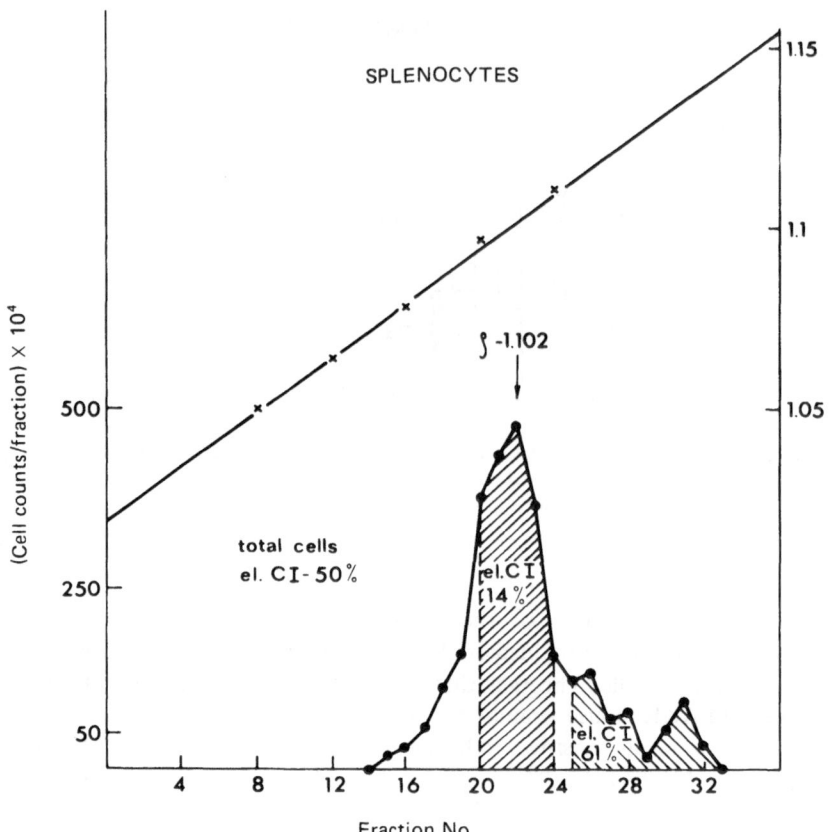

Figure 3. Distribution of A.BY splenocytes after isopycnic sedimentation in a percoll linear density gradient. Fractions 20–24 and 25–33 were pooled and tested for sensitivity to CdL mediated by SEYF-a eluates. CI was determined by dye exclusion. The CI value for the unfractionated splenocyte population was 50%. The major subpopulation was relatively resistant to CdL mediated by the eluates, whereas a minor subpopulation (fractions 25–33) seemed to be enriched for cells sensitive to eluate-mediated CdL.

sRBC, was inhibited by SEYF-a and Sa-601 eluates plus complement. Neither complement alone nor S-19 eluates plus complement inhibited EA rosetting. This suggested that the TALCA were directed against receptors for 7 S immuno-globulin or against an antigen located very close to this receptor.

The fact that active complement was required for inhibition (experiment II, Table IV) indicated that EA-rosette inhibition was mediated by antibodies rather than by a nonspecific factor. The fact that anti-Thy 1 and complement also inhibited EA rosettes (experiment II, Table IV) indicates that the EA ro-settes forming cells were in fact FcR-positive T cells.

Table III. Inhibition by Tumor Eluates of EA Rosettes Formed by Cultured L5178Y Cells[a]

Experiment	Group	Inhibitor	Complement	Rabbit anti-s-RBC (7 S) Counted	Percent	Mouse anti-s-RBC (serum) Counted	Percent
I	Control[b]	–	–	13/143	9.0	11/138	8.0
		–	+[c]	11/157	7.0	15/152	9.9
	Experimental[b]	S-19[d] eluate	+	8/107	7.4	NT	
		SEYF-a eluates					
		1	+	1/33	3.0	4/80	5.0
		2	+	NT		4/90	4.4
		3	+	2/109	1.8	1/63	1.5
II	Control[b]	Normal spleen[d] eluate	–	NT		21/325	6.4
		S-19[d] eluate	+	NT		15/287	5.2
			+	NT		18/336	5.3
			+	12/243	4.9	16/272	5.9
	Experimental[b]	SEYF-a eluates					
		1	+	3/164	1.8	NT	
		2	+	2/155	1.2	3/180	1.6
		3	+	6/205	3.0	8/234	3.4

[a] 10^6 L5178Y cells were incubated at 37°C for 45 min with tumor eluates and complement. Cells were then washed three times, suspended, and mixed with sheep red blood cells (s-RBC) sensitized with a subagglutinating dilution of an anti-sRBC serum. Sensitization of the s-RBC with a rabbit 7 S fraction or mouse unfractionated antiserum was performed at 37°C for 30 min with gentle shaking. Rosetting was performed by incubating L5178Y cells with s-RBC in a volume of 0.25 ml at 37°C for 45 min with very gentle shaking. The mixture was diluted 1:4, kept overnight at 4°C, and then counted. L5178Y cells surrounded by at least three s-RBC were scored as rosettes.

[b] The percentage of rosettes in the control mixtures was significantly higher than in eluate-treated mixtures ($p < 0.005$ in Student's t test), in both experiments I and II.

[c] Complement-fresh rabbit serum was used as source of complement.

[d] Eluates from S-19 tumors and from normal spleen did not contain lymphocytotoxic antibodies.

Table IV. Inhibition by Tumor Eluates of EA Rosettes Formed by Activated T cells[a]

Experiment	Group	Inhibitor	Complement	EA rosettes/cell			
				Rabbit anti-s-RBC (7 S)		Mouse anti-s-RBC (serum)	
				Counted	Percent	Counted	Percent
I	Control[b]	—	—	13/134	10.0	58/224	25.0
		—	+[c]	10/132	8.0	47/221	21.0
		S-19 eluate[d]	+	NT		36/228	15.0
	Experimental[b]	SEYF-a eluates					
		1	+	3/92	3.0	15/166	9.0
		2	+	3/128	2.3	24/236	10.0
		3	+	4/121	3.0	21/194	10.0
		Sa-601 eluate[e]	+	3/127	2.3	22/236	9.0
II	T-cell control	Anti-Thy 1	+			2/85; 1/75	2.4; 1.3
	Control[b]	None	–[f]			11/172; 16/206	6.7; 7.7
		Anti-Thy 1	+			18/189; 19/185	9.5; 10.0
		Eluates of thymocytes[d]	–[f]			16/149; 17/170	10.8; 10.0
		SEYF-a eluate 1	+			14/217; 13/200	6.4; 6.5
	Experimental[b]	SEYF-a eluates					
		1	+			7/171; 8/204	4.0; 3.9
		2	+			7/182; 6/170	3.8; 3.5
		Sa-601 eluate[e]	+			8/220	3.6
		AS[g] precipitate of Sa-601 eluate	+			9/251	3.5

[a] Rosetting was performed as described for L5178Y culture cells in Table III. Activated T cells (ATC) were prepared according to Leclerc *et al.* (1977).

[b] The percentage of rosettes in the negative control mixture was significantly higher than in the mixtures treated with eluate plus complement ($p < 0.005$ in Student's t test).

[c] Complement-fresh rabbit serum was used as source of complement (C').

[d] Eluates from normal thymocytes or from S-19 tumors did not contain lymphocytotoxic antibodies.

[e] Sa-601 tumor eluates contained lymphocytotoxic antibodies as described.

[f] Inactivated normal rabbit serum was added as a C' control.

[g] AS, ammonium sulfate.

D. The Nature of Interaction between TALCA and the Target Cells

TALCA is an induced antibody appearing in tumor bearers following tumor inoculation. This was concluded from the fact that CdL of lymphocytes was detected in eluates from late, but not from early, tumors. The observation that antibody activity is associated with the IgG class (Ran *et al.*, 1978), in contrast to naturally occurring thymocytotoxic antibodies that are of the IgM class (W. J. Martin and Martin, 1975), also supported this contention. The induced TALCA are also different from natural antibodies in their reactivity spectrum (compare the reactivity spectrum of normal sera of mice of the 129 strain with that of serum drawn from tumor bearers, Table II).

The question whether TALCA were induced by a cross-reacting antigen that induced antibodies to tumor antigens was partially resolved by the fact that TALCA could be induced in SEYF-a-bearing mice without the concomitant induction of antitumor antibodies (Table V). Eluates from SEYF-a cells were prepared by two methods: low-pH treatment of freshly harvested cells or incuba-

Table V. Complement-Dependent Cytotoxicity Mediated by SEYF-a Tumor Eluates[a]

Group No.	Eluate No.	Elution procedure[b]	Dilution:	CI against: SEYF-a cells 1:2	1:4	Thymocytes 1:2	1:4
I	1	Low pH		0.66	0.51	0.15	0.00
	2	Low pH		0.40	0.22	0.13	0.05
	3	Low pH		0.52	0.31	0.10	0.06
	4	Low pH		0.32	0.06	0.10	0.04
	5	Low pH		0.51	0.31	0.20	0.09
	6	Low pH		0.26	0.03	0.27	0.14
	7	60 min at 37°C		0.34	0.22	0.05	0.00
	8	120 min at 37°C		0.40	0.12	0.17	0.09
II	1	Low pH		0.00	0.00	0.29	0.14
	2	Low pH		0.00	0.00	0.22	0.11
	3	Low pH		0.00	0.00	0.23	0.12
	4	Low pH		0.00	0.00	0.29	0.14
	5	Low pH		0.00	0.00	0.24	0.13
	6	Low pH		0.00	0.00	0.11	0.04
	7	60 min at 37°C		0.00	0.00	0.20	0.06
	8	120 min at 37°C		0.00	0.00	0.15	0.13

[a] Eluates were prepared from SEYF-a cells propagated in A.BY mice. Two groups of mice were used. The mice in group I developed cytotoxic anti-SEYF-a antibodies detected in their sera, while those belonging to group II did not.
[b] Eluates were prepared by two methods: low-pH treatment, or incubation at 37°C of freshly harvested cells.

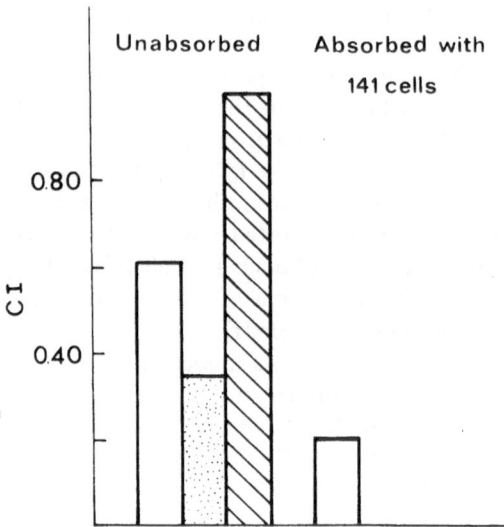

Figure 4. CdL of thymocytes (▭), 141 B-cell lymphoma (▦), and EL4 cells (◺) mediated by a rabbit antiserum directed against a low-pH tumor eluate. The serum was assayed prior to absorption and following exhaustive absorption with the 141 cells. The ^{51}Cr release assay was used. CI values before and after absorption with the B cells are shown.

tion at 37°C of such cells. The eluates were tested for ability to mediate CdL of SEYF-a cells and of thymocytes. Two types of reactivities were obtained: some eluates reacted with both cell types (group I), whereas other eluates (for as yet unknown reasons) reacted with thymocytes but not with SEYF-a cells (group II). These results supported the possibility that the antigens inducing the formation of cytotoxic antibodies for lymphocytes and for SEYF-a cells are distinct entities.

We have previously shown that neither small lymphocytes nor adherent cells are those cells that are coated with TALCA (Ran *et al.*, 1978). This tentative conclusion was based on the observation that a higher percentage of small lymphocytes is present in early tumors than in late tumors, while TALCA are present in eluates of late, but not of early, tumors. This observation argues against the possibility that TALCA are contributed to eluates by tumor-seeking T cells, which have been found to be smaller than splenocytes (Holden *et al.*, 1976). TALCA were also not contributed to tumor eluates by adherent cells, since eluates from tumor cell populations from which adherent cells were depleted did not have reduced CdL titers toward thymocytes.

The possibility that tumor-infiltrating, host-derived plasma cells contributed the TALCA to tumor eluates cannot yet be excluded. However, preliminary cell separation did not reveal the presence of plasma cells in tumor cell populations.

Although it is not clear whether or not the antigen inducing the formation of TALCA is present on tumor cells *per se* or on an as yet unknown type of host cells, we have some indirect evidence that the antigen inducing the formation of TALCA may be present in tumor cell populations in an immunogenic form. This was shown by the ability of tumor eluates to induce the formation of anti-T-cell antibodies in rabbits. The results presented in Figure 4 show that the unabsorbed rabbit antiserum reacted with thymocytes as well as with EL4 cells and with 141 cells (a NZB/NZW murine B-cell lymphoma, Sugai *et al.*, 1974). After exhaustive and complete absorption with the latter cells, the antiserum still reacted with thymocytes but the reactivity against EL4 cells also disappeared. This indicated that tumor eluates contained an antigen specific for thymocytes. The question of whether this antigen is identical with the one inducing the formation of TALCA in tumor bearers is still open.

III. DISCUSSION

T-cell autoantigens are probably normally present in various strains of mice, since one can detect naturally occurring IgM thymocytotoxic antibodies in these strains (W. J. Martin and Martin, 1975). However, lymphocytotoxic antibodies of the IgG class were found to be induced in mice bearing nonlymphoid tumors. The neo-induction of such IgG antibodies could be explained by one of the following:

1. Slightly modified T-cell-associated antigens may be expressed on non-lymphoid tumor cells in immunogenic form. The antigens may induce antilymphocyte antibodies, which are then bound by tumor cells. This possibility is supported by findings on the expression of an antigen cross-reactive with T cells on nonlymphoid tumors (DeLeo *et al.*, 1977).

2. Modification of T cells by a virus or a chemical carcinogen (Allison *et al.*, 1971) may render them autoimmunogenic, resulting in the induction of lymphocytotoxic autoantibodies. It is not unlikely that following the infiltration of the T cells into the tumor the corresponding anti-T-cell antibodies follow and also localize there.

3. A soluble factor released by T cells may be bound by nonlymphoid tumor cells. The binding site (or receptor) for the soluble factor on the tumor cell membrane acts as a modifying carrier for the otherwise nonimmunogenic factor thus rendering it able to induce antibodies against itself. These autoantibodies may in turn react against the factor when still bound by the tumor cells and/or when expressed on its cell of origin—the T cell. It is not unlikely that this factor is FcR released by activated T cells and bound by tumor cells, as suggested previously (Braslawsky *et al.*, 1976a,b; Witz, 1977).

The presence, and furthermore the induction, of TALCA in tumor bearers might have very important implications for tumor growth. If, indeed, those antibodies are directed against the FcR of T cells or even against an antigen closely associated with FcR, they might play a role in regulating the immune response of the host. FcR-bearing cells compose 20–30% of T cells, and these cells express various fundamental roles in immunity such as amplifier or effector cells participating in cell-mediated killing (Stout et al., 1977), killing by antibody-dependent cellular cytotoxicity (Kimura et al., 1977), or suppression of antibody-forming cells against sRBC (Fridman et al., 1978). It is possible that the decrease in FcR-positive suppressor cells occurring in tumor bearers (Whitney et al., 1978) might be caused by TALCA. In support of this hypothesis are findings obtained in our laboratory indicating that TALCA-sensitive cells have a decreased representation in the spleen of tumor bearers.

ACKNOWLEDGMENTS

This study was supported by Public Health Service Contract N01-CB-74134 from the Division of Cancer Biology and Diagnosis; by Grant 1R01 CA20088 awarded by the National Cancer Institute, National Institutes of Health, USA; and by a grant from the Israel Cancer Association.

We thank Mrs. Tamar Natanel and Mrs. Margot Lakonishuk for their excellent technical assistance. We thank engineer Mario Kuszpet from the Research Institute, Environmental Health, Tel Aviv University, School of Medicine, for animal irradiation.

IV. REFERENCES

Allison, A. C., Denman, A. M., and Barnes, R. D., 1971, Cooperating and controlling functions of thymus-derived lymphocytes in relation to auto immunity, Lancet 2:135.

Andersen, P., and Andersen, H. K., 1975, Smooth-muscle antibodies and other tissue antibodies in cytomegalovirus infection, Clin. Exp. Immunol. 22:22.

Braslawsky, G. R., Ran, M., and Witz, I. P., 1976a, Tumor-bound immunoglobulins: The relationship between the in vivo coating of tumor cells by potentially cytotoxic antitumor antibodies, and the expression of immune complex receptors, Int. J. Cancer 18:116.

Braslawsky, G. R., Serban, D., and Witz, I. P., 1976b, Receptors for immune complexes on cells within a polyoma-virus-induced murine sarcoma, Eur. J. Immunol. 6:579.

Brooks, W. H., Nesby, M. G., Normansell, D. E., and Horwitz, D. A., 1972, Depressed cell mediated immunity in patients with primary intracranial tumors. Characterization of humoral immunosuppression factor, J. Exp. Med. 136:1631.

Cooke, A., Hutchings, P. R., and Playfair, J. H. L., 1978, Suppressor T cells in experimental autoimmune haemolytic anaemia, Nature (London) 273:154.

DeLeo, A. B., Shiku, H., Takahaski, T., John, M., and Old, L. J., 1977, Cell surface antigens and chemically induced sarcomas of the mouse. I. murine leukemia virus-related antigens and alloantigens on cultured fibroblasts and sarcoma cells. Description of a unique antigen in Balb/c metho A sarcoma, *J. Exp. Med.* 146:720.

Ehrlich, R., and Witz, I. P., 1979, The elution of antibodies from viable murine tumor cells, *J. Immunol. Methods* 26:345.

Forbes, A. P., Lake, J. F., and Bloch, K., 1976, Circulating antibody to renal collecting ducts in patients with hepatoma or renal cell carcinoma, *Clin. Exp. Immunol.* 26:426.

Fridman, H., Fradelizi, D., Guinezanes, A., Plater, C., and Leclerc, J. C., 1978, The role of the Fc receptor (FcR) of thymus-derived lymphocytes. II. Presence of FcR on suppressor cells and direct involvement in suppression, *Eur. J. Immunol.* 8:549.

Fujimoto, S., Green, M. I., and Sehon, A. H., 1976, Regulation of the immune response to tumor antigens. II. The nature of immunosuppressor cells in tumor-bearing hosts, *J. Immunol.* 116:800.

Furnie, G. J., Lambert, P. H., and Miescher, P. A., 1974, Release of DNA in circulating blood and induction of anti DNA antibodies after injection of bacterial lypopolysaccharide, *J. Exp. Med.* 140:1189.

Gabbioni, G., Trencher, P., and Holborrow, E. J., 1975, Increase of contractile proteins in human cancer cells, *Lancet* 2:796.

Galili, N., Naor, D., Asjo, B., and Klein, G., 1976, Induction of immune responsiveness in a genetically low-responsive tumor host combination by chemical modification of the immunogen, *J. Immunol.* 6:473.

Garrido, F., Schirrmacher, V., and Festenstein, M., 1976, H-2 like specificities of foreign haplotypes appearing on mouse sarcoma after vaccine virus injection, *Nature (London)* 259:228.

Haba, S., Hamaoka, T., Takatsu, K., and Kitogawa, M., 1976, Selective suppression of T-cell activity in tumor-bearing mice and its improvement by lentinan, a potent antitumor polysaccharide, *Int. J. Cancer* 18:93.

Holden, H. T., Haskill, J. S., Kirchner, H., and Herberman, R. B., 1976, Two distinct antitumor effector cells isolated from primary murine sarcomavirus-induced tumors, *J. Immunol.* 117:440.

Humphrey, L. J., Volenec, P. J., Volenec, F. J., and Cross, D., 1977, Autoantibodies to an altered IgG in human breast cancer, *J. Surg. Oncol.* 9:29.

Ioachim, H. L., 1976, The stromal reaction of tumors. An expression of immune surveillance, *J. Natl. Cancer Inst.* 57:465.

Jacquemin, P. C., Saxinger, C., and Gallo, R. C., 1978, Surface antibodies of human myelogenous leukemia leukocytes reactive with specific type-C viral reverse transcriptases, *Nature (London)* 276:230.

Kerbel, R. S., and Davies, A. J. S., 1974, The possible biological significance of Fc receptors in mammalian cells lymphocytes and tumor cells, *Cell* 3:105.

Kerbel, R. S., Pross, H. F., and Elliot, E. V., 1975, Origin and partial characterization of Fc receptor-bearing cells found within experimental carcinomas and sarcomas, *Int. J. Cancer* 15:918.

Kimura, A. K., Rubin, B., and Anderson, L. C., 1977, Evidence of K-cell killing by alloreactive Fc receptor-bearing cytotoxic T lymphocytes, *Scand. J. Immunol.* 6:787.

Klein, G., Ehlin, B., and Witz, I. P., 1977, Serological detection of a polyoma-tumor-associated membrane antigen, *Int. J. Cancer* 23:683.

Leclerc, J. C., Platen, C., and Fridman, W. H., 1977, The role of the Fc receptor (FcR) of thymus-derived lymphocytes. I. Presence of FcR on cytotoxic lymphocytes and absence of direct role in cytotoxicity, *Eur. J. Immunol.* 8:543.

Martin, W. J., and Martin, S. E., 1975, Thymus reactive IgM autoantibodies in normal mouse sera, *Nature (London)* 254:716.

McMaster, R., Buhler, K., Whitney, R., and Levy, J. G., 1977, Immunosuppression of T lymphocyte function by fractionated serum from tumor bearing mice, *J. Immunol.* 118:218.

Milgrom, F., Humphrey, L., Tønder, O., Yasuda, J., and Witebsky, E., 1968, Antibody mediated hemadsorption by tumor tissues, *Int. Arch. Allergy Appl. Immunol.* 33:478.

Moav, N., and Witz, I. P., 1978, Characterization of immunoglobulins eluted from murine tumor cells. Binding patterns of cytotoxic anti-tumor IgG, *J. Immunol. Methods* 22:51.

Müller, N., and Koenig, U. D., 1977, Cold lymphocytotoxic antibodies in sera of patients with cervical carcinoma, *Blut* 34:479.

Nelson, D. S., 1977, Autoantibodies in cancer patients, *Pathology* 9:155.

Nepom, J. T., Hellström, I., and Hellström, K. E., 1976, Purification and partial characterization of a tumor-specific blocking factor from sera of mice with growing chemically induced sarcomas, *J. Immunol.* 117:1846.

Profitt, M. R., Hirsh, M. S., Ellis, D. A., Gheridian, B., and Black, P. H., 1975, Immunological mechanisms in the pathogenesis of virus-induced murine leukemia. II. Target cell specificity of auto reactive thymocytes, *J. Immunol.* 117:11.

Quan, P. C., and Burtin, P., 1978, Demonstration of nonspecific suppressor cells in the peripheral lymphocytes of cancer patients, *Cancer Res.* 38:288.

Ran, M., and Witz, I. P., 1970, Tumor-associated immunoglobulins. The elution of IgG2 from mouse tumors, *Int. J. Cancer* 6:361.

Ran, M., Klein, G., and Witz, I. P., 1976, Tumor-bound immunoglobulins. Evidence for the *in vivo* coating of tumor cells by potentially cytotoxic antitumor antibodies, *Int. J. Cancer* 4:90.

Ran, M., Yaakubowicz, M., and Witz, I. P., 1978, Lymphocytotoxic autoantibodies eluted from *in vivo* propagating sarcoma cells: Brief communication, *J. Natl. Cancer Inst.* 60:1509.

Rand, R. J., Henkins, D. M., and Bulmer, R., 1977, T and B lymphocyte subpopulations in preinvasive and invasive carcinoma of the cervix, *Clin. Exp. Immunol.* 30:421.

Shiku, H., Takahasi, T., Resnick, L. A., Oettgen, H. R., and Old, L. T., 1977, Cell surface antigens of human malignant melanoma. III. Recognition of autoantibodies with unusual characteristics, *J. Exp. Med.* 145:784.

Sjörgren, H. A., 1964a, Studies on specific transplantation resistance to polyoma-virus-induced tumors. I. Transplantation resistance induced by polyoma-virus injection, *J. Natl. Cancer Inst.* 32:361.

Sjörgren, H. A., 1964b, Studies on specific transplantation resistance to polyoma-virus-induced tumors. II. Mechanism of resistance induced by polyoma-virus injection, *J. Natl. Cancer Inst.* 32:375.

Steinberg, A. K., Gershwin, M. E., and Gerber, N. L., 1975, Role of suppressor cells in the pathogenesis of autoimmunity in New Zealand mice, in: *Immune Depression and Cancer* (G. W. Siskind, C. L. Christian, and S. D. Litwin, eds.), p. 42, Grune and Stratton, New York.

Stout, R. D., Murphy, D. B., McDevitt, H. O., and Herzenberg, L. A., 1977, The Fc receptor on thymus-derived lymphocytes. IV. Inhibition of binding of antigen–antibody complexes to Fc receptor-positive T cells by anti-Ia sera. *J. Exp. Med.* 145:187.

Succi-Foca, N., Buda, J., McManus, J., Threpp, T., and Rumsta, K., 1973, Impaired responsiveness of lymphocytes and serum inhibitory factors in patients with cancer, *Cancer Res.* 33:2373.

Sugai, S., Palmer, D. W., Talal, W., and Witz, I. P., 1974, Protective and cellular immune responses to idiotypic determinants on cells from a spontaneous lymphoma of NZB/NZW F1 mice, *J. Exp. Med.* 140:1547.

Talal, N., and Steinberg, A. K., 1974, The pathogenesis of autoimmunity in New Zealand black mice, *Curr. Top. Microbiol. Immunol.* 64:79.

Thunold, S., Abeyounis, C. J., Milgrom, F., and Witebsky, E., 1970, Anti-γ-globulin factors in serum and tissue of cancer patients, *Int. Arch. Allergy Appl. Immunol.* **38**:260.

Toh, B. H., and Müller, H. K., 1975, Smooth muscle-associated antigen in experimental cutaneous squamous cell carcinoma, keratoacantoma and papilloma, *Cancer Res.* **33**:3741.

Tønder, O., and Thunold, S., 1973, Receptors for immunoglobulin Fc in human malignant tissues, *Scand. J. Immunol.* **2**:207.

Tønder, O., Krishman, E. C., Jewell, W. R., Morse, P. A., Jr., and Humphrey, L. J., 1976, Tumor Fc receptors and tumor-associated immunoglobulins, *Acta. Pathol. Microbiol. Scand. Sect. C* **84**:105.

Waksman, B. H., and Tada, T., 1977, Specific and nonspecific suppressed T-cell factors derived from thymic lymphocytes, *Cell. Immunol.* **30**:189.

Wasserman, J., Glass, U., and Blomgren, H., 1975, Autoantibodies in patients with carcinoma of the breast. Correlation with prognosis, *Clin. Exp. Immunol.* **19**:417.

Whitney, R. B., Kelly, D. B., and Levy, J. C., 1978, Immunosuppression in mice bearing primary tumors, *Eur. J. Cancer* **14**:699.

Witz, I. P., 1977, Tumor-bound immunoglobulins. *In situ* expression of tumor immunity, *Adv. Cancer Res.* **25**:95.

Witz, I. P., Lee, W., and Klein, G., 1976, Serologically detectable specific and cross reactive antigens on the membrane of a polyoma-virus-induced murine tumor, *Int. J. Cancer* **18**:243.

Wood, A. W., Gillespie, G. V., and Barth, R. F., 1975, Receptor sites for antigen–antibody complexes on cells derived from solid tumors. Detection by means of antibody sensitized sheep erythrocytes labeled with technetium 99m, *J. Immunol.* **114**:950.

Yasuda-Yasaki, Y., and Yoshida, T. O., 1975, Isolation of a "speckled" nuclear antigen reactive with autoantibodies in patients with cancer and autoimmune diseases, *Scand. J. Immunol.* **21**:357.

Chapter 10

Correlations between Tumor Antigenicity, Malignant Potential, and Local Host Immune Response

Harry L. Ioachim

Department of Pathology   and   *Department of Pathology*
Lenox Hill Hospital   *College of Physicians and Surgeons*
New York, New York 10021   *Columbia University*
                                     New York, New York 10032

I. INTRODUCTION

In the process of induction and growth of tumors, complex interrelationships are established between tumor and host. Among the multiple participating factors, some are particularly important in determining the outcome of tumor growth. To understand this complex interrelationship, it is therefore necessary to identify the determinant factors of tumor–host interaction and to study their functions.

In an experimental tumor system, we have explored various parameters that influence the growth of tumors and came to the conclusion that three major factors played a determinant role: the malignant potential of a tumor, the tumor antigenicity, and the immune response of the host.

In the study of human tumors an analysis of all these parameters is not entirely feasible, since essential qualities of tumor cells such as antigenic expression still cannot be fully evaluated. However, progress is being made by exploring new, previously neglected aspects of host–tumor relationship such as the local immune response to neoplasia (Black and Leis, 1971; Baldwin *et al.*, 1972; Ran and Witz, 1972; Underwood, 1972; Thunold *et al.*, 1973; von Kleist *et al.*, 1974; Irie *et al.*, 1975; Dorsett *et al.*, 1975; Zeromski *et al.*, 1975; Dorval *et al.*, 1976; Ioachim *et al.*, 1976; Lewis *et al.*, 1976; Koneval *et al.*, 1977).

In the present review, the correlations between major parameters of host–tumor interaction will be examined in both animal and human systems. Data regarding such correlations obtained from the study of experimental virus-

213

induced rat leukemia will be presented first. In a second part, observations and experiments indicating the presence of cellular and humoral immune responses in human tumors will be described. Finally, the conclusions obtained from animal experiments will be applied to the interpretation of human cancer in an attempt to better understand the role of host–tumor relationships in the process of neoplasia.

II. MALIGNANT POTENTIAL AND ANTIGENICITY OF TUMOR CELLS

Some tumors are more malignant than others. Tumors expressing a high malignant potential grow progressively when transplanted in suitable hosts, rapidly invade the surrounding tissues, and are able to disseminate and establish distant metastases. Numerous attempts have been made to properly assess the malignant potential of tumors, and well-known correlations have been established between the behavior of tumors and their histological, cytological, and karyotypical features. More recently, new correlations have been uncovered linking the malignant potential of tumor cells to their antigenic expression (Baldwin *et al.*, 1972; Alexander, 1974; Ioachim *et al.*, 1974*b,c*; Kobayashi *et al.*, 1975; Lewis *et al.*, 1976; G. Klein and Klein, 1977). In some tumor systems, such as the one to be described, an absence of antigenicity was the determinant factor of tumor transplantability, invasiveness, and metastatic capacity (Alexander, 1974; Iochim *et al.*, 1974*b,c*, 1975, 1977*a*; Kim *et al.*, 1975; Kobayashi *et al.*, 1975; G. Klein and Klein, 1977; Jamasbi and Nettesheim, 1977; Kuzumaki *et al.*, 1978).

Tissue culture line LT_1 was established from a Gross murine leukemia virus (G-MuLV)-induced thymoma in a W/Fu rat and continuously maintained *in vitro* since 1962 (Ioachim *et al.*, 1966). The LT_1 cells have the morphological appearance of neoplastic lymphoblasts and a short doubling time, and they replicate continuously the original G-MuLV. Abundant virus particles bud and mature at the plasma membrane of LT_1 cells, being subsequently released in the medium as mature virions (Fig. 1). As a result, the cells express strong, specific virus antigenicity at both cytoplasmic and membrane levels. This can be readily revealed in immunofluorescence assays (Ioachim and Sabbath, 1979), using anti-G-MuLV sera prepared in syngeneic rats and FITC-labeled goat antirat sera. Specific granular cytoplasmic fluorescence and granular, ringlike membrane fluorescence (Fig. 2) are easily demonstrated, while with similar specific sera and horseradish-peroxidase-labeled rabbit antirat sera, the location of G-MuLV antigens on the cell membrane can be visualized under the electron microscope (Ioachim and Sabbath, 1979). Cytotoxicity tests using rat anti-G-MuLV sera against LT_1 cells accordingly show cytotoxicity indexes of over 90% (Ioachim and Sabbath, 1979).

Transplantation attempts with LT_1 cells in normal adult, syngeneic rats have

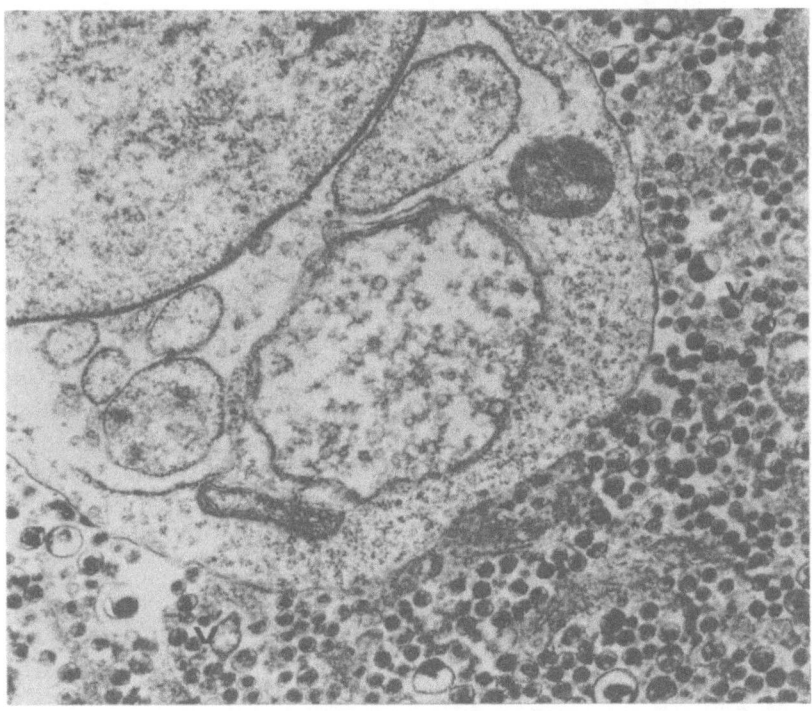

Figure 1. LT$_1$ cell in tissue culture showing abundant production of Gross murine leukemia virus (V) ($\times$16,000).

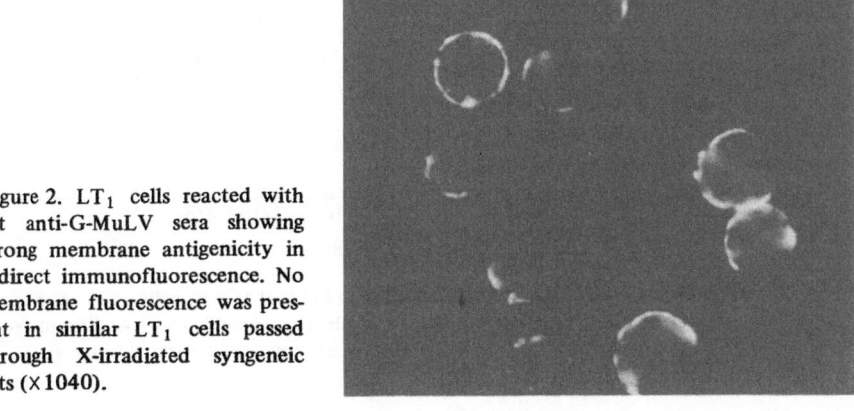

Figure 2. LT$_1$ cells reacted with rat anti-G-MuLV sera showing strong membrane antigenicity in indirect immunofluorescence. No membrane fluorescence was present in similar LT$_1$ cells passed through X-irradiated syngeneic rats ($\times$1040).

been consistently negative; however, the same cells grow progressively and kill the recipients when transplanted in rats up to 10 days of age or in rats treated with 300 R total body X irradiation (Ioachim *et al.*, 1965, 1977*a*). By various manipulations, to be later detailed, we have been able to originate antigenically negative lines of LT$_1$ cells. Although morphologically identical to the original LT$_1$-G-MuLV+ cells, the new lines of LT$_1$-G-MuLV- cells were totally areactive in immunofluorescence and resisted killing in cytotoxicity tests (Fig. 3) (Ioachim *et al.*, 1974*b*, 1975). When transplantation was attempted with these cells, a sharp increase in malignant potential was recorded. The negative LT$_1$ cells grew progressively in all normal adult W/Fu rats, killing the recipients (Table I) (Ioachim *et al.*, 1974*b*, 1975, 1977*a*). There was local as well as extensive distant invasion (Fig. 4). Not only were the lymph nodes and spleen, which are occasionally involved in primary thymomas, affected, but large masses of metastatic tumors were present in the liver, kidneys (Fig. 5), lungs (Fig. 6), and adrenals, organs which are rarely the site of lymphoid tumors. Regardless of the site of injection, subcutaneous, intraperitoneal, or intravenous, the antigenically positive cells were consistently rejected whereas equal numbers of antigenically negative

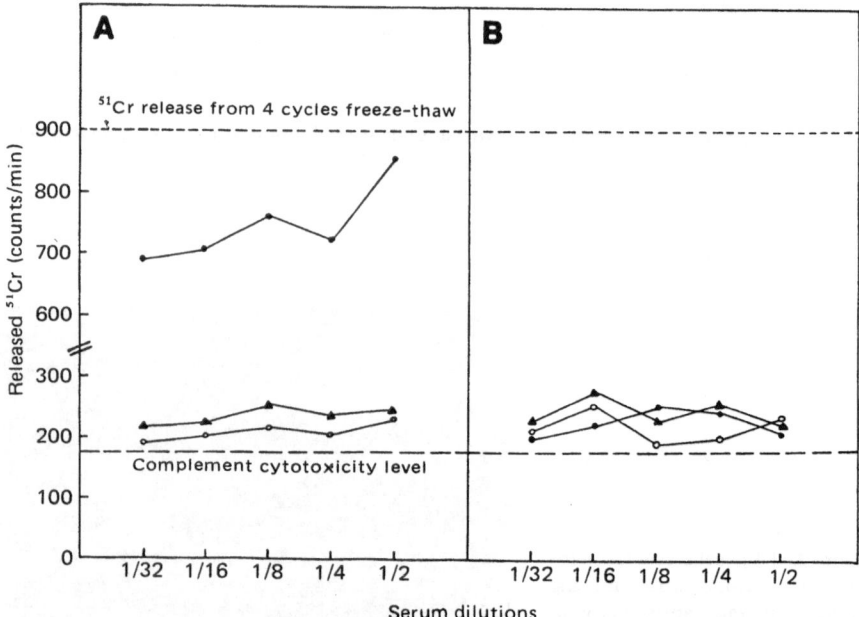

Figure 3. Serum cytotoxicity against G-MuLV+ (A) and G-MuLV- (B) cells. (●——●) Serum from W/Fu rat grafted s.c. with G-MuLV+ cells. Cells are rejected. (▲——▲) Serum from W/Fu rat grafted s.c. with G-MuLV- cells. Cells are accepted and form tumors. (○——○) Serum from W/Fu rat nongrafted (control).

Table I. Antigenic Conversion of G-MuLV+ Cells Grafted in X-Irradiated
W/Fu Rats

Generation	Treatment	Tumors (%)		Metastases (%)		Antigens		Antibodies
1	350R	7/9	(77)	6/9	(66)	+	-	144 (8–512)
2	None	18/21	(85)	12/21	(57)	-	-	684 (32–4096)
3	None	20/21	(95)	20/21	(95)	-	-	72 (16–256)
4	None	18/20	(90)	18/20	(90)	-	-	25 (4–64)
5	None	14/14	(100)	14/14	(100)	-	-	14 (4–64)
Controls	None	0/23	(0)	0/23	(0)	+	+	83 (32–128)

cells established tumors and killed the recipients every time. Finally, the difference in malignant potential of G-MuLv+ and G-MuLV- cells was again demonstrated when a similar number of cells of both lines was injected subcutaneously on opposite sides of the same recipient (Ioachim et al., 1974b, 1975). All rats grew huge tumors on the side injected with MuLV- cells, whereas no trace of the injected MuLV+ cells was found on the opposite side when the rats were sacrificed 3 months later (Fig. 7).

In these experiments, the change in membrane antigenicity was induced by transfer of cells in vivo -in vitro (Ioachim et al., 1972, 1974c). Although the antigenic changes were reversible and the two lines of cells were different only in regard to their antigenic expression, the malignant potential of these cells was totally reversed and appeared to depend directly on the lack of membrane antigenicity of the tumor cells.

Supported by these (Ioachim et al., 1974b,c, 1975, 1977a) and other experiments reported in the literature (Fenyö et al., 1968; Baldwin et al., 1972; Bartlett, 1972; Kim et al., 1975; Cikes, 1975; Kobayashi et al., 1975; G. Klein and Klein, 1977; Mora et al., 1977; Jamasbi and Nettesheim, 1977; Alexander, 1977; Kuzumaki et al., 1978), an inversely proportional correlation can thus be established between the membrane antigenicity of tumor cells and their malignant potential.

III. ANTIGENICITY OF TUMOR CELLS AND HOST IMMUNE RESPONSE

As mentioned earlier, G-MuLV+ cells obtained either from thymomas or from our permanent LT_1 cell line are not accepted when transplanted into normal adult, immunocompetent syngeneic rats, whereas they establish invasive tumors in immunodeficient newborn and X-irradiated recipients. While this behavior appears expectable, it was discovered in the course of our experiments that the G-MuLV+ cells growing in X-irradiated rats had undergone fundamental

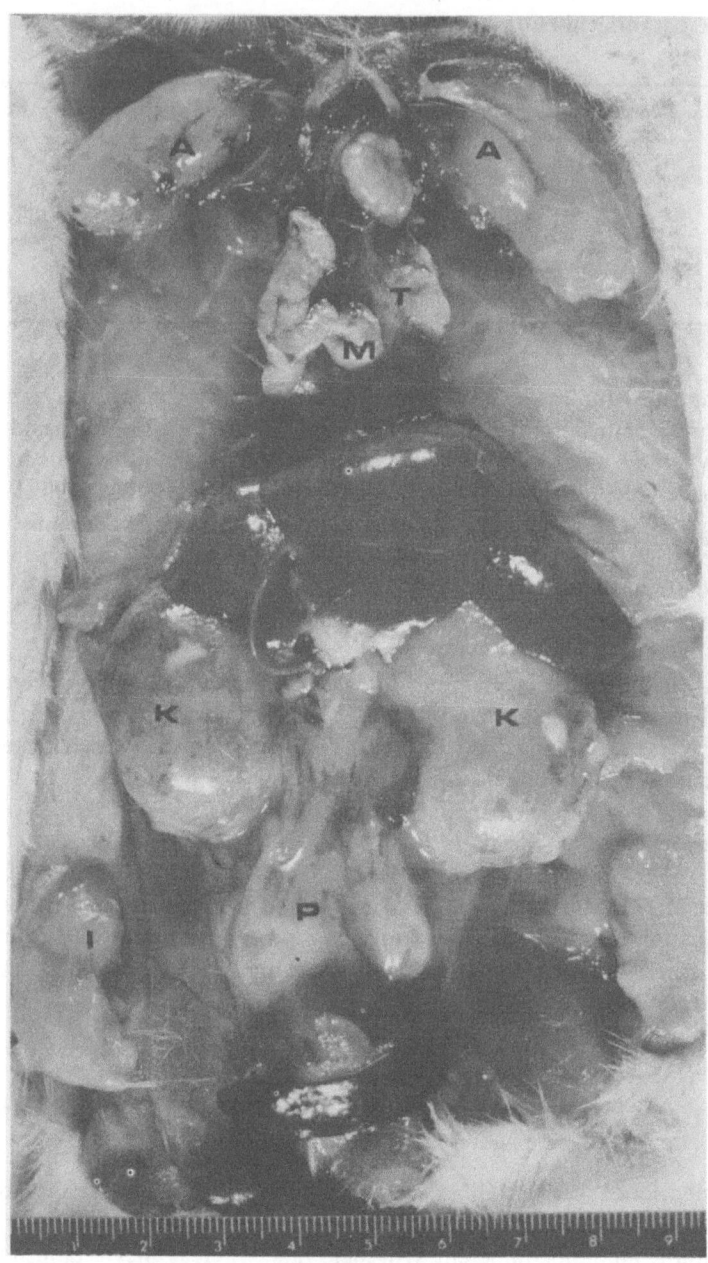

Figure 4. W/Fu rat grafted s.c. with G-MuLV– lymphoma cells showing extensive metastases in both kidneys (K), axillary (A), mediastinal (M), peritoneal (P), and inguinal lymph (I) nodes. Thymus (T), spleen, and liver not involved.

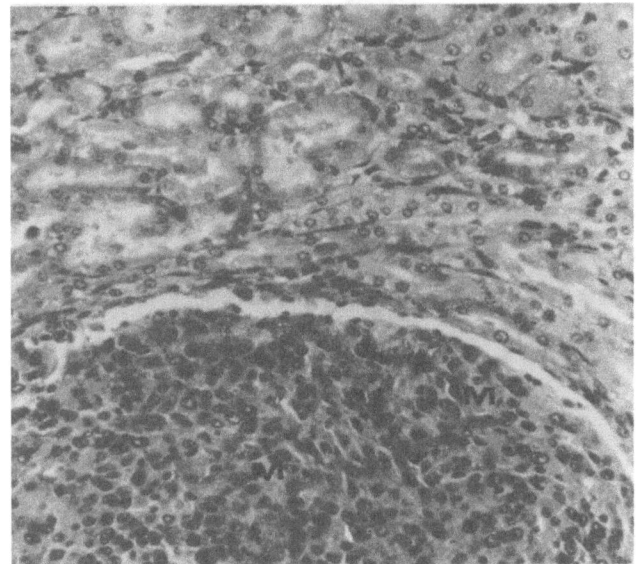

Figure 5. Renal metastasis (M) in W/Fu rat grafted s.c. with G-MuLV– lymphoma cells (×240).

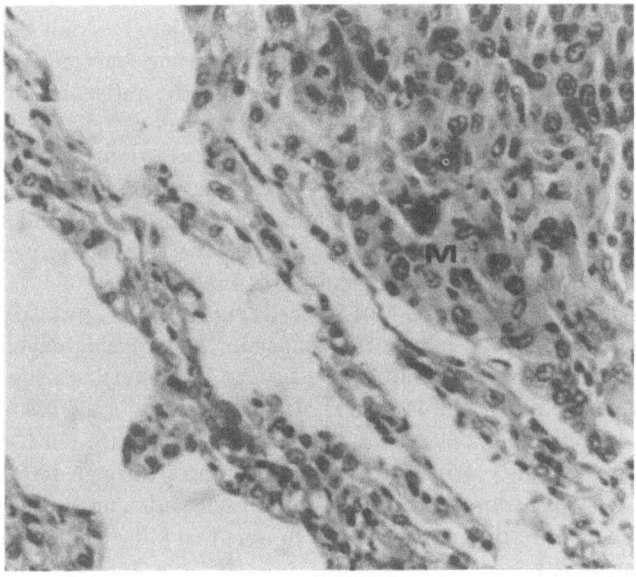

Figure 6. Lung metastasis (M) in W/Fu rat grafted s.c with G-MuLV– lymphoma cells (×320).

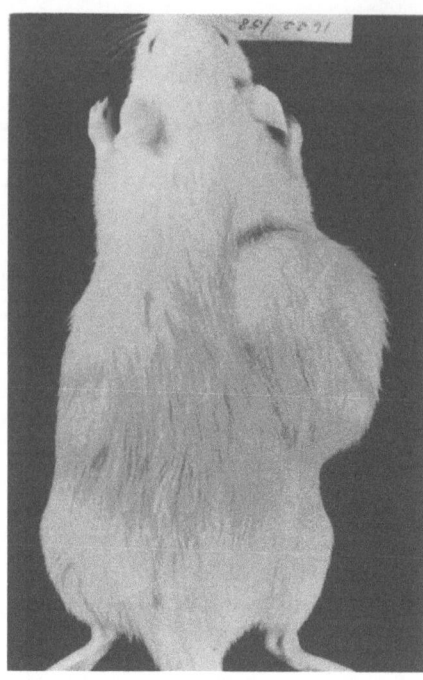

Figure 7. W/Fu rat grafted s.c. with 5×10^5 G-MuLV+ cells on left side (no tumor) and with 5×10^5 G-MuLV– cells on right side (large, growing tumor).

changes in both antigenicity and malignant potential (Ioachim *et al.*, 1977*a*). Examined in indirect immunofluorescence after being reacted with rat anti-G-MuLV serum, the cells showed a total loss of membrane antigenicity subsequently confirmed by a substantial drop in the cytotoxicity index (Fig. 3). Even more surprising, when these now negative G-MuLV cells were transplanted into normal adult rats, they were not only accepted but displayed unusual malignant potential, growing rapidly at the site of injection and metastasizing widely to various organs (Figs. 4–6). After these initial changes, the cells became serially transplantable in any number of normal adult rats (Table I).

Thus a single passage of G-MuLV+ cells through an X-irradiated, immunodeficient host was able to induce the conversion of antigenic expression as well as the change in transplantability, invasiveness, and metastasizing capacity of these cells (Ioachim *et al.*, 1977*a,b*). In more recent experiments, a similar cellular conversion was obtained by successive transplantation of G-MuLV+ cells in 1- to 6-day-old rats. When after several passages through immunodeficient infant rats the cells were transplanted into normal adults, most cells had become G-MuLV– and as a result grew into large tumors that killed the recipients (Pearse and Ioachim, 1978).

Finally, a third means of converting antigenically positive to antigenically negative cells and consequently increasing their malignant potential was by passage of leukemia cells through hosts made immunologically unresponsive at birth (Ioachim et al., 1974b,c, 1975). A soluble antigen from G-MuLV+ cells was prepared (Ioachim et al., 1974c) and injected into 1- to 3-day-old syngeneic W/Fu rats. When 3 months old, the rats conditioned at birth were grafted with G-MuLV+ cells. In contrast to the unconditioned controls, which all rejected the transplants, the cells grew in the conditioned rats, underwent antigenic conversion, and subsequently became transplantable in all normal, nonconditioned adult rats.

Thus, by apparently different means we succeeded in inducing an antigenic conversion in leukemia cells that increased substantially their malignant potential and was permanently carried in further generations (Ioachim et al., 1975). However, when G-MuLV- cells were explanted in vitro, antigenic reversion was obtained and the cells resumed viral replication and antigenic expression (Ioachim et al., 1972). Even cells lines that had been serially transplanted in normal adults for up to 2 years reverted to become G-MuLV+ after grown in vitro for variable periods of time.

These experiments led to remarkable conclusions. They showed that the host immune response can produce a spectrum of results ranging from the complete eradication of tumor cells to the induction of substantial alterations in their antigenic expression and consequently in their malignant potential. The inducers of antigenic changes of tumor cells are the specific antibodies directed against these cells as part of the host immune response (Table I). Tumor cells under the effect of specific antibodies are able to modulate their antigenic expression as a modality of escape from destruction (Klein, 1975; Ioachim, 1976; Alexander, 1977). We have demonstrated the occurrence of modulation of G-MuLV antigens of leukemia cells under the effect of specific antibodies not only in vivo as previously described but also in vitro when anti-G-MuLV antisera were added to the cultures of G-MuLV+ LT$_1$ cells (Ioachim and Sabbath, 1979).

The conclusions of these experiments indicate that antigen-positive tumor cells can be consistently destroyed by immunocompetent hosts. However, immunoincompetent hosts (newborns, infants, X-irradiated, tolerant) usually mount an inadequate response, in which an excess of antibodies may induce antigenic modulation of tumor cells, thus insuring their escape from destruction. Even more unfortunate, the modulated tumor cells, lacking antigenic expression, exhibit a considerably higher malignant potential. Thus, an inadequate immune response, instead of leading to tumor cell eradication, may achieve the opposite effect of selecting for the least antigenic and consequently the most malignant clones of tumor cells.

IV. THE LOCAL CELLULAR ANTITUMOR IMMUNE RESPONSE

Long before the present concepts of tumor immunology were developed, changing this field of oncology into one of the fastest growing areas of medical research, pathologists were puzzled by the presence of inflammatory cells within the tumor tissues. Russel (1908), Murphy (1921), and Ewing (1940), among others, observed the infiltration of various tumors by lymphocytes, termed it "stromal reaction" (Russel, 1908), and regarded it as an indication of host resistance to tumor invasion.

In the succeeding years, the stromal reaction of tumors was studied by different authors (Berg, 1959; Takahashi, 1961; Black and Leis, 1971; E. R. Fisher and Fisher, 1972; Lauder and Aherne, 1972; Underwood, 1972; Barber *et al.*, 1975) in an attempt to find significant correlations with tumor prognosis and patients' survival. Although such investigations were contributory, direct histological–clinical correlations were not revealed, which resulted in a lack of interest for similar studies. It is reasonable to assume that the many variables affecting the complex processes of tumor growth do not allow the formulation of simple bifactorial correlations. Yet the cellular infiltrates of tumors remain an intriguing reality that is consistently present and appears to reflect the immune mechanisms of host defense.

To investigate the cellular reactions of neoplasms, we examined histologic sections of a variety of malignant tumors, including different organs, different histological types, different grades of differentiation, early and advanced stages, and primary and metastatic.

One of our studies was concerned with the immune response at the tumor site in lung carcinoma (Ioachim *et al.*, 1976). The morphology of the local cellular reactions was comparatively examined in 50 lung tumors that were diagnosed as squamous cell carcinoma (21 cases), adenocarcinoma (14 cases), bronchiolo–alveolar carcinoma (2 cases), small-cell (oat cell) carcinoma (5 cases), large-cell undifferentiated carcinoma (6 cases), and metastatic carcinoma (2 cases). The degrees of differentiation were evaluated on a scale from 1 to 4 as undifferentiated and poorly, moderately, and well differentiated, and the capacity for tumor invasion was estimated in relation to the invasion of pulmonary tissues, blood vessels, and hilar lymph nodes. The invasion of local tissues was recorded as (1) round tumor nodules, (2) tumor cords, (3) monocellular tumor files, and (4) single-tumor-cell invasion, which were considered to indicate increasing degrees of aggresssiveness. The cellular reactions in the tumor tissues were estimated in relation to three parameters: amount, distribution, and composition. The latter was characterized as predominantly lymphocytic, predominantly plasmacytic, or mixed. The amount of cellular infiltration was graded on a scale from 1 to 4, and the distribution was considered in relation to the tumor cords as well as to bronchi and blood vessels.

The results of these studies showed that the amount of cellular infiltrates in and around lung carcinomas, clearly correlated with their histological types and degrees of differentiation. When the estimates of cellular amounts were averaged, it was noted that well-differentiated tumors had significantly more cellular infiltrates than poorly differentiated or undifferentiated tumors. Squamous

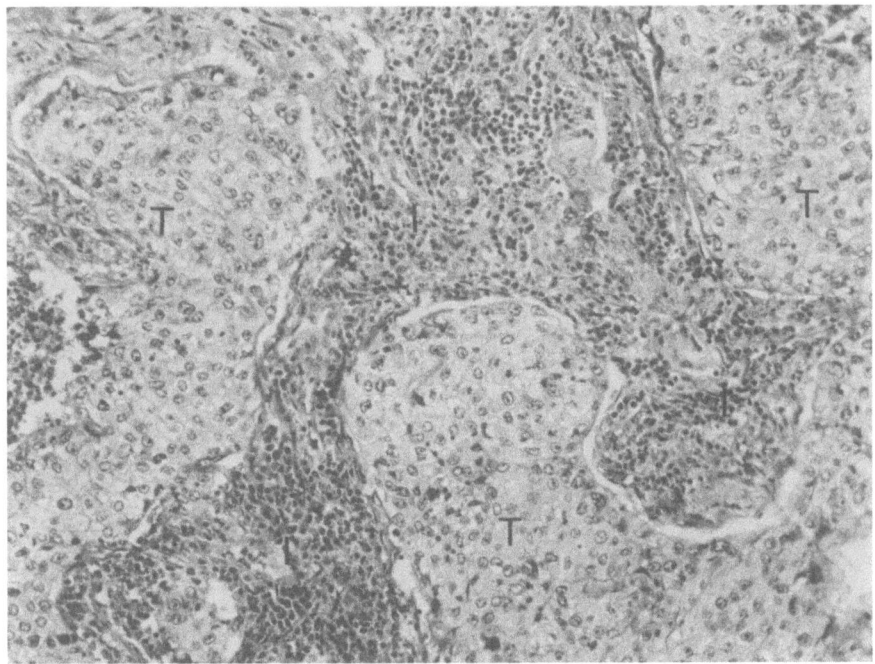

Figure 8. Squamous cell carcinoma of the lung. Broad cords of tumor cells (T) separated by abundant cellular infiltrates (I) of plasma cells and lymphocytes (×100, reproduced at 80%).

cell carcinomas, well differentiated, had the largest amounts of cellular infiltrates (Fig. 8), whereas oat cell carcinomas were almost entirely devoid of cellular infiltrates (Fig. 9). This contrast between the very large cellular infiltrates of squamous cell carcinomas, which sometimes exceeded the amount of tumor tissue, and their absence in oat cell carcinomas was striking and consistent.

The distribution of reactive cells was mostly at the periphery of tumor nodules in the less differentiated tumors and in between tumor cords and tumor cells in the squamous cell carcinomas. When the amount of cellular infiltration was high, such as in squamous cell carcinomas, lymphocytes were often seen within tumor cells.

Destruction of tumor cells, singly or in groups, surrounded by abundant agglomerates of lymphocytes and plasma cells was frequently noted in these tumors. The appearance of single tumor cell death due to lymphocytic activity was entirely distinct from the ischemic necrosis of tumor tissue that involved larger areas and was not accompanied by lymphoplasmacytic infiltration.

Of all parameters used, the composition of cellular infiltrates correlated best with the histological type of lung carcinoma. Plasma cells were present in large amounts in the squamous cell carcinomas (Fig. 10), while few or none were

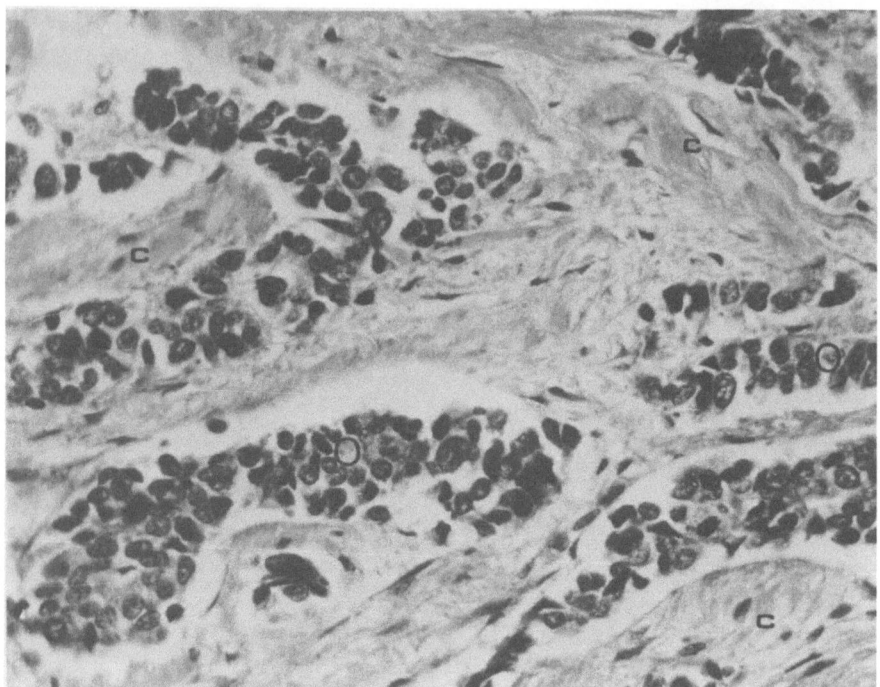

Figure 9. Small (oat) cell carcinoma of lung (O). Almost total absence of cellular reaction (C) (×250, reproduced at 80%).

seen in other histologic types. The well-differentiated squamous cell carcinomas that included the formation of keratin, exhibited the greatest numbers of plasma cells. Not unusually in such tumors, plasma cells were the only constituent of stromal cellular reactions, occasionally forming huge sheets of cells that sometimes exceeded the size of tumor cords (Figs. 8 and 10). It appeared that a direct correlation existed between the presence of keratin or keratin precursors in squamous cell carcinomas and the amount of plasma cells in the surrounding stroma. In the adenocarcinomas, plasma cells were present mostly in areas of squamous metaplasia. In lymph nodes with tumor metastases, numerous plasma cells were present in contact with the tumor, particularly when this was squamous cell carcinoma. On occasion, huge areas of lymph nodes invaded by metastatic squamous cell carcinoma were transformed in sheets of plasma cells. Fibrosis was noted in almost all lung carcinomas; however, its degree and distribution were variable. In general the amount of fibrocollagenous tissue around and within the tumor nodules was inversely proportional to the amount of cellular infiltrates. Tumors with abundant cellular reaction showed little proliferation of collagen fibers, whereas tumors with few or no cellular infiltrates contained broad, dense

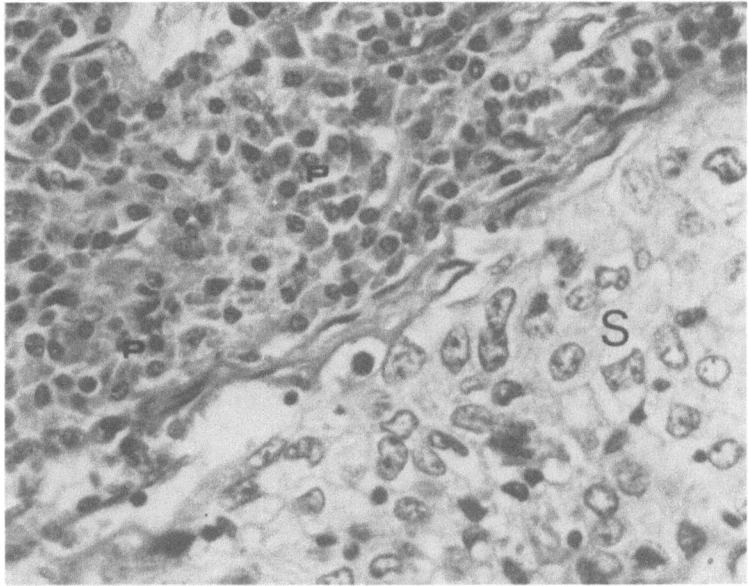

Figure 10. Squamous cell carcinoma of the lung (S) with cellular infiltrate composed exclusively of plasma cells (P) (×250).

bands of collagen. Even within the same tumor there were areas of fibrosis with poor cellularity, in contrast to areas of abundant cellular reaction that did not include a sizable fibrous component. Metastatic carcinomas to the lung showed patterns of cellular infiltrates similar in size and composition to those of primary carcinomas of same histological type.

In subsequent studies we examined the local cellular reaction in tumors of the tongue, breast (Fig. 11), esophagus, cervix (Fig. 12), endometrium, anus, and skin (Fig. 13) (Ioachim, 1976) and found that the squamous cell carcinomas (Fig. 12) were accompanied by the largest amounts of cellular infiltrates and that these types of tumors were consistently associated with plasma cells. Not infrequently the lymph nodes draining such tumors and including metastatic squamous cell carcinoma were also populated by masses of plasma cells replacing the normal population of lymphocytes. We were thus able to recognize patterns of cell reaction that were characteristic for different histologic types of tumors regardless of their organ location. The lymphoplasmacytic infiltrates of tumors did not appear to represent a nonspecific reaction in response to infected or necrotic tissues, because the cells usually responding to infection or necrosis were polymorphonuclears, not lymphocytes or plasma cells, and because our studies indicated clearly that carcinomas with the greatest amount of necrosis (e.g., oat cell carcinomas of the lung, undifferen-

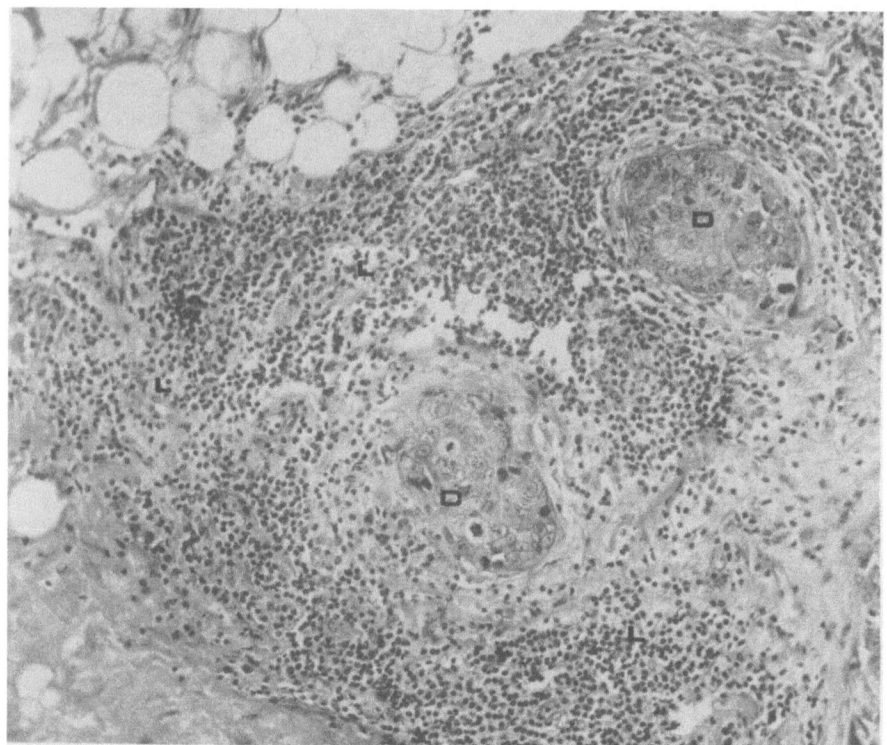

Figure 11. Mammary duct cell carcinoma. Two ducts (D) obliterated by carcinoma cells with atypical nuclei and frequent mitoses. Abundant lymphocytic infiltrate (L) surrounds the neoplastic ducts (×100, reproduced at 90%).

tiated carcinomas of various organs) comprised the least amount of cellular infiltration.

Considering that the cellular stromal reaction is an expression of immune surveillance against tumors (Ioachim, 1976), we investigated comparatively its presence in early and late stages of tumor growth as well as in primary and metastatic tumors. We were thus able to note the occurrence of heavy lymphocytic aggregates bordering the foci of various carcinomas *in situ*. In such neoplastic processes as carcinoma *in situ* of the bronchial epithelium, uterine cervix (Fig. 12), and vaginal mucosa; intraductal mammary carcinoma (Fig. 11); Bowen's disease of the skin; and Paget's disease of the nipple, although the tumor cells had not crossed the basement membranes and were still strictly intraepithelial, large collections of lymphocytes usually bordered the lesions and separated the epithelial cancer from the underlying stroma. Even when the epi-

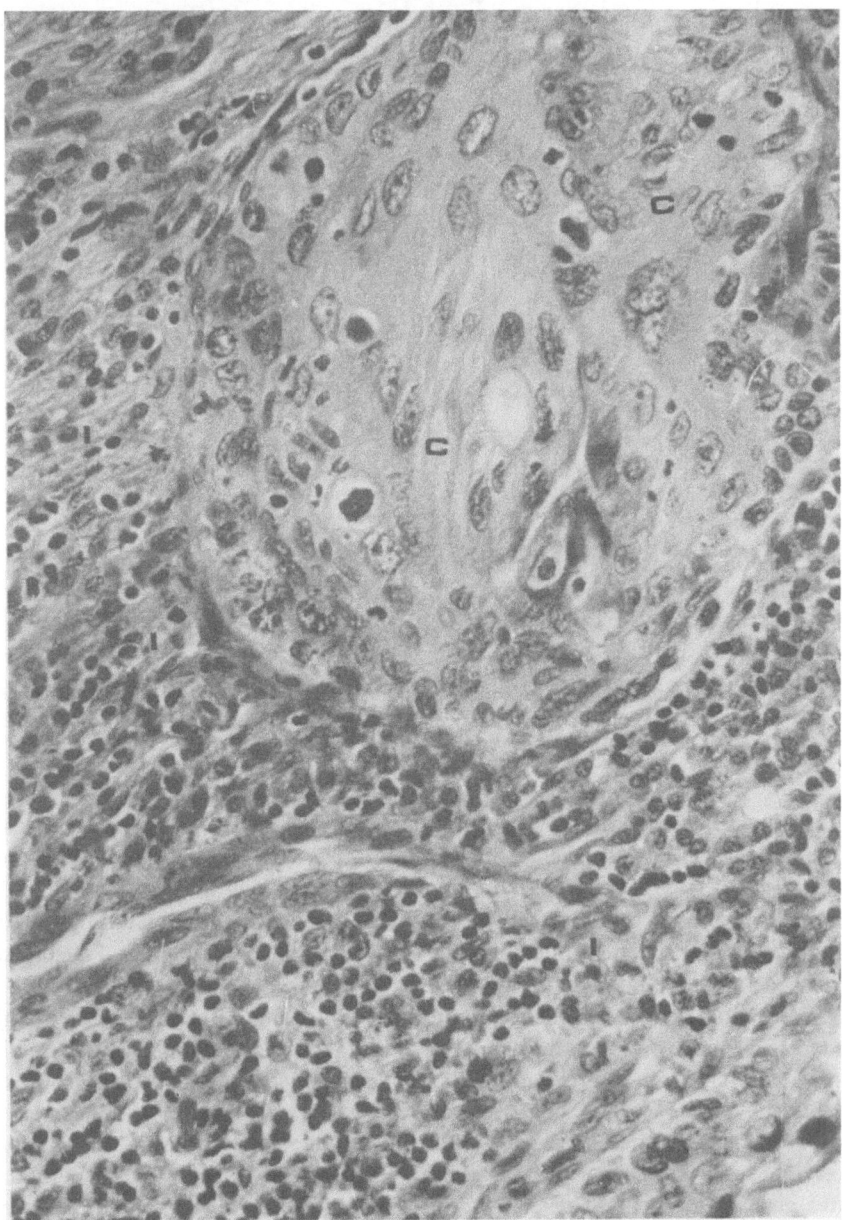

Figure 12. Squamous cell carcinoma *in situ* of uterine cervix. Although not yet invasive, the cancer cells (C) are surrounded by large amounts of plasma cells and lymphocytes (I) (×250).

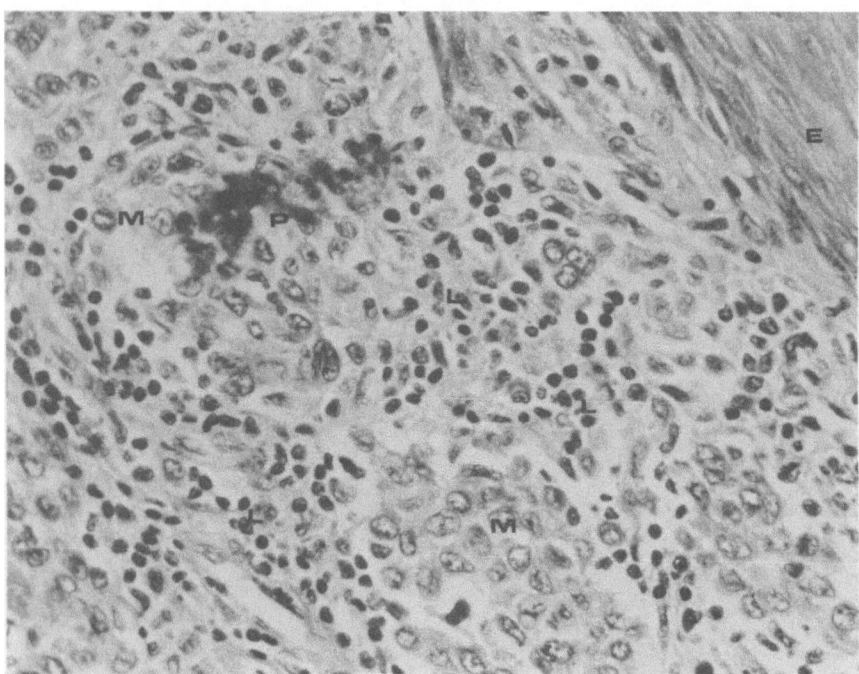

Figure 13. Melanoma of skin. Unaffected epidermis (E), nests of malignant melanoma cells (M), melanin-laden macrophages (P), and numerous lymphocytes (L) (×250, reproduced at 80%).

thelial changes were only preneoplastic, like those of dysplasia of laryngeal, bronchial, or cervical epithelia, numerous lymphocytes were selectively aggregated below the affected areas. In superficially spreading melanomas (Fig. 13) as well as in incipient basal cell carcinomas of the skin, the accumulation of lymphocytes consistently accompanied the tumors and in doubtful instances furnished a reliable indicator of neoplastic change.

The histology of precancerous and early cancerous lesions compared with that of advanced, invasive, recurrent, or metastatic carcinomas almost invariably showed a significantly greater cellular stromal reaction in the first group of neoplasms.

In conclusion, our histologic studies showed that the growth of most tumors is accompanied by a local cellular reaction represented by infiltrates of lymphocytes and plasma cells. The cellular infiltrates are generally greater in primary than in metastatic tumors, greater in early than in advanced tumors, and greater in differentiated than in undifferentiated tumors. A consistent association, not previously reported, between plasma cells and squamous cell carcinomas of various organs was also described (Ioachim et al., 1974a, 1976).

V. THE LOCAL HUMORAL ANTITUMOR IMMUNE RESPONSE

A great number of experimental and clinical studies have demonstrated the presence of circulating tumor-associated antibodies in tumor-bearing animals (Klein and Sjögren, 1960; Hellström *et al.*, 1970; Herberman and Oren, 1971; Baldwin *et al.*, 1973) and man (Gold, 1967; Morton *et al.*, 1968; Herberman *et al.*, 1968; Bubenick *et al.*, 1970; Henle *et al.*, 1973; Lewis *et al.*, 1973) and have attempted to assess their beneficial (Essex *et al.*, 1971; Alexander, 1974; Lewis *et al.*, 1978) and detrimental (Hellström *et al.*, 1970; Baldwin *et al.*, 1972; Witz, 1973; Lewis *et al.*, 1978) effects.

Fewer studies have been concerned with the presence of immunoglobulins at the tumor site, although it is reasonable to assume that more tumor-specific antibodies will be found in contact with the tumor than in the general circulation. Indeed, lower animal (Sobczac and De Vaux Saint Cyr, 1971; Dorval *et al.*, 1976) and human (Sjögren *et al.*, 1972; Ran and Witz, 1972; Thunold *et al.*, 1973; Gupta and Morton, 1975; Dorsett *et al.*, 1975; Irie *et al.*, 1975; Koneval *et al.*, 1977; Paluch and Ioachim, 1978) studies showed that immunoglobulins are associated with various malignant tumors and that their presence in tumor tissues as either free or tumor-bound antibodies can be demonstrated. The selective accumulation of plasma cells and lymphocytes (Fig. 14) in and around tumor tissues (Ioachim, 1976; Ioachim *et al.*, 1974*a*, 1976) further supported

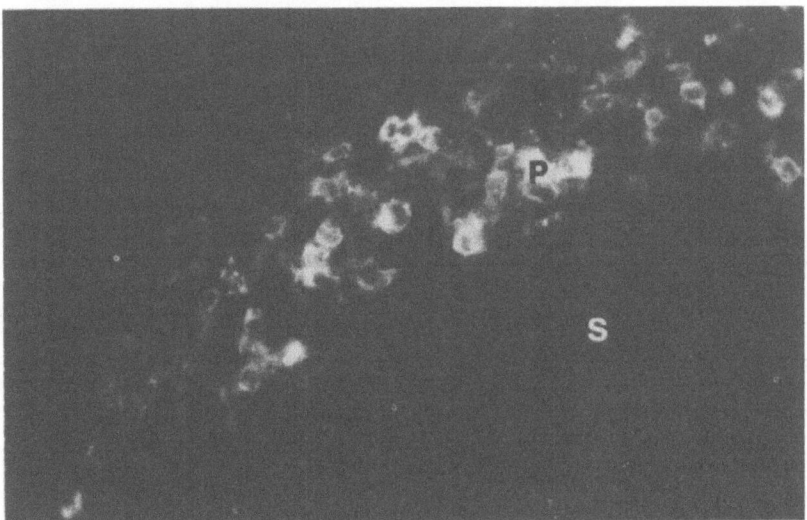

Figure 14. Squamous cell carcinoma of lung (S) reacted in direct immunofluorescence with FITC-labeled antihuman polyvalent Ig serum. Peritumoral plasma cells (P) show intra-cytoplasmic fluorescence (× 400).

the idea that tumor-specific antibodies are produced and released at the tumor site, which consequently appears to be the most favorable place for their isolation and identification.

In addition to the elution of free antibodies from tumors of ovary (Dorsett *et al.*, 1975) and lung (Ioachim *et al.*, 1976; Paluch and Ioachim, 1978), we noted that peritoneal and pleural effusions of patients with these types of tumors contain sizable amounts of both free and complexed immunoglobulins. Using low-pH elution techniques that facilitate the dissociation of antigen-antibody complexes (Phillips and Lewis, 1971), we were able to obtain immunoglobulins that after purification and concentration displayed a high degree of specificity when tested against cells of the tumor or origin. We showed in earlier work (Dorsett *et al.*, 1975) that immunoglobulins isolated from peritoneal effusions and from eluates of ovarian carcinomas react with cells of all major types of ovarian carcinomas in both membrane and cytoplasmic indirect immunofluorescence tests but not with cells of normal fetal and adult ovaries, benign ovarian tumors, or malignant tumors of other organs.

More recently (Paluch and Ioachim, 1978), we used similar dissociation techniques on lung carcinoma eluates and were able to obtain sizable amounts of IgG and small amounts of IgA and IgM from all tumors as determined by radial immunodiffusion. Immunoglobulins were also obtained from pleural effusions of patients with squamous cell and adenocarcinomas of lung and assayed against various target cells in indirect immunofluorescence tests. They were shown to react positively in significant titers only with cells of squamous cell carcinomas and adenocarcinomas of the lung both in tissue cultures and in fresh cell suspensions (Table II). The fluorescence (Fig. 15) was bright, granular, and strictly intracytoplasmic. Cells of normal adult and fetal lung or of nonpul-

Table II. Indirect Immunofluorescence Assays of Immunoglobulins Isolated from Pleural Effusions of Patients with Squamous Cell Carcinoma of the Lung[a]

Cells tested	Effusions						
	1	2	3	4	5	6	7
Squamous cell carcinoma of lung	4/5[b]	5/5	3/3	2/3	4/4	5/5	3/4
Adenocarcinoma of lung	3/3	2/3	3/5	4/4	2/2	5/5	2/2
Normal adult lung	0/4	0/2	0/3	0/4	0/4	0/3	0/2
Normal fetal lung	0/2	0/1	0/1	0/2	0/2	0/1	0/1
Carcinoma of ovary	0/2	0/1	0/2	0/1	1/2	0/2	0/2
Carcinoma of cervix	0/1	0/1	−	0/1	1/1	−	−
Carcinoma of colon	0/3	0/2	0/2	1/3	0/1	0/2	0/3
Carcinoma of breast	0/2	0/2	0/1	0/2	−	0/1	0/2

[a]Positive results with eluates in dilutions less than 1 : 8 were disregarded. Dashes, not done.
[b]No. positive/No. tested.

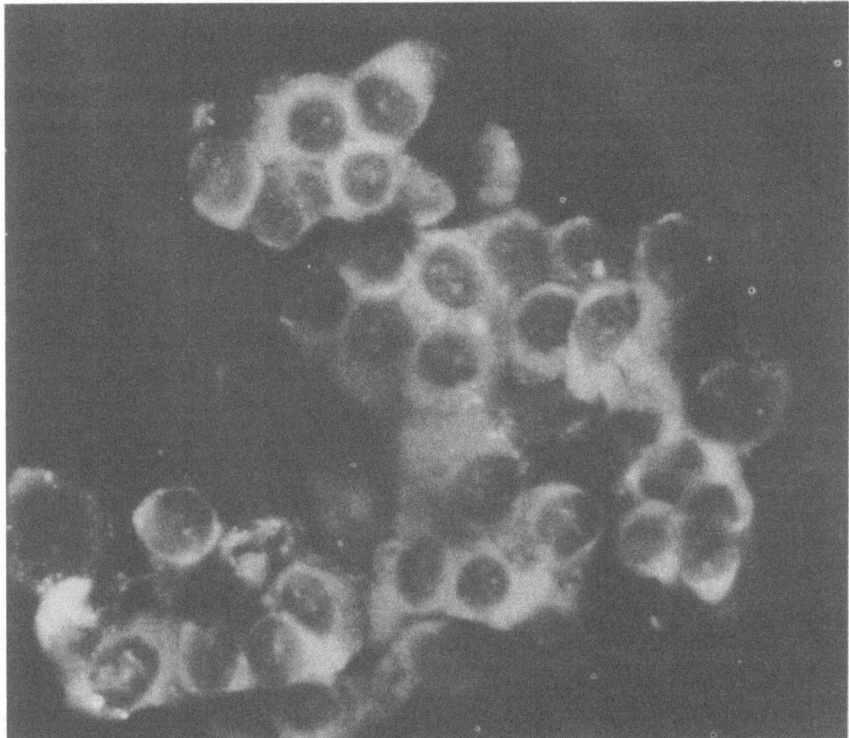

Figure 15. Adenocarcinoma of lung in tissue culture reacted with immunoglobulin fractions isolated from lung cancer effusion and stained with FITC-labeled antihuman polyvalent Ig serum. Tumor cells show bright intracytoplasmic fluorescence (× 1200).

monary tumors did not react. Similarly, no reaction was obtained with immuno-globulins dissociated from tumor effusions of other organs. Small-cell carcinomas of the lung were areactive in these assays for both cells and immunoglobulin fractions, indicating perhaps that squamous cell carcinomas and adenocarcinomas, but not small-cell carcinomas of the lung, share cross-reacting antigens.

As these results indicated the presence of tumor specific antibodies in tumor tissues, we investigated the bronchial washings of patients with various lung tumors (Paluch and Ioachim, 1979) for the presence of similar antibodies that could be advantageously used in immunodiagnostic tests. After antigen–antibody complexes were dissociated, we recovered significantly greater amounts of immunoglobulins from the bronchial washings of lung cancer patients than from those of both normal individuals and patients with various inflammatory lung diseases. Comparing histological types of lung cancer, squamous cell carcinomas were associated with highest levels of immunoglobulins in bronchial washings, which appears to be in accordance with our previous findings (Ioachim *et al.*, 1974*a*, 1976) that squamous cell carcinomas are also accompanied by the largest local cellular reaction, predominantly composed of plasma cells. The specificity of immunoglobulins isolated from bronchial washings was tested as before in indirect immunofluorescence against a spectrum of lung normal and cancer cells of various histological types in tissue cultures and fresh suspensions. The results were entirely similar to those previously obtained with immunoglobulins isolated from lung tumor eluates and effusions.

The accessibility of bronchial washings makes the estimation of lung-cancer-associated antibodies relatively easy and raises the possibility of its eventual conversion into a screening test. A more general conclusion of these studies on the local humoral immune reactions in tumors of the ovary and the lung is that specifically reactive antibodies are commonly produced at the tumor site, representing a part of the immune response to the growth of tumors.

VI. MODULATION AND SELECTION OF TUMOR CELLS

The conflict between tumor and host is a process of long duration and constant change. By necessity, our investigations can only examine samples of this broad, organismic process. In time, the observations we make are similarly limited as we are only able to probe, at fixed intervals, a dynamic process characterized by continuous evolution.

A tumor growth begins with biochemical and morphologic cellular changes below our capacity of recognition. It is perhaps at this incipient stage that the mechanisms of immunological surveillance are activated and that the first immune responses of the host occur. In support of this assumption are the observations of lymphocytes selectively accumulated at the site of dysplastic or of other so-called precancerous lesions (Ioachim, 1976). A step further in tumor progression is the stage of carcinoma *in situ*, which can be generally recognized by morphological criteria. Here, a lymphocytic reaction is frequently present, suggesting that special, possibly antigenic qualities of the neoplastic cells have permitted their recognition as abnormal or foreign (Ioachim, 1976). As the tumor growth increases its volume and begins to invade the local tissues, more lymphocytes aggregate around the cords of tumor cells, sometimes assuming a peripheral, barrierlike distribution (Ioachim, 1976; Iochim *et al.*, 1976). In some tumors, plasma cell transformation takes place; in others, abundant deposition of collagen is noted; and in still others, no stromal reaction of any kind is present (Ioachim 1976; Ioachim *et al.*, 1976). The observation that particular types of stromal reaction are associated with particular types of tumors in itself suggests that the response of the host is not haphazard but, rather, adapted to the antigenic expression of the tumor cells.

In animal systems in which the tumor cells are associated with strong antigenic expression, such as in the one previously described in the present paper, a consistent correlation has been established between malignant potential and tumor antigenicity (Ioachim *et al.*, 1974*b*, 1975, 1977*a*; Kim *et al.*, 1975; Cikes, 1975; Jamasbi and Nettesheim, 1977; Klein and Klein, 1977; Kuzumaki *et al.*, 1978). These two qualities of a tumor vary in indirect proportion with each other (Ioachim *et al.*, 1974*b*; Klein, 1975; Alexander, 1977). As a result of host immune response, the more antigenic tumor cells are destroyed, favoring the progressive selection of the least antigenic. Thus, during multiple successive generations, new clones of tumor cells emerge, endowed with superior qualities of resistance among which the lack of membrane antigenicity is of utmost importance. Concomitantly, the newly selected, less antigenic tumor cells now able to avoid immune recognition and destruction exhibit progressively increased malignant potentials for local invasion and distant metastasis (Ioachim *et al.*, 1974*b*, 1977*a*; Alexander, 1977).

In human neoplasia, a similar progression from tumors *in situ* to highly invasive and metastatic tumors is generally observed. Since the antigenicity of human tumors cannot be adequately measured, correlations between these two parameters, similar to those established in animal systems, are not apparent. However, another property of human cancers shows consistent changes during tumor progression, suggesting here, too, the presence of selective mechanisms.

The microscopic features of human tumors, including both histological patterns and cytological characteristics, undergo regressive changes as the tumors increase their rates of multiplication. The process of cellular dedifferentiation that takes place during tumor growth is associated with an increase in the malignant potential of tumors that is similarly expressed by local invasion and distant metastasis. The parallel evolution of these two properties of tumors occurs consistently enough to have permitted the establishment of clinical prognostic criteria based on the degrees of tumor morphologic differentiation.

As earlier described, the lymphoid infiltrates that accompany the tumor tissues appear to steadily decrease during the progression of tumors (Ioachim, 1976). Thus, the lymphocytic reaction, representing the local antitumor immune response of the host, varies inversely proportional with the process of cellular dedifferentiation. Less differentiated tumor cells emerging during the progression of tumors seem to attract fewer lymphocytes, suggesting that their surface antigenicity is also expressed to a lesser degree. If the lymphoid infiltration of human tumors is a reflection of their antigenicity, we may assume that like their animal counterparts, human tumors by continuous selection similarly undergo a progressive loss of antigenic expression. It is thus tempting to conclude that morphologic and antigenic dedifferentiation of tumors are simultaneous if not complementary processes that occur as a result of tumor cell selection under the constant pressure of the local host immune response.

In following this reasoning, it appears that the host immune response at the site of a tumor is efficient only if all the tumor cells are eventually destroyed. By contrast, if total eradication has not been achieved, the local host immune reaction becomes a strong promoter of tumor cell selection that will inevitably result in the emergence of new clones of tumor cells that are less differentiated, less antigenic, and thus more apt to survive and invade.

In the treatment of cancer, it has been often observed that tumors recurring after radio- and/or chemotherapy exhibit morphological dedifferentiation accompanied by marked increase in their malignant potential (Dao *et al.*, 1962, 1967; Fisher 1970; Stjernsward *et al.*, 1972). Extending our previous conclusions to this situation, we may assume that, similarly to the immune defenses of the host, the failure of therapy to eradicate all tumor cells is inducive of tumor cell selection, resulting in increased incidence of tumor recurrence and metastasis.

VII. SUMMARY

Correlations between three major parameters of host–tumor interaction were examined in both animal and human neoplasia. The relationship between the malignant potential and the antigenicity of tumor cells was studied in a virus-induced murine leukemia system. It was concluded that the transplantability, invasiveness, and ability of tumor cells to metastasize vary inversely proportional to their expression of membrane antigenicity.

In the same system, it was shown that immunocompetent rats are able to reject transplanted tumor cells, whereas recipients rendered immunoincompetent induce antigenic changes in tumor cells that considerably increase their malignant potential. Thus, an inadequate immune response, instead of leading to tumor eradication, may achieve the opposite effect of selecting for tumor cells that are less antigenic and therefore more malignant.

In human tumors, histological studies demonstrated the presence of local cellular reactions represented by infiltrates of lymphocytes and plasma cells. The cellular infiltrates were generally greater in primary than in metastatic tumors, greater in early than in advanced tumors, and greater in differentiated than in undifferentiated tumors. A consistent association between plasma cells and squamous cell carcinomas of various organs was also described.

The humoral immune response at the tumor site in carcinomas of lung and ovary was revealed by the isolation of immunoglobulins from tumor tissues and effusions and by the demonstration of their tumor-specific reactivity. Bronchial washings of lung tumor patients also contained immunoglobulins with similar properties.

It was concluded that tumor cells under the pressure of local host immune response are subjected to continuous selection, generally resulting in new cell clones endowed with superior malignant potential. The progression to increased malignancy is commonly associated with loss of antigenic expression in animal tumors and with loss of morphologic differentiation in human tumors. Possible correlations between antigenic and morphological differentiation of tumor cells remain to be explored.

VIII. REFERENCES

Alexander, P., 1974, Escape from immune destruction by the host through shedding of surface antigens: Is this a characteristic shared by malignant and embryonic cells? *Cancer Res.* 34:2077–2082.

Alexander, P., 1977, Back to the drawing board—The need for more realistic model systems for immunotherapy, *Cancer* 40:467–470.

Baldwin, R. W., Price, M. R., and Robins, R. A., 1972, Blocking of lymphocyte-mediated cytotoxicity for rat hepatoma cells by tumor-specific antigen-antibody complexes, *Nature (London) New Biol.* 238:185–187.

Baldwin, R. W., Embleton, M. J., and Robins, R. A., 1973, Cellular and humoral immunity to rat hepatoma-specific antigens correlated with tumor status, *Int. J. Cancer* 11:1–10.

Barber, H. R. K., Sommers, S. C., Snyder, R., and Kwon, T. H., 1975, Histologic and nuclear grading and stromal reactions as indices for prognosis in ovarian cancer, *Am. J. Obstet. Gynecol.* 121:795–804.

Bartlett, G. L., 1972, Effect of host immunity on the antigenic strength of primary tumors, *J. Natl. Cancer Inst.* 49:493–504.

Berg, J. W., 1959, Inflammation and prognosis in breast cancer—A search for host resistance, *Cancer* 12:714–720.

Black, M. M., and Leis, H. P., 1971, Cellular responses to autologous breast cancer tissue, *Cancer* 28:263–273.

Bubenick, J., Perlman, P., Helmstein, K., and Moberger, G., 1970, Cellular and humoral immune responses to human urinary bladder carcinomas, *Int. J. Cancer* 5:310–319.

Cikes, M., 1975, Antigenic changes in cultured murine lymphomas after retransplantation into syngeneic hosts, *J. Natl. Cancer Inst.* 54:903–906.

Dao, T. L., and Kovaric, J., 1962, Incidence of pulmonary and skin metastases in women with breast cancer who received postoperative irradiation, *Surgery* 52:203–212.

Dao, T. L., and Yogo, H., 1967, Enhancement of pulmonary metastases by x-irradiation in rats bearing mammary cancer, *Cancer* 20:2020–2025.

Dorsett, B. H., Ioachim, H. L., Stolbach, L., Walker, J., and Barber, H. R. K., 1975, Isolation of tumor-specific antibodies from effusions of ovarian carcinomas, *Int. J. Cancer* 16:779–786.

Dorval, G., Witz, I. P., Klein, E., and Wigzell, H., 1976, Tumor-bound immunoglobulins: An *in vivo* phenomenon of masked specificity, *J. Natl. Cancer Inst.* 56:523–527.

Essex, M., Klein, G., Snyder, S. P., and Boyd Harrold, J., 1971, Correlation between humoral antibody and regression of tumors induced by feline sarcoma virus, *Nature (London)* 233:195–196.

Ewing, J., 1940, *Neoplastic Diseases*, W. B. Saunders, Philadelphia.

Fisher, B., 1970, Postoperative radiotherapy in the treatment of breast cancer—Results of the NSABP clinical trial, *Ann. Surg.* 172:711–732.

Fisher, E. R., and Fisher, B., 1972, Local lymphoid response as an index of tumor immunity, *Arch. Pathol.* 94:137–146.

Fenyö, E. M., Klein, E., Klein, G., and Swiech, K., 1968, Selection of an immunoresistant Moloney lymphoma subline with decreased concentration of tumor-specific surface antigens, *J. Natl. Cancer Inst.* 40:69–89.

Gold, P., 1967, Circulating antibodies against carcino-embryonic antigens of the human digestive system, *Cancer* 20:1663–1667.

Gupta, R. K., and Morton, D. L., 1975, Suggestive evidence for *in vivo* binding of specific antitumor antibodies of human melanomas, *Cancer Res.* 35:58–62.

Hellström, I., Hellström, K. E., Sjogren, H. O., 1970, Serum-mediated inhibition of cellular immunity to methylcholanthrene-induced murine sarcomas, *Cell Immunol.* 1:18–30.

Henle, W., Henle, G., Gunven, P., Klein, G., Clifford, P., and Singh, S., 1973, Patterns of antibodies to Epstein–Barr virus-induced early antigens in Burkitt's lymphoma, *J. Natl. Cancer Inst.* **50:**1163–1173.

Herberman, R. B., and Fahey, J. L., 1968, Cytotoxic antibody in Burkitt's tumor and normal human serum reactive with cultures of lymphoid cells, *Proc Soc. Exp. Biol. Med.* **127:**938.

Herberman, R. B., and Oren, M. E., 1971, Immune response to Gross virus-induced lymphoma. I. Kinetics of cytotoxic antibody response, *J. Natl. Cancer Inst.* **46:**391–396.

Ioachim, H. L., 1976, The stromal reaction of tumors: An expression of immune surveillance —Guest editorial, *J. Natl. Cancer Inst.* **57:**465–475.

Ioachim, H. L., and Sabbath, M., 1979, Redistribution and modulation of Gross murine leukemia virus antigens induced by specific antibodies, *J. Natl. Cancer Inst.* **62:**169–180.

Ioachim, H. L., Cali, A., and Sinha, D., 1965, Age-dependent transplantability in rats of virus-induced thymic lymphoma cultured *in vitro, Cancer Res.* **25:**132–139.

Ioachim, H. L., Berwick, L., and Furth, J., 1966, Replication of Gross leukemia virus in long-term cultures of rat thymomas. Bioassays and electron microscopy, *Cancer Res.* **20:**803–811.

Ioachim, H. L., Dorsett, B., Sabbath, M., and Keller, S., 1972, Loss and recovery of phenotypic expression of Gross leukemic virus, *Nature (London) New Biol.* **237:**215–218.

Ioachim, H. L., Dorsett, B. H., and Paluch, E., 1974a, Cellular and humoral immune reactions to squamous cell carcinomas of the lung, in: *Proceedings of the XIth International Cancer Congress*, Vol. 2, p. 104, Florence.

Ioachim, H. L., Keller, S., Sabbath, M., and Dorsett, B. H., 1974b, Antigenic expression as a determining factor of tumor growth in Gross virus lymphoma, *Prog. Exp. Tumor Res.* **19:**284–296.

Ioachim, H. L., Keller, S., Dorsett, B., and Pearse, A., 1974c, Induction of partial immunologic tolerance in rats and progressive loss of cellular antigenicity in Gross virus lymphoma, *J. Exp. Med.* **139:**1382–1394.

Ioachim, H. L., Keller, S., and Dorsett, B., 1975, Transplantability, immunological unresponsiveness, and loss of cellular antigenicity in Gross virus lymphoma, in: *Comparative Leukemia Research, 1973. Leukemogenesis* (Y. Ito, and R. M. Dutcher, eds.), pp. 301–310, University of Tokyo Press, Tokyo.

Ioachim, H. L., Dorsett, B., and Paluch, E., 1976, The immune response at the tumor site in lung carcinoma, *Cancer* **38:**2296–2309.

Ioachim, H. L., Pearse, A., and Keller, S., 1977a, Antigenic deletion and malignant enhancement induced in lymphoma cells by passage through x-irradiated hosts, *Nature (London)* **265:**55–57.

Ioachim, H. L., Pearse, A., and Keller, S., 1977b, Patterns of metastases in hemopoietic neoplasms: Immunologic correlations, in: *Cancer Invasion and Metastasis* (S. B. Day, ed.), pp. 333–345, Raven Press, New York.

Irie, K., Irie, R. F., and Morton, D. L., 1975, Detection of antibody and complement complexed *in vivo* on membranes of human cancer cells by mixed hemadsorption techniques, *Cancer Res.* **35:**1244–1248.

Jamasbi, R. J., and Nettesheim, P., 1977, Increased immunogenicity of a pulmonary squamous cell carcinoma, propagated *in vitro, Int. J. Cancer* **20:**817–823.

Kim, U., Baumler, A., Corruthers, C., and Bielat, K., 1975, Immunological escape mechanism in spontaneously metastasizing mammary tumors, *Proc. Natl. Acad. Sci. USA* **72:**1012–1016.

Klein, G., 1975, Immunological surveillance against neoplasia, *Harvey Lect.* **69:**71–102.

Klein, G., and Klein, E., 1977, Rejectability of virus-induced tumors and non-rejectability of spontaneous tumors: A lesson in contrasts, *Transplant Proc.* **9:**1095–1104.

Klein, G., and Sjögren, H. O., 1960, Humoral and cellular factors in homograft and isograft immunity against sarcoma cells, *Cancer Res.* 20:452–461.

Kobayashi, H., Gotohda, E., Hosokawa, M., and Kodama, T., 1975, Inhibition of metastasis in rats immunized with xenogenized autologous tumor cells after excision of the primary tumor, *J. Natl. Cancer Inst.* 54:997–999.

Koneval, T., Applebaum, E., Popovic, D., Gill, L., Sissou, G., Wood, G. W., and Anderson, B., 1977, Demonstration of immunoglobulin in tumor and marginal tissues of squamous cell carcinomas of the head and neck, *J. Natl. Cancer Inst.* 59:1089–1093.

Kuzumaki, N., Fënyo, E. M., Giovanella, B. C., and Klein, G., 1978, Increased immunogenicity of low-antigenic rat tumors after superinfection with endogenous murine C-type virus in nude mice, *Int. J. Cancer* 21:62–66.

Lauder, I., and Aherne, W., 1972, The significance of lymphocytic infiltration in neuroblastoma, *Br. J. Cancer* 26:321–330.

Lewis, M. G., McCloy, E., and Blake, J., 1973, The significance of humoral antibodies in the localization of human malignant melanoma, *Br. J. Surg.* 60:443–446.

Lewis, M. G., Proctor, J. W., Thompson, D. M. P., Rowden, G., and Phillips, T. M., 1976, Cellular localization of immunoglobulin within human malignant melanoma, *Br. J. Cancer* 33:260–266.

Lewis, M. G., Phillips, T. M., and Rowden, G., 1978, Beneficial and detrimental effects of humoral immunity in malignancy, in: *Pathobiology Annual*, Vol. 8 (H. L. Ioachim, ed.), pp. 217–239, Appleton-Century-Crofts, Englewood Cliffs, New Jersey.

Mora, P. T., Chang, C., Couvillion, L., Kuster, J. M., and McFarland, V. W., 1977, Immunological selection of tumor cells which have lost SV40 antigen expression, *Nature (London)* 269:36–40.

Morton, D. L., Malmgren, R. A., Holmes, F. C., and Ketcham, A. S., 1968, Demonstration of antibodies against human malignant melonomas by immunofluorescence, *Surgery* 64:233–240.

Murphy, J. B., Nakahara, W., and Sturm, E., 1921, Studies on lymphoid activity. V. Relation between the time and extent of lymphoid stimulation induced by physical agents and the degree of resistance to cancer in mice, *J. Exp. Med.* 33:423–428.

Paluch, E., and Ioachim, H. L., 1978, Lung carcinoma-reactive antibodies isolated from tumor tissues and pleural effusions of lung cancer patients, *J. Natl. Cancer Inst.* 61:319–325.

Paluch, E., and Ioachim, H. L., 1979, Reactive antibodies in the bronchial washings of lung cancer patients, *Int. J. Cancer* 23:42–46.

Pearse, A., and Ioachim, H. L., 1978, Effect of host immunity on tumor cell antigenic variability, *Proc. Am. Assoc. Cancer Res.* 18:175.

Phillips, T. M., and Lewis, M. G., 1971, A method for elution of immunoglobulin from the surface of living cells, *Rev. Eur. Etud. Clin. Biol.* 16:1052–1055.

Ran, M., and Witz, I. P., 1972, Tumor-associated immunoglobulins. Enhancement of syngeneic tumors by IgG_2-containing tumor eluates, *Int. J. Cancer* 9:242–247.

Russel, B. R. G., 1908, The nature of resistance to the inoculation of cancer, *Third Scientific Rep. Imperial Cancer Res. Fund.* 3:341–358.

Sjögren, H. O., Hellström, I., Bansal, S. C., Warner, G. A., and Hellström, K. E., 1972, Elution of "blocking factors" from human tumors capable of abrogating tumor-cell destruction by specifically immune lymphocytes, *Int. J. Cancer* 9:274–283.

Sobczac, E., and De Vaux Saint Cyr, C., 1971, Study of the *in vivo* fixation of antibodies on tumors provoked in hamsters by injection of SV40-transformed cells (TSV_5Ci_2), *Int. J. Cancer* 8:47–52.

Stjernsward, J., Jondal, M., Vanky, F., Wigzell, H., and Sealy, R., 1972, Lymphopenia and change in distribution of human B and T lymphocytes in peripheral blood induced by irradiation for mammary carcinoma, *Lancet* 1:1352–1356.

Takahashi, K., 1961, Squamous cell carcinoma of the esophagus. Stromal inflammatory cell infiltration as a prognostic factor, *Cancer* **14**:921-933.

Thunold, S., Tønder, O., and Larsen, O., 1973, Immunoglobulins in eluates of malignant human tumors, *Acta Pathol. Microbiol. Scand. Sect. A* (Suppl.) **236**:97-100.

Underwood, J. C. E., 1972, Lymphoreticular infiltration in human tumors—Prognostic and biological implications, a review. *Br. J. Cancer* **30**:538-547.

von Kleist, S., King, M., and Burtin P., 1974, Characterization of a normal tissular antigen extracted from human colonic tumors, *Immunochemistry* **11**:249-253.

Witz, I. P., 1973, The biological significance of tumor-bound immunoglobulins. *Curr. Top. Microbiol. Immunol.* **61**:151-171.

Zeromski, J., Gorny, M. K., Wruk, M., and Sapula, J., 1975, Behaviour of local and systemic immunoglobulins in patients with lung cancer, *Int. Arch. Allergy Appl. Immunol.* **49**:548-563.

Chapter 11

Host Cell Analysis of a Rapidly Metastasizing Mouse Tumor and Derived Low-Metastatic Variant Lines

R. S. Kerbel and R. R. Twiddy

National Cancer Institute of Canada Research Group
Division of Cancer Research
Department of Pathology
Queen's University
Kingston, Ontario, Canada K7L 3N6

and

P. Frost

Department of Immunology and Microbiology
Wayne State University
Detroit, Michigan 48201

I. INTRODUCTION

Pathologists have been aware for decades that malignant tumors can become infiltrated with significant numbers of nonmalignant stromal and lymphoreticular host cells. For certain types of malignancies, e.g., breast carcinoma, it has been claimed that the prognosis may correlate with the extent of host cell infiltration (reviewed by Underwood, 1974, and Ioachim, 1976). However, it is obvious that the light microscope has certain serious limitations when it comes to screening neoplasms for host cells. It cannot, for example, discriminate between a T or a B lymphocyte, nor can it be used as a reliable tool, as Alexander has stressed (1975), to detect certain kinds of host cells, in particular, macrophages. This fact, combined with the increasing awareness of the existence of functional subclasses of lymphocytes and macrophages (e.g., helper, killer, and suppressor

239

Table I. Examples of Descriptive Studies of Intratumor Lymphoreticular
Host Cells

System	Key findings	References
Analysis of tumors of varying immunogenicity	Highly immunogenic experimental tumors contain more host cells and macrophages than poorly immunogenic tumors	K. Moore and Moore (1977), Eccles and Alexander (1975)
Analysis of primary versus serially transplanted chemically induced tumors	Relative host cell content of all cell types, including macrophages, drops with increasing sequential passage	Kerbel and Pross (1976)
Analysis of progressing versus regressing tumors	Host cells can make up predominant population in spontaneously regressing tumors but only a minor component in same type of tumor growing progressively	Haskill *et al.* (1975)

T-cell subclasses), has made quantitative and qualitative studies of host cell infiltration an important feature of current tumor biology research.

As the papers in this volume attest, there are two basic approaches to the study of intratumor host cell infiltration: (1) descriptive, in which different types of tumors in various growth situations are analyzed for their relative contents of different types of host cells; and (2) analytical, in which the object is the isolation and functional *in vitro* testing of host cells. Some examples of the first approach are given in Table I. The idea behind this approach is reasonably simple: the host cell contents of tumors showing particular growth characteristics, e.g., regression, metastasis, excessively fast or slow growth, are analyzed in an attempt to correlate a particular pattern of host cell infiltration with a particular growth characteristic. Although this approach is not without its obvious problems, it should nevertheless prove useful, especially when used in conjunction with the "functional" approach.

II. Fc RECEPTORS AND TUMOR CELL POPULATIONS

Previous work in our laboratory has concentrated on developing methods to easily quantitate the level of host cells in transplantable carcinomas and sarcomas. Our specific area of interest has been the Fc-receptor-positive (FcR^+) cell. As reviewed by Tønder (this volume) and Kerbel and Davies (1974), tissue sections of tumors or single-cell preparations made from solid tumors invariably contain FcR^+ cells. A study was devoted to ascertaining the nature of these cells, and the evidence obtained from experimental tumor studies appeared unequivical: The

FcR$^+$ cells were of "host" origin and consisted of a mixture of different cell types including macrophages and lymphocytes (Kerbel et al., 1975). Further studies using a variety of progressively growing syngeneic mouse tumors revealed that a majority (>80%) of infiltrating host cells were FcR$^+$, thus enabling one to exploit the FcR as an index of host cell infiltration (Kerbel and Pross, 1976).

The situation with human tumors is not so well defined, but the picture that is emerging seems very similar to that with experimental tumors. Thus, analysis of over 30 long-term established human carcinoma tissue culture cell lines clearly revealed that all were FcR$^-$ (Kerbel et al., 1977). This finding is consistent with the notion that the FcR$^+$ cells observed in human carcinomas are infiltrating host cells. Nonetheless we have tried to refrain from being dogmatic on this issue. There are still several reasonable possibilities to account for FcR$^+$ tumor cells, as we have previously discussed (Kerbel and Pross, 1976; Kerbel et al., 1977). This issue is discussed in detail elsewhere in this volume by Tønder and his associates.

Having shown that the FcR could be exploited as a convenient host cell marker, we embarked on a program to ascertain how the types of levels of FcR$^+$ cells varied in certain tumor growth situations in vivo (Pross and Kerbel, 1976). Our primary goal remains to establish how these cells might influence— or be made to influence—the process of metastasis.

III. HOST CELLS AND METASTASIS

The literature on host cell responses in metastasizing tumors is quite small, but a nucleus of papers exists that incriminate certain types of intratumor host cells in the metastatic process. Most notable is the claim of Eccles and Alexander (1974) that there exists an inverse relationship between the levels of macrophages in various rat tumors and the tendency of these same tumors to metastasize in immunosuppressed hosts. Similarly, Wood and Gillespie (1975) have shown that injection of macrophage-depleted mouse tumor cells obtained from solid tumors resulted in an increased incidence of metastases.

In an earlier study, Gershon et al. (1967), examined two transplantable hamster lymphomas, only one of which metastasized, for their content of infiltrating macrophages. Using light-microscope histological methods, they concluded that the nonmetastasizing tumor contained significant numbers of macrophages (during the middle stages of tumor growth), while the metastasizing tumor lacked such cells. However, later studies using the electron microscope revealed that the metastasizing tumor did in fact contain macrophages, but that these cells—in contrast to the macrophages found in the nonmetastasizing tumor— appeared to be in a nonstimulated state (Birbeck and Carter, 1972).

A very recent functional study of intratumor macrophages by Mantovani

(1978) revealed results that paralleled the ultrastructural studies of Carter and his colleagues. Macrophages were isolated from a strongly immunogenic, non-metastasizing mouse sarcoma and a presumptive, spontaneously metastasizing (to the lungs) variant of the same tumor. Freshly harvested macrophages from the nonmetastasizing sarcoma inhibited growth of tumor cells *in vitro* in a non-specific fashion, while macrophages isolated from the variant actually enhanced tumor cell growth *in vitro*.

These intriguing observations are difficult to interpret, but they certainly imply that tumor-associated macrophages can, at least in some cases, influence metastasis (see Alexander, 1975). But equally important, they also imply that tumors (and in particular, tumors that have a strong tendency to metastasize) can affect the physiological status of the resident macrophages themselves.

Less is known about the possible effects intratumor lymphocytes may have on metastasis. Although the evidence seems to be increasing for various regulatory roles being played by T lymphocytes in metastasis (Graham *et al.*, 1978), such studies have not yet been extended to the local tumor environment. One exception is the study of Husby *et al.*, (1976). These authors found an inverse relationship between the level of T lymphocyte infiltration of various human tumors and their tendency to metastasize.

IV. METASTASIZING MOUSE TUMORS

One of the more obvious problems in attempting to study biological parameters that may affect metastasis is the relative lack of experimental tumors showing rapid and widespread spontaneous metastases. In fact, it sometimes would seem to appear that most experimental tumors do not metastasize at all. However, the incidence of spontaneous metastases can be significantly increased by the rather simple procedure of removing the primary tumor after it has reached a certain critical size (Sugarbaker *et al.*, 1977; Mellgren, 1976).

The reasons for this are not clear. It has been speculated that many experimental tumors grow so quickly that they kill the host before significant visible metastases have a chance to develop (Mellgren, 1976). In addition, the primary tumor, although itself the ultimate source of metastatic foci, may somehow actively inhibit the growth of distant micrometastases (Sugarbaker *et al.*, 1976). This may be due to the action of tumor-associated chalones, or nutrient "depletion," to list but a few possible mechanisms.

Removal of the primary tumor, however, provides only a limited solution to many of the problems associated with studying certain aspects of metastasis. First, metastases are often restricted to one site, the lungs (Mellgren, 1976), and these can often take a considerable time to manifest themselves. Second, there is the problem of what one uses as controls for such studies.

In an effort to overcome these obstacles, several ingenious approaches have been devised, some of which involve the isolation of "variant" tumor lines. Such lines have an increased or decreased capacity to metastasize, in comparison to the "wild-type" line from which they derived. Fidler has been the pioneer in this field and has found that metastatic variants can be obtained by progressive selection *in vivo* (Fidler, 1973) or by random, single-cell cloning procedures (Fidler and Kripkie, 1977). Tao and Burger (1977) have found that making the cells of a moderately metastasizing tumor line resistant to the toxic effects of wheat germ agglutinin (WGA) can severely impair their ability to metastasize, even though their tumorigenic potential at the site of injection remained intact.

The object of this paper is to summarize results involving a somewhat unique metastasizing mouse tumor and to present new results pertaining to the host cell characteristics of this tumor in comparison to several types of derived variants, all of which have a greatly reduced metastasizing capacity.

V. ORIGIN AND PROPERTIES OF MDAY-D2: A MOUSE TUMOR SHOWING RAPID AND WIDESPREAD SPONTANEOUS METASTASES

Features of this tumor system have recently been described in detail (Kerbel *et al.*, 1978) and are summarized here. In 1960 the Kleins induced a number of tumors in $(A \times DBA/2)F_1$ hybrids with methylcholanthrene, one of which, a sarcoma, was designated MDAY (Klein *et al.*, 1960). It was later adapted for growth as an ascites tumor, and we received a sample of the tumor, which had been frozen down after 373 passages.

In our hands, MDAY grows progressively in syngeneic AD_2F_1 recipients so that animals start dying of tumor within 4–5 weeks of subcutaneous injection of 10^6 cells. If MDAY cells are injected subcutaneously into DBA/2 parental-strain recipients, no growth is observed. This is to be expected, since A-strain mice are H-2 recombinants, being H-2K^k and H-2D^d (see Klein, 1975). Hence, the MDAY cells should not grow in the H-2^d-incompatible DBA/2 parent. Serotyping of MDAY cells confirmed the presence of H-2.23, the private H-2 specificity of the K end of the H-2^k haplotype; and the absence of H-2.32, the private specificity of the D end of the H-2^k haplotype (Klein, 1975).

However, we found that if MDAY cells were inoculated intraperitoneally into DBA/2 recipients they gave rise to a transient ascites. A typical growth curve is shown in Fig. 1. Rejection of the cells was eventually observed after a peak of about $2–3 \times 10^8$ cells was attained, usually by day 8 or day 9. If the cells were still harvested at day 8 (they were found to be H-2K^k-positive) and repeatedly reinjected into new DBA/2 recipients, it was found that the cells eventually lost their H-2^k alloantigens. An example of this is shown in Table II. In three out of four experiments, complete loss of H-2K^k antigen was noted by

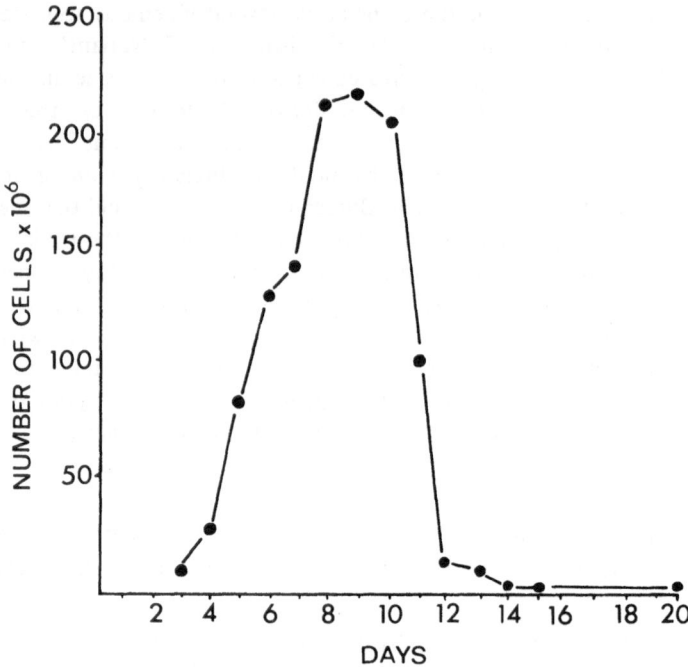

Figure 1. Growth curve of MDAY ascites tumor in DBA/2 H-2 incompatible recipients. A large group of DBA/2 mice were injected with 10^6 MDAY ascites tumor cells obtained from an AD_2F_1 doner. On the indicated days two mice were killed and the cells harvested from the peritoneal cavity. They were counted and analyzed for FcR^+ cells and macrophages. By day 12 the majority of cells were of host origin, of which at least 30% were macrophages.

the 9th passage. The loss was confirmed by absorption experiments in which anti-H-2.23 serum was absorbed with large numbers of the cells. It will be noted that in one experiment, loss of $H-2^k$ was not observed, even after 14 passages. This is unusual, since in five previous experiments loss of $H-2^k$ was always attained within 5-9 passages. However, the cells in this experiment were harvested every 7 days, instead of every 8.

When these $H-2^k$-negative cells were injected into DBA/2 or AD_2F_1 recipients we were surprised at the growth characteristics of the tumor cells: extremely rapid and widespread dissemination of tumor was observed after subcutaneous, intradermal, intravenous, or intramuscular injection (Kerbel *et al.*, 1978). Total replacement of liver tissue was often noted by day 16. Widespread growth was also observed in the spleen, lungs, and kidneys. In contrast, the original $H-2^k$-positive MDAY cells showed limited metastatic growth potential in their syngeneic AD_2F_1 hosts: in many animals no metastases were observed. When they were present, they were confined to the liver (Kerbel *et al.*, 1978). If the tumor

Table II. Effect of Serial Passage of H-2K^k-Positive
MDAY Cells in DBA/2 Parental Strain Hosts on the
Percentage of H-2K^k-Positive Cells

Passage No.[a]	Percent H-2K^k-positive cells[b]			
	Exp. I	Exp. II	Exp. III	Exp. IV[c]
1	>99	>99	>99	>99
2	>99	>99	>99	>99
3	>99	>99	>99	>99
4	94	80	>99	>99
5	40	52	>99	>99
6	31	8	>99	97
7	0	0	96	90
8	0	0	42	98
9	–	–	0	95
10	–	–	0	91
11	–	–	–	98
12	–	–	–	90
13	–	–	–	>99
14	–	–	–	97

[a]10^6 or 0.5×10^6 MDAY ascites cells were inoculated intraperitoneally into successive DBA/2 recipients.
[b]Assessed with anti-H-2.23 antiserum (Kerbel et al., 1978).
Once cells lost their H-2^k antigens there was no reexpression
of the antigens if the cells were injected into "neutral"
AD$_2$F$_1$ hosts or placed into tissue culture.
[c]Cells harvested every 7 days.

was surgically removed 10 days after an intradermal injection, the incidence of
liver metastases showed a definite increase. In addition, brain metastases were
observed. Nonetheless, metastatic growth of the tumor was far more limited
than seen with MDAY-D2.

A. Is MDAY-D2 an H-2 Loss Variant of the MDAY Tumor?

The most likely explanation for the origin of MDAY-D2 is that it is a so-
called "H-2 loss variant" of the original H-2 heterozygous MDAY tumor. This
is a well-known phenomenon and has been observed by many laboratories (e.g.,
Bayreuther and Klein, 1958; Bjaring and Klein, 1968; and reviewed by J. Klein,
1975). The mechanism of H-2 loss variant formation remains somewhat obscure.
Obviously one possibility is the selection of preexisting rare variant cells that
lack the H-2-incompatible antigen. It appears from recent results by Rajan and
Flores (1977) that the selection process may follow a primary genetic event

(e.g., gene or chromosome loss, somatic crossing over). In the case of epigenetic or induced H-2 alterations, the variant may or may not exist before the actual selection (Rajan and Flores, 1977).

The origin of MDAY-D2 is not clear, but several results make the explanation of selection of a preexisting variant very unlikely. These include:

1. Subcutaneous injection of MDAY cells into DBA/2 recipients does not lead to any growth of tumors: If H-2K^k-negative variant cells preexisted, such growth would be expected.
2. Although variants eventually arose after intraperitoneal injection, many passages were required, i.e., the process appeared to be a multistep one that presumably would not have been necessary if the variant cells preexisted. The fact that a series of passages was required argues for an induction event prior to selection, or that MDAY-D2 is in fact a newly derived DBA/2 host tumor.
3. The alloantigen and receptor profiles of the MDAY and MDAY-D2 tumor lines were quite different (Kerbel *et al.*, 1978). A summary of the results is given in Table III. Most notable is the fact that MDAY is FcR⁻ while MDAY-D2 is FcR⁺. This is true also for cells obtained from long-term established tissue culture lines of these cells. In our experience, only lymphoreticular tumors have Fc receptors (Kerbel *et al.*, 1975; Kerbel *et al.*, 1977). This raised the possibility, in our view, that MDAY-D2 may be a newly induced tumor, and not a variant of MDAY. In any case, it is difficult to see how the selection process exerted *in vivo* could result in the emergence of Fc receptors on MDAY-D2.

Table III. Summary of Cell Surface Properties of MDAY and MDAY-D2[a]

Property	MDAY	MDAY-D2
H-2^d antigens	+	+
H-2K^k antigens	+	−
Thy-1.2 antigen	+	−
Ly-1.2 antigen	+	−
Ly-2.2 antigen	+	−
Ia antigens	−	−
Surface Ig	−	−
C3 receptor	−	+
Fc receptor	−	+

[a]The assays used to test for the above receptors and antigens were done on both tissue-culture-derived and ascites lines of MDAY and MDAY-D2 (Kerbel *et al.*, 1978).

4. On the assumption that H-2K^k-negative variant cells preexisted, we treated MDAY cells *in vitro* with anti-H-2^k antiserum and rabbit complement. We obtained cells after four cycles of treatment that lacked H-2^k antigens, as assessed by cytotoxicity testing (Kerbel, unpublished observations). However, when these cells were injected into DBA/2 recipients we never observed any progressive tumor growth. In most instances no takes were observed. When there was tumor growth, it was quickly followed by regression. This implied the presence of very low levels of H-2K^k antigens, and this was subsequently confirmed by absorption studies (Kerbel *et al.*, 1980). In summary, we have not yet succeeded in obtaining a true H-2^k loss variant of MDAY *in vitro* with antiserum and complement.

5. The results of certain genetic marker experiments: In one experiment an artificial genetic marker was inserted into the MDAY cells, namely resistance to the membrane-active (toxic) drug ouabain (Mankovitz *et al.*, 1974). Ouabain resistance is a genetically stable dominant genetic marker (Baker and Ling, 1978). The rationale was to inject ouabain-resistant MDAY cells into successive DBA/2 hosts and check to see if ouabain resistance was retained or lost when the cells lost their H-2^k antigens and gained their unusual metastatic properties. The results, published elsewhere (Kerbel *et al.*, 1980), were quite unequivocal: When the cells became H-2^k-negative, they were also found to concomitantly lose all of their ouabain resistance. In contrast, repeated passage of ouabain-resistant MDAY cells in syngeneic AD$_2$F$_1$ hosts did not result in any precipitous decline in ouabain resistance. The most reasonable explanation for these results is that MDAY-D2 is a newly induced DBA/2 tumor. This is discussed in more detail in a recent publication (Kerbel *et al.*, 1980) which also includes detailed H-2 serotyping analysis.

If MDAY-D2 is in fact a newly induced tumor, the only possible oncogenic agent we can think of would be the presence of potentially oncogenic passenger viruses in the MDAY cells. Indeed, there is a precedent for such a situation (Pasqualini *et al.*, 1970). However karyotypic analysis of several MDAY-D2 lines (five altogether) has revealed that they all have very similar or identical karyotypes, including the presence of three metacentric marker chromosomes. Such an occurrence would not have been predicted for virus-induced tumors (Koller, 1972), where chromosomal variation between tumors is to be expected.

Whatever its origin, the results make it clear that we cannot assume MDAY-D2 is an H-2 loss variant of MDAY. Therefore, comparison of intratumor host cell responses between MDAY and MDAY-D2 may be meaningless. Instead, we have attempted to derive low- or nonmetastatic variants of the high-metastatic MDAY-D2 cells. Several procedures were adopted, as outlined in the next section.

B. Production of Low-Metastatic Variants of the High-Metastatic MDAY-D2 Tumor

Three methods were used to derive variants of MDAY-D2 showing reduced metastatic capacity. The first method, based on Fidler and Kripkie (1977), consisted of deriving multiple clones of MDAY-D2 by single cell cloning at limiting dilution. We derived 20 different clones, and each was tested individually for its relative growth rate and capacity to metastasize in DBA/2 hosts. We found that 18 of the clones showed no change, or even an increased metastatic growth potential. However, 2 of the clones, D2-7 and D2-13, displayed a greatly reduced capacity to metastasize. Animals injected with these cells often died of massive primary tumor growth at the site of injection. There was usually no evidence of metastases. When metastatic growth was evident, it was usually confined to the liver. These results confirm those of Fidler and Kripkie (1977), who showed by cloning procedures that cells with greatly altered metastatic capacity preexisted within heterogeneous tumor cell populations.

The second method, after Tao and Burger (1977), involved the testing of lectin-resistant variants of MDAY-D2. We tested clones of PHA-, Con-A-, and WGA-resistant variants. Thus far, a Con-A-resistant variant, D2-Con A^R-2 (MC-2), has demonstrated reduced metastatic growth potential. Tao and Burger (1977) found that WGA-resistant variants of the B16 melanoma did not metastasize. In our hands MDAY-D2 variants resistant to very high concentrations of WGA, although maintaining their malignant growth properties *in vitro*, were often nontumorigenic *in vivo*, although we have found many lines that were both tumorigenic and metastatic.

A third method was based on experiments performed by one of us (P. F.) in which the growth pattern of MDAY-D2 in immunodeficient BALB/c nude mice versus reconstituted BALB/c mice was assessed. It was found that MDAY-D2 metastasized widely and rapidly in BALB/c nude mice. In one mouse that had been previously reconstituted with normal BALB/c spleen cells, the tumor grew at the site of injection but did not metastasize (Frost and Wiltrout, unpublished observations). This characteristic appeared to be maintained when these cells were injected into DBA/2 recipients for at least the first three passages. This line is called ND3.

The low-metastatic behavior of the various randomly cloned MDAY-D2 variants has been found to be unstable (Kerbel, 1980). This obviously constitutes a limitation on the interpretation of the results obtained using these sorts of variants.

C. Host Cell Analysis of MDAY-D2 versus Low- and High-Metastatic Variants Obtained by Single Cell Cloning

As discussed here and shown previously, MDAY-D2 normally metastasizes extensively to liver, lungs, kidneys, and spleen within 16–18 days (Kerbel *et al.*,

1978). A number of clones of MDAY-D2, almost all of which behaved like MDAY-D2, were obtained by limiting cell dilution procedures. However, two clones that metastasized poorly, D2-7 and D2-13, were obtained. The primary tumors of these and other clones were tested for their relative host cell contents. In addition, we occasionally found that some of the other clones would show limited metastasis, although this was an exception. Only the solid tumor at the injection site was tested.

Three different assay procedures were performed, namely: (1) assessment for complement receptor-positive cells by rosetting with sheep erythrocytes coated with rabbit IgM antibody and mouse complement, i.e., EAC indicator cells; (2) assessment of T cells by anti-Thy-1.2 serum and guinea pig complement; and (3) assessment of macrophages by phagocytosis of IgG-antibody-coated sheep erythrocytes. We used EAC rosettes as a partial host cell marker instead of Fc rosettes, since the MDAY-D2 cells are themselves FcR^+, as discussed in a pre-

Table IV. Host Cell Analysis of High-Metastatic MDAY-D2 Solid Tumors versus Cloned Variants with Low or High Metastatic Capacity

Tumor	Days[a]	Metastatic pattern				Host cell analysis[b]		
		Liver	Spleen	Lungs	Kidneys	% EAC[+]	% Thy-1.2[+]	% MΦ
D2-clone 13	28	±	–	–	–	6	7	0
D2-clone 13	28	±	–	–	–	1	0	4
D2-clone 13	28	–	–	–	–	6	6	2
D2-clone 13	28	–	–	–	–	6	0	0
D2-uncloned	16	++++	++++	+++	++	6	28	1
D2-uncloned	16	++++	–	+++	+++	4	1	0
D2-clone 7	31	±	–	–	–	4	0	1
D2-clone 6	32	–	–	–	–	5	11	2
D2-clone 6	28	–	–	–	–	11	10	0
D2-clone 7	28	±	–	–	–	5	0	1
D2-clone 7	28	–	–	–	–	7	4	1
D2-clone 17	24	–	–	–	–	9	5	6
D2-clone 13	24	+++	++	–	–	2	3	0
D2-clone 13	24	–	–	–	–	7	2	0
D2-clone 13	24	–	–	–	–	23	35	0
D2-clone 13	23	±	–	–	–	0	NT[c]	0
D2-clone 17	23	±	–	–	+	7	NT	0
D2-clone 17	23	++++	++++	+++	++	4	NT	0
D2-clone 19	23	++++	++++	+++	++	2	NT	0
D2-clone 6	30	++++	++++	++	++	8	4	2
D2-clone 6	31	++++	++++	+++	++	4	4	1

[a] Refers to the time period the tumor was growing before removal. Tumors were generally 1.5–3 cm in diameter.
[b] Refers to analysis of solid tumor obtained at site of subcutaneous injection.
[c] NT, not tested.

vious section. Because the EAC (C3) receptor is trypsin-sensitive, we attempted analysis on solid tumor disaggregated by mechanical means in the absence of any proteolytic enzymes. This was feasible because the MDAY-D2 tumor does not contain much dense fibrous connective tissue and is relatively easy to disaggregate by mechanical means. The cell suspensions obtained were treated to remove dead cells and debris by centrifugation on ficoll–urovison solutions as described by Nagy *et al.* (1976). This is a modification of the method of Davidson and Parish (1975).

The results in Table IV demonstrate that no significant differences could be found between high- and low-metastatic variants of MDAY-D2. In general, the proportion of EAC-positive (C3R$^+$) cells was less than 8%, whether or not there was evidence of metastasis. Similarly, the percentages of macrophages and T cells were usually very low, even nondetectable in most cases. Only rarely were more than 2% macrophages found.

These results certainly do not incriminate a role of host cells in influencing the metastatic process of this tumor.

D. Host Cell Analysis of Lectin-Resistant Variants of MDAY-D2

The results obtained with some of our cloned lectin-resistant MDAY-D2 lines provided a refreshing change from the results described in the last section. An example of this is shown in Table V, in which the host cell responses of MC-2, a Con-A-resistant variant of MDAY-D2, are shown. It will be noted that the level of EAC-positive cells was markedly higher than that obtained with the cloned variants of MDAY-D2. Although the level of macrophages was still not high, it was at least higher than that obtained with lectin-sensitive MDAY-D2 cell lines. Levels of T cells remained low. We have not yet ascertained the nature of the EAC-positive cells. However, they do not represent the MC-2 cells, since tissue-culture-derived MC-2 cells were shown to be EAC-negative.

Table V. Host Cell Analysis of MC-2, a Con-A-Resistant Variant of MDAY-D2[a]

Tumor	Size of tumor (cm)	Metastatic pattern				Host cell response		
		Liver	Spleen	Lungs	Kidneys	% EAC$^+$	% Thy-1.2$^+$	% MΦ
1	2.5 × 2.8	+	–	–	–	23	–	3
2	2.0 × 2.7	+++	–	–	–	14	–	2
3	2.2 × 2.0	+++	–	–	–	15	–	3
4	2.3 × 2.0	+	–	–	–	19	–	4
5	2.2 × 1.8	–	–	–	–	18	–	3

[a]DBA/2 mice were injected subcutaneously 30 days previously with 10^6 M-C2 cells. When liver metastases were observed they tended to be large, oval, and discrete.

Table VI. Host Cell Analysis of ND3, a Low-Metastatic Variant of MDAY-D2[a]

Tumor size (cm)	Days	Metastatic pattern				Host cell response		
		Liver	Spleen	Lungs	Kidney	% EAC[+]	% Thy-1.2[+]	% MΦ
4 × 3	20	+	−	+	−	2	0	0
4 × 3.5	20	−	−	−	−	3	0	0
4 × 3	20	−	−	−	−	10	0	0
4 × 3	20	−	−	−	−	4	4	0
2 × 2.5	20	−	−	+	−	9	10	0
2.5 × 2.7	20	+++	−	−	−	5	2	1
2 × 3	20	+++	−	−	−	2	5	0
3 × 2	18	−	−	−	−	5	0	0
3 × 3.5	18	−	−	−	−	7	0	0
2.5 × 3	23	−	−	−	−	6	1	2

[a]ND3 was derived by injecting a BALB/c nude mouse (that had been reconstituted with normal BALB/c spleen cells) with MDAY-D2 cells. The tumor did not metastasize and was passaged at least three times in DBA/2 hosts prior to testing.

In another experiment we analyzed one WGA-resistant variant line and again found elevated host cell responses, including macrophages. However, the tumor was metastatic despite the fact that it grew more slowly. In attempting to repeat these results, we made a number of new WGA-resistant variants. When we analyzed them we found that two of them, MDW1 and MDW3, were not tumorigenic, i.e., no tumors arose, even at the site of injection, using a dose of 10^6 cells (Kerbel, 1980).

In Table VI are recorded the results obtained with the ND3 low-metastatic variant cell line. As with the cloned variants no significant host cell responses were observed.

VI. SUMMARY

With the possible exception of the lectin-resistant variant tumor line results, the studies here do not indicate a significant role for intratumor host cells in affecting the metastic process. We recognize, however, that there are certain limitations to the model and approach, one of the most important being the uncertainty of the nature of the MDAY-D2 tumor line. If, for example, this tumor is in fact a newly induced DBA/2 lymphoreticular tumor, then it would be difficult to compare these results with those obtained with carcinomas and sarcomas in which intra tumor macrophages have been implicated, in some cases, in altering the metastatic process.

ACKNOWLEDGMENTS

This work was supported by grants from the National Cancer Institute of Canada. Ms. M. S. Man, Ms. Ingrid Louwman, and Mrs. Marie Florian provided excellent technical assistance, and Mrs. Monika Conley provided excellent secretarial help.

VII. REFERENCES

Alexander, P., 1975, The role of macrophages in the host defense cancer, in: *Host Defense against Cancer and its Potentiation* (D. Mizuno, ed.), pp. 113–123, University of Tokyo Press, Tokyo.

Baker, R. M., and Ling, V., 1978, Membrane mutants of mammalian cells in culture, *Methods Membrane Biol.* 9:337–384.

Bayreuther, K., and Klein, E., 1958, Cytogenetic, serologic, and transplantation studies on a heterozygous tumor and its derived variant sublines, *J. Natl. Cancer Inst.* 21:885–923.

Birbeck, M. S. C., and Carter, R. L., 1972, Observations on the ultrastructure of two hamster lymphomas with particular reference to infiltrating macrophases, *Int. J. Cancer* 9:249–257.

Bjaring, B., and Klein, G., 1968, Antigenic characterization of heterozygous mouse lymphomas after immunoselection *in vivo*, *J. Natl. Cancer Inst.* 4:1411–1429.

Davidson, W. F., and Parish, C. R., 1975, A procedure for removing red cells and dead cells from lymphoid cell suspensions, *J. Immunol. Methods* 7:291–300.

Eccles, S., and Alexander, P., 1974, Macrophage content of tumors in relation to metastatic spread and host immune reaction, *Nature (London)* 250:667–669.

Fidler, I. J., 1973, Selection of successive tumor lines for metastasis, *Nature (London)* 242:148–149.

Fidler, I. J., and Kripkie, M., 1977, Metastasis results from pre-existing variant cells within a malignant tumor, *Science* 197:898–895.

Gershon, R. K., Carter, R. L., and Lane, N. J., 1967, Studies on homotransplantable lymphomas in hamsters, *Am. J. Pathol.* 51:1111–1113.

Graham, S. D., Mickey, D. P., and Paulson, D. F., 1978, Detection of metastatic tumors in nude mice, *J. Natl. Cancer Inst.* 60:715–716.

Haskill, J. S., Yamamura, Y., and Radov, L., 1975, Host responses within solid tumors: Non-thymus-derived specific cytotoxic cells within a murine mammary adenocarcinoma, *Int. J. Cancer* 16:798–809.

Husby, G., Hoagland, P. M., Strickland, R. C., and Williams, R. C., 1976, Tissue T and B cell infiltration of primary and metastatic cancer, *J. Clin. Invest.* 3:465–475.

Ioachim, H. L., 1976, The stromal reaction of tumors: An expression of immune surveillance, *J. Natl. Cancer Inst.* 3:465–475.

Kerbel, R. S., 1980, Immunologic studies of membrane mutants of a highly metastic murine tumor, *Am. J. Pathol.* 97:609–622.

Kerbel, R. S., and Davies, A. J. S., 1974, The possible biological significance of Fc receptors in mammalian cells lymphocytes and tumor cells, *Cell* 3:105–112.

Kerbel, R. S., and Pross, H. F., 1976, Fc receptor-bearing cells as a reliable marker for quantitation of host lymphoreticular infiltration of progressively growing solid tumors, *Int. J. Cancer* 18:432–438.

Kerbel, R. S., Pross, H. F., and Elliott, E. V., 1975, Origin and partial characterization of Fc receptor-bearing cells found within experimental carcinomas and sarcomas, *Int. J. Cancer* 15:918-932.

Kerbel, R. S., Pross, H. F., and Liebovitz, A., 1977, Analysis of established human carcinoma cell lines for lymphoreticular-associated membrane receptors, *Int. J. Cancer* 20:673-679.

Kerbel, R. S., Twiddy, R. R., and Robertson, D. M., 1978, Induction of a tumor with greatly increased metastatic growth potential by injection of cells from a low-metastatic H-2 heterozygous tumor cell line into an H-2 incompatible parental strain, *Int. J. Cancer* 22:583-594.

Kerbel, R. S., Florian, M., Man, M. S., Dennis, J., and McKenzie, I. F. C., 1980, On the carcinogenicity of tumor cell populations: Studies on the origin of a putative H-2 isoantigenic loss variant tumor, *J. Natl. Cancer Inst.* **64.**

Klein, J., 1975, *Biology of the Mouse Histocompatability-2 Complex*, Springer-Verlag, New York.

Klein, G., Sjögren, H. O., Klein, E., and Hellström, K. E., 1960, Demonstration of resistance against methylcholanthrene-induced sarcomas in the primary autochthonous host, *Cancer Res.* 20:1561-1572.

Koller, P. C., 1972, The role of chromosomes in cancer biology, in: *Recent Results in Cancer Research*, pp. 89-96, Springer-Verlag, New York.

Mankovitz, R., Buchwald, M., and Baker, R. M., 1974, Isolation of ouabain-resistant human diploid fibroblasts, *Cell* 3:221-226.

Mantovani, A., 1978, Effects on *in vitro* tumor growth of murine macrophages isolated from sarcoma lines differing in immunogenicity and metastasizing capacity, *Int. J. Cancer* 22: 741-746.

Mellgren, J., 1976, Quantitation of metastases in experimental animals, in: *Fundamental Aspects of Metastasis* (L. Weiss, ed.), pp. 243-252, Elsevier-North Holland, New York.

Moore, K., and Moore, M., 1977, Intra-tumor host cells of transplanted rat neoplasms of different immunogenicity, *Int. J. Cancer* 19:803-813.

Nagy, Z., Elliott, B. E., and Nabholz, M., 1976, Specific binding of K- and I- region products of the H-2 complex to activated thymus-derived (T) cells belonging to different Ly subclasses, *J. Exp. Med.* 144:1545-1553.

Pasqualini, C. D., Saal, F., Braylan, R. C., and Rabasa, S. L., 1970, Induction of leukemia in BALB/c mice by allogeneic AKR leukemic cells, *Int. J. Cancer* 5:338-345.

Pross, H. F., and Kerbel, R. S., 1976, An assessment of intratumor phagocytic and surface marker-bearing cells in a series of autochthonous and early passaged chemically induced murine sarcomas, *J. Natl. Cancer Inst.* 57:1157-1167.

Rajan, R. V., and Flores, C., 1977, H-2 antigen variants in a cultured heterozygous mouse leukemia cell line. III. Effect of selection against a D-end gene, *Immunogenetics* 5:585-596.

Sugarbaker, E. V., Thornthwaite, T., and Ketcham, A. S., 1977, Inhibitory effect of a primary tumor on metastasis, in: *Cancer Invasion and Metastasis: Biologic Mechanisms and Therapy* (S. B. Day, W. P. L. Meyers, P. Stansly, S. Garattini, and M. G. Lewis, eds.), pp. 227-241, Raven Press, New York.

Tao, T. W., and Burger, M. M., 1977, Non-metastasizing variants selected from metastasizing melanoma cells, *Nature (London)* 270:437-438.

Underwood, J. C. E., 1974, Lymphoreticular infiltration in human tumors: Prognostic and biological implications: A review, *Br. J. Cancer* 30:353-547.

Wood, G. W., and Gillespie, G. Y., 1975, Studies on the role of macrophages in regulation of growth and metastasis of murine chemically induced fibrosarcomas, *Int. J. Cancer* 16: 1022-1029.

Chapter 12

Cellular Basis for Regulation of Tumor Growth

Robert Evans

The Jackson Laboratory
Bar Harbor, Maine 04609

I. INTRODUCTION

The association of host-derived cells with progressing transplantable tumors raises several important issues. For example, the relevance of the host cells to tumor growth is not clear, and the mechanisms that determine whether macrophages, lymphocytes, or granulocytes infiltrate the tumor mass are not understood. Similarly, it is not clear whether tumor-associated host cells (TAHC) play a role in therapy-induced regression, and to what extent manipulation of TAHC is possible either within the tumor or before they reach the tumor (see review by Evans, 1977c). Other questions arise from these, such as whether any influence that TAHC may appear to exert on tumor growth (induced regression or stimulation) is mediated directly, by soluble mediators or by acting in cooperation with other cell types. Moreover, while an effect may appear to occur locally, that is, progression or regression may be associated with the presence of particular cell types, the effect may actually be mediated from a distance, for example, by soluble mediators that originate at a distant site and circulate through the tumor and react directly with the neoplastic cells or with tumor-associated host effector cells. Dissection of the wide array of reactions that probably occur is obviously difficult and complex, but as a starting point it is a reasonable assumption that some of the answers may lie at the site of tumor growth, not necessarily to the exclusion of reactions occurring peripherally but perhaps in concert with them. This is not a comprehensive review and will cover only certain aspects of the cellular basis for regulation of tumor growth, having special reference to events occurring at the level of the tumor mass. Some experiments on the accumulation of host cells will be described, together with a discussion on the implications of

255

such accumulation. The review will explore the possibility that tumor progression might be associated with cells able to enhance neoplastic cell proliferation directly, or indirectly by preventing cells generally associated with graft rejection from expressing cytotoxicity. Finally, the effects of drugs on the cellular composition of tumors during regression and regrowth following a period of remission will be discussed.

II. ACCUMULATION OF HOST CELLS IN TUMORS

A number of experimental protocols utilize the findings that tumors of man and experimental animals may contain the whole spectrum of leukocytes found in the blood and various tissues and organs (Evans, 1977c). The objective of some forms of therapy, e.g., bacillus Calmette–Guerin (BCG), *Corynebacterium parvum*, or glucan injection, is to enhance immunity against the tumor and/or to provoke an accumulation of certain types of cells, e.g., lymphocytes or macrophages, at the tumor site. Such therapeutic approaches are limited, to a certain extent, in that little is known about the kinetics of movement or accumulation of host-derived cells at the tumor site, how long particular categories of cell reside in the tumor mass, whether cells die or move away, what their precise relationship is with leukocytes in the peripheral circulation, and, when using the above-mentioned (re)agents, whether stimulation of particular cell types is likely to result in preferential homing to the tumor mass. Certainly, intralesional injection of therapeutic agents has resulted in tumor regression, and this has been associated with accumulation of host cells, particularly macrophages. Nevertheless, when applied systemically, these agents frequently show no antitumor effects, indicating a failure of cells to accumulate or to act at the site of tumor growth. For reasons such as these, kinetic studies are of basic importance.

The mechanisms that control the accumulation of TAHC or that determine the level of any particular category of host cells are far from being understood. For example, in a series of recent experiments with C57BL mice involving a syngeneic fibrosarcoma designated FS6, it was shown that this tumor contained a relatively high proportion of macrophages and that depletion of macrophages by whole body irradiation (WBI) (Evans, 1977a) or azathioprine treatment (Evans, 1977b) impaired the subsequent growth of implanted tumor cells. Experiments designed to repopulate the tumors with macrophages resulted in normal tumor growth and suggested a requirement for bone-marrow-derived monocytes or macrophages (Evans, 1978a).

In another series of experiments, involving three chemically induced transplantable immunogenic C57BL ($\female$) fibrosarcomas (designated FS6, FS25, and FS28), we assessed the numbers of cells accumulating at the site of tumor cell implantation after an intramuscular (im) injection of 10^6 neoplastic cells into control and X-irradiated (400 R WBI 24 previously) mice, with a view to showing whether an intact marrow system was required for tumor growth (Evans, 1979). At daily intervals, the whole of the musculature of the tibia was excised (this contained the tumor cell inoculum), and dissociated with a mixture of trypsin, collagenase, and DNase. Table I summarizes the overall results of a representative experiment. Only selected time points (days 1-7) are given. Results are expressed as average yield of cells per tumor mass. The first point of note is that the total tumor cell yield is clearly reduced in mice receiving WBI, compared with the control counterparts. The second point is that each tumor showed a different response, the FS6 tumor showing the lowest in terms of cell numbers present throughout, the FS28 showing the highest. It should also be noted that each fibrosarcoma showed a well-defined rate of growth in that after 10^6 cells were injected, tumors became palpable at different times. The FS6 tumors showed the longest latent period, the FS28 tumors the shortest. Table II subdivides the results of Table I into neoplastic and host cell yields (containing cumulative data on macrophages, lymphocytes, and granulocytes). On the basis of neoplastic cell yields, it is seen that the rate of increase from days 1-7 was more or less identical with all three control tumors, each undergoing about seven population doublings in this time. This indicated that in fact there was no difference in tumor growth rates, even though tumors became palpable at different times. The explanation for this apparent paradox lies in the cell yields noted on day 1, when it is seen that there was only a low level of FS6 cells (8% of the starting inoculum) but a much higher level of FS28 cells (50% of the starting inoculum). Whether these levels reflect variable sensitivity of neoplastic cells to the enzyme procedures used to disaggregate the tumor fragments or to transplantation into syngeneic recipients, or to both, is not known. These results provide a good explanation

Table I. Total Tumor Cell Yields from FS6, FS25, and FS28 Fibrosarcomas Growing in Control or Irradiated C57BL Mice[a]

		Total cell yield ($\times 10^6$)/tumor[b]			
Tumor	Day:	1	2	4	7
FS6 in control mice		0.88	3.7	5.9	24.9
FS6 in irradiated mice		0.37	0.8	2.9	5.2
FS25 in control mice		1.0	3.5	8.8	48.6
FS25 in irradiated mice		0.7	1.1	7.1	17.6
FS28 in control mice		3.1	9.7	29.4	215.4
FS28 in irradiated mice		0.8	3.2	13.4	58.4

[a] Mice received 400 R WBI 24 h prior to injection of 10^6 neoplastic cells.
[b] Mean of 3-5 tumors.

Table II. A Comparison of the Cellular Composition of FS6, FS25, and FS28 Fibrosarcomas Growing in Normal or Irradiated C57BL Mice[a]

| | | Cellular composition ($\times 10^6$) per tumor mass[b] | | | | | | | |
| | | Neoplastic cells[c] | | | | Normal host cells | | | |
Tumor	Day: 1	2	4	7	1	2	4	7
FS6 in control mice	0.08	0.3	1.5	8.6 ± 2.4	0.8	3.4	4.4	16.30
FS6 in irradiated mice	0.07	0.3	1.4	3.2 ± 1.8	0.3	0.5	1.5	2.0
FS25 in control mice	0.2	0.8	4.3	18.7 ± 3.9	0.8	2.7	4.5	29.9
FS25 in irradiated mice	0.2	0.5	4.3	11.9 ± 1.9	0.5	0.6	2.8	5.7
FS28 in control mice	0.5	3.3	9.7	67.7 ± 3.7	2.6	6.4	19.7	147.7
FS28 in irradiated mice	0.4	2.5	8.0	41.6 ± 2.4	0.4	0.7	5.4	16.8
Muscle injected with TC 199 alone	−	−	−	−	0.7 ± 0.3	−	−	0.8 ± 0.1
Muscle not injected	−	−	−	−	0.4 ± 0.2	−	−	0.4 ± 0.1

[a]10^6 Neoplastic cells implanted i.m. 24 h after 400 R WBI.
[b]Mean of 3–5 tumors.
[c]SD included only for those points showing apparent difference in neoplastic cell numbers.

for the relatively high number of FS6 cells needed for a 50% take (5×10^3 to 10^4 cells) and for the lower numbers of FS25 cells (10^3) and FS28 cells (10^2) needed for a take.

Of interest was the finding that although the level of neoplastic cells was different for each control tumor on day 7, the number of TAHC was proportional, that is there was a ratio of approximately two TAHC to one neoplastic cell (this tended to shift to about 1:1 by day 10). The major host cells at these times were macrophages and neutrophils. These results suggested that the level of TAHC was determined either by the extent of neoplastic cell proliferation or by the actual number of neoplastic cells.

When considering cell yields from tumors growing in irradiated mice, it is seen that there were fewer neoplastic cells compared with control counterparts, larger differences being seen with FS6 tumors and smaller, but reproducible, differences seen with FS25 and FS28 tumors. However, although it is clear that the level of TAHC was markedly lower than in controls, the actual levels again appeared to be related to the number of neoplastic cells. Thus, since all mice received identical WBI treatment before tumor cell implantation, it is evident that differences in the level of TAHC were due to the presence of the particular tumor. In this regard it was of interest that the FS28 tumor appeared to stimulate bone marrow recovery faster than the FS6 or FS25 tumors (see Table III). It is well established that some tumors induce a monocytosis and granulocytosis (Lappat and Cawein, 1964; Hibbard and Metcalf, 1971; Baum and Fisher, 1972; Eccles et al., 1976),

Table III. Bone Marrow Cell Counts (BMC) after i.m. Implantation of Fibrosarcoma Cells[a] into Control and Irradiated Mice

| | Days after | BMC per tibia $(\times 10^6) \pm SD^b$ | | |
Tumor	implantation: 2	4	7
Control C57 black mice;			
no tumors	6.7 ± 0.9	7.7 ± 0.7	7.6 ± 0.3
FS6 in control mice	5.7 ± 1.4	7.8 ± 1.3	7.4 ± 0.7
FS25 in control mice	4.2 ± 1.6	7.3 ± 0.9	7.9 ± 0.8
FS28 in control mice	4.9 ± 0.8	6.8 ± 1.2	9.6 ± 1.6
Irradiated mice;			
no tumors	1.6 ± 0.3	2.0 ± 0.7	5.3 ± 0.9
FS6 in irradiated mice	1.3 ± 0.3	3.6 ± 1.3	4.8 ± 1.3
FS25 in irradiated mice	1.0 ± 0.2	4.3 ± 1.2	4.0 ± 0.8
FS28 in irradiated mice	2.0 ± 0.3	1.3 ± 0.3	8.7 ± 1.8

[a] 10^6 Neoplastic cells injected i.m. in 0.1 ml TC 199.
[b] Mean of 6–10 samples.

but it is not clear in some cases whether this is due to a defective capacity for the monocytes, for example, to move out of the circulation (Eccles *et al.*, 1976; Meltzer and Stevenson, 1977; Normann and Cornelius, 1978; Snyderman and Pike, 1976), hence resulting in elevated blood levels, or to hyperactive cell production by bone marrow. The reports that the so-called "monocyte-defect" is a possible reason for progressive tumor growth (Snyderman and Pike, 1976; Rhodes *et al.*, 1979) on the basis that monocytes might destroy the neoplastic cells if they reached the tumor are a generalization, for it is evident that not all tumors induce this defect in migration properties (Normann *et al.*, 1977), and it has been reported that the macrophage numbers may continue to increase as the tumor increases in size (Evans, 1972, 1977c).

III. MECHANISMS CONTROLLING HOST CELL ACCUMULATION

The conclusion from the above experiments was that progressive increase in tumor growth was associated with a progressive increase in the level of tumor-associated host cells. What remains to be resolved is whether the accumulation of these cells is determined solely by the extent of neoplastic cell proliferation, or by other factors, such as chemotactic stimuli, that may be related to the properties of the tumor itself (see Evans, 1977c). For example, it has been suggested that the level of macrophages is related to the immunogenicity of the tumor (Eccles and Alexander, 1974) such that strongly immunogenic tumors should have a high macrophage content, and weakly immunogenic tumors a low content. One might speculate at this point that strongly immunogenic tumors might invoke the appearance of antibodies directed against tumor-associated antigens, which may react with soluble antigen to form complexes that are chemotactic for macrophages and perhaps granulocytes. The presence of antichemotactic or antiinflammatory substances in the blood of tumor bearers (Snyderman and Pike, 1976; Fauve et al., 1974; Brozna and Ward, 1975) suggests a regulatory mechanism for host cell accumulation. Indeed, the fact that for a given tumor the level of macrophages is reported to be predictable at any given time (Evans, 1972) supports the notion of control. These exciting and potentially important aspects of tumor–host relationships warrant high-priority investigation, since one would suggest that an understanding of the nature of the mechanisms controlling accumulation of host cells is fundamental to our understanding how to use these cells to best effect in therapy programs.

IV. TUMOR-ASSOCIATED HOST CELLS, CYTOTOXICITY, AND GROWTH STIMULATION

The accumulation of host cells at the site of tumor growth has led to the notion that this is possibly an indication of immune reactivity towards the tumor. The evidence for this is slight and mostly speculative, based in the main on findings in vitro. For example, a number of investigators have reported that tumor-associated macrophages, monocytes, and lymphocytes can destroy neoplastic cells in vitro directly or indirectly in the presence of antibody (see review by Evans, 1977c). The obvious problem with findings in vitro is proving that they hold in vivo significance, and this is particularly noteworthy in the case of tumor-associated host cells showing cytotoxicity in vitro. The best correlate in vivo–in vitro is seen in cases of spontaneously regressing tumors, which contain cytotoxic host cells, as demonstrated by tests in vitro (Haskill et al., 1975; Holden et al., 1976; Russell et al., 1977b). The major problems arise when cytotoxic host cells are derived from progressing tumors, for in these situations it is evident that their effectiveness in situ is minimal or negligible. However, host cells from progressing tumors are frequently not cytotoxic in culture (Evans and Alexander, 1976), which, if one is looking for an explanation for progressive tumor growth in terms of cell-mediated stimulation, is what one might expect. In other words, it is the reverse of what one would expect, and finds, with spontaneously regressing tumors. This is not to say, however, that such cells may not have an important role to play in tumor rejection under well-defined conditions. Macrophages from tumors can be rendered cytotoxic by incubation with endotoxin, lipid A, Poly I:Poly C, or dsRNA (Evans, 1973), and Russell et al. (1977a) have recently shown that they are very sensitive to low doses of LPS. The relevance of these studies is seen when tumors are induced to regress as a result of the antitumor action of the tumor-necrotizing factor (TNF). Whether the macrophages are involved in the destruction *in situ* is not clear. It has been suggested that in fact macrophages may only secrete the TNF, while sensitized T lymphocytes destroy the neoplastic cells (Berendt *et al.*, 1978*a*,*b*).

The evidence that host cells stimulate tumor growth is mostly of an indirect nature, but it is strong enough to support the possibility. There is ample evidence from the literature that lymphoid cells from control or sensitized mice can stimulate tumor cells to grow both *in vivo* and *in vitro*. Whether this is due to immunostimulation (Prehn, 1976) or to nonspecific mechanisms is not clear. For example, the murine fibrosarcoma FS6 has been shown to grow less well in irradiated mice (see also Table I) (Evans 1977*a*). This was associated with a lack of macrophage infiltration and vascularization. Reconstitution of irradiated mice with syngeneic bone marrow cells before injecting FS6 cells or mixing the FS6 cells with macrophages prior to implantation resulted in tumor growth comparable to that seen in control mice (Evans, 1978*a*). Table IV compares the number of neoplastic cells and host cells (Fc-receptor-positive and -negative) on day 10 after injection of FS6 cells. It is clear that growth was depressed in irradiated mice but was stimulated after bone marrow reconstitution. These data do not constitute direct evidence that the macrophages were stimulating growth, but the requirement for these cells was apparent. It is possible, in this context, that bone-marrow-derived macrophages (or monocytes) were required to restore immune competence or lymphocyte reactivity or perhaps to process tumor-associated antigen. These data would then lend themselves to the suggestion that stimulation of tumor growth was dependent on induction of immunity.

There are other lines of evidence suggesting that tumor-associated macro-

Table IV. Cellular Composition of FS6 Fibrosarcomas Growing in Control of Irradiated (400 R WBI) C57BL Mice[a]

| Mice | Total cell yield ($\times 10^6$)/tumor | | |
	Neoplastic	Fc-receptor-positive[b]	Remainder[c]
Controls	13.6 ± 1.1	12.3 ± 1.7	9.6 ± 1.0
WBI	3.6 ± 0.6	1.3 ± 0.1	2.0 ± 0.1
WBI + BMC[d]	12.7 ± 1.5	11.0 ± 1.2	8.9 ± 0.9

[a] Mice injected with 10^6 neoplastic cells 5 days after WBI.
[b] Fc-receptor-positive refers to cells able to rosette antibody-coated SRBC.
[c] Referred to as Fc-receptor-negative cells in text.
[d] BMC, bone marrow cells (10^7) injected i.v. within 5 h of WBI and 5 days before i.m. injection of 10^6 FS6 cells.

phages can stimulate normal, transformed, or neoplastic cells *in vitro*. In a previous report (Evans, 1976) it was shown that tumor macrophages (both cytotoxic and noncytotoxic from progressing tumors) conditioned culture fluids, in which was later found a low-molecular-mass material (<10,000 daltons) that stimulated neoplastic cells to proliferate in the absence of serum (Evans, 1979). Using macrophages from the FS6 fibrosarcoma, Mantovani (1979) also showed that these could stimulate proliferation *in vitro*, and Salmon and Hamburger (1978) have reported similar findings with macrophages for human tumors.

V. CELLULAR BASIS OF TUMOR REGRESSION FOLLOWING DRUG THERAPY

There is evidence to suggest that some therapeutic agents exert an antitumor effect best, or only, in the presence of established antitumor immunity (Mathé *et al.*, 1974; Moore and Williams, 1973; Radov *et al.*, 1976; Steele and Pierce, 1974; Ziegler *et al.*, 1970). In this particular context there appears to be some confusion concerning the nature of the antitumor effect, whether this is defined as the ability of drug treatment to cause tumor regression or to result in total tumor eradication. In a recent report (Evans, 1978b), we showed that tumor regression was not dependent on established immunity when mice bearing a strongly or nonimmunogenic tumor were treated with cyclophosphamide (CY). Indeed, total tumor eradication was achieved in the absence of overt immunity as long as CY was given within a few days of tumor cell implantation. This effect was almost certainly due to the alkylating potential of the drug. However, regression without eradication was obtained with relatively large tumor burdens, and this was seen whether tumors were immunogenic or not, regardless of whether tumors were implanted into irradiated or control mice. Nevertheless, eradication of large tumors was not achieved, even when concomitant immunity could be demonstrated. Table V shows the results of concomitant immunity studies, in which 80 FS6-tumor-bearing mice, treated with CY, went into remission for 2–3 weeks. During this period 60 mice were challenged in the contralateral limb with an inoculum of 10^6 FS6 cells. Tumor incidence was assessed 14 days later and compared with controls. It was seen that 12/60 regressed tumors regrew very rapidly when mice were challenged in the other limb, and only one of these was challenge-tumor free on day 14. It was also seen that 44/60 tumors regrew within 2–3 weeks of CY treatment and that of these 42/44 showed no growth of the challenge inoculum. A small number of mice (4/80) showed no recurrence of tumor, and these also showed no growth of the challenge inoculum.

The obvious question to arise from experiments of this nature is why a challenge inoculum was rejected, while in most cases the regressed tumors recurred. The problem of eradicating residual tumor is a problem central to therapy

Table V. Expression of Concomitant Immunity
after CY-Induced Regression of the FS6
Fibrosarcoma: Incidence of Challenge Tumors[a]

Rate of recurrence after CY treatment	Incidence of challenge tumors on day 14
Fast	92% (11/12)
Delayed	5% (2/44)
No recurrence	0% (0/4)
Control mice	100% (30/30)

[a]FS6-tumor-bearing mice injected i.p. with 4 mg cyclophosphamide: 10 days later mice received a challenge injection of 10^6 FS6 cells in opposite hind limb.

in general; thus any observations on changes that occur in cell populations within the tumor site might help in understanding why neoplastic cells survive, even when the host shows antitumor immunity. Very few studies have been reported at this particular level (Evans, 1978b; Radov et al., 1976; Szymaniec and James, 1976). The possibility was suggested that this site, unlike that of the challenge, might have been refractile to infiltration by cells normally associated with graft rejection, but it was later shown that macrophages, T lymphocytes, and granulocytes appeared at the site, particularly when the tumors were regrowing after the period of remission (Evans, 1979). Whether these cells possessed cytotoxic capacity or suppressor activity, or whether they were stimulating recurrence is currently under investigation. One possibility is that the neoplastic cells remaining after regression represent a minority population of cells antigenically different from the majority of parental cells, which are, moreover, frequently resistant to further CY treatment. These speculative remarks indicate the general lack of information concerning changes in the cellular events taking place in the tumor mass and emphasize the need for research in depth into these various aspects.

VI. CONCLUSIONS

During the last decade it has become clear that host blood leukocytes and those in various tissues and organs can destroy neoplastic cells in a direct manner, and those that cannot kill can be rendered cytotoxic by antibody or other soluble factors. Such cytotoxic reactions have been demonstrated in many different systems, but of particular interest is the presence of cytotoxic cells in the tumor-bearing host. Concomitant immunity attests to the presence of effector mechanisms. However, the primary tumor that elicits this response invariably escapes destruction and overcomes the host. The reasons for this escape are probably numerous. Although it is evident that while those cells with the potential to reject the neoplasm do in fact enter the tumor mass, their antitumor effect is clearly negligible, and the question is why this should be. The study of TAHC, the kinetics of infiltration, their functional capacities, and their interactions with other cell types are aspects requiring investigation, for it is this level at which any changes that may be induced in the host with a view to causing tumor rejection are ultimately seen. Without the knowledge of what events occur at the tumor site, we may retard the development of potentially useful protocols aimed at tumor eradication.

ACKNOWLEDGMENTS

This research was supported by a grant from the Medical Research Council, England.

VII. REFERENCES

Baum, M., and Fisher, B., 1972, Macrophage production by the bone marrow of tumor-bearing mice, *Cancer Res.* **32**:2813.

Berendt, M. J., North, R. J., and Kirstein, D. P., 1978a, The immunological basis of endotoxin-induced tumor regression. Requirement for T-cell mediated immunity, *J. Exp. Med.* **148**:1550.

Berendt, M. J., North, R. J., and Kirstein, D. P., 1978b, The immunological basis of endotoxin-induced tumor regression. Requirement for a pre-existing state of concomitant anti-tumor immunity, *J. Exp. Med.* **148**:1560.

Brozna, J. P., and Ward, R. A., 1975, Antileukotactic properties of tumor cells, *J. Clin. Invest.* **56**:616.

Eccles, S. A., and Alexander, P., 1974, Macrophage content of tumors in relation to metastatic spread and host immune reactions, *Nature (London)* **250**:667.

Eccles, S. A., Bandlow, G., and Alexander, P., 1976, Monocytosis associated with growth of transplanted syngeneic sarcomas differing in immunogenicity, *Br. J. Cancer* **34**:20.

Evans, R., 1972, Macrophages in syngeneic animal tumors, *Transplantation* **14**:468.

Evans, R., 1973, Macrophages and the tumor-bearing host, *Br. J. Cancer* **22**(i):19.

Evans, R., 1976, Tumor macrophages in host immunity to maligancies, in: *The Macrophage in Neoplasia* (M. A. Fink, ed.), p. 27, Academic Press, New York.

Evans, R., 1977a, The effect of X-irradiation on host cell infiltration and growth of a murine fibrosarcoma, *Br. J. Cancer* **35**:557.

Evans, R., 1977b, The effect of azathioprine on host cell infiltration and growth of a murine fibrosarcoma, *Int. J. Cancer* **20**:120.

Evans, R., 1977c, Macrophages in solid tumors, in: *The Macrophage and Cancer* (K. James, B. McBride, and A. Stuart, eds.), p. 321, Econoprint, Edinburgh.

Evans, R., 1978a, Macrophage requirement for growth of a murine fibrosarcoma, *Br. J. Cancer* **36**:1086.

Evans, R., 1978b, Failure to relate the anti-tumor action of cyclophosphamide with the immunogenicity of two murine fibrosarcomas, *Int. J. Cancer* **21**:611.

Evans, R., 1979, Host cells in transplanted murine tumors and their possible relevance to tumor growth, *J. Reticuloendothel. Soc.* **26**:427–437.

Evans, R., and Alexander, P., 1976, Mechanisms of extracellular killing of nucleated mammalian cells by macrophages, in: *Immunobiology of the Macrophage* (D. S. Nelson, ed.), p. 536, Academic Press, New York.

Fauve, R. M., Hevin, B., Jacob, H., Guillard, J. A., and Jacob, F., 1974, Anti-inflammatory effects of murine malignant cells, *Proc. Natl. Acad. Sci. USA* **71**:4052.

Haskill, J. S., Yamamura, Y., and Radov, L. A., 1975, Host responses within solid tumors: Non-thymus derived specific cytotoxic cells within a murine mammary adenocarcinoma, *Int. J. Cancer* **16**:798.

Hibbard, A. D., and Metcalf, D., 1971, Proliferation of macrophage and granulocyte precursors in response to primary and transplanted tumors, *Isr. J. Med. Sci.* **7**:202.

Holden, H. T., Haskill, J. S., Kirchner, H., and Herbermann, R. B., 1976, Two functionally distinct anti-tumor effector cells isolated from primary murine sarcoma virus-induced tumors, *J. Immunol.* **117**:440.

Lappat, E. J., and Cawein, M., 1964, A study of the leukemoid response to transplantable A-280 tumor in mice, *Cancer Res.* **24**:302.

Mantovani, A., 1979, Effects on *in vitro* tumor growth of murine macrophages isolated from sarcoma line differing in immunogenicity and metastasizing capacity, *Int. J. Cancer* **22**:741.

Mathé, G., Halle-Panneko, O., and Bourut, C., 1974, Immune manipulation by BCG administered before or after cyclophosphamide chemo-immunotherapy of L1210 leukemia, *Eur. J. Cancer* **10**:661.

Meltzer, M. A., and Stevenson, M. M., 1977, Macrophage function in tumor-bearing mice: Tumoricidal and chemotactic responses of macrophages activated by infection with *Mycobacterium bovis*, strain BCG, *J. Immunol.* **118**:2176.

Moore, M., and Williams, D. E., 1973, Contribution of host immunity to cyclophosphamide therapy of a chemically-induced murine fibrosarcoma, *Int. J. Cancer* **11**:358.

Normann, S. J., and Cornelius, J., 1978, Concurrent depression of tumor macrophage infiltration and systemic inflammation by progressive cancer growth, *Cancer Res.* **38**:3453.

Normann, S. J., Schardt, M., and Sorkin, E., 1977, Do tumors escape suveillance by depression of macrophage inflammation? in: *The Macrophage and Cancer* (K. James, B. McBride, and A. Stuart, eds.), p. 247, Econoprint, Edinburgh.

Prehn, R. T., 1977, Immunostimulation of the lymphodependent phase of neoplastic growth, *J. Natl. Cancer Inst.* **59**:1043.

Radov, L. A., Haskill, J. S., and Korn, J. H., 1976, Host immune potentiation of drug responses to a murine mammary adenocarcinoma, *Int. J. Cancer* **17**:773.

Rhodes, J., Bishop, M., and Benfield, J., 1979, Tumor surveillance: How tumors may resist macrophage-mediated host defense, *Science* **203**:179.

Russell, S. W., Doe, W. F., and McIntosh, A. T., 1977a, A non-cytolytic stage of macrophage activation in Maloney sarcomas, in: *The Macrophage and Cancer* (K. James, B. McBride, and A. Stuart, eds.), p. 341, Econoprint, Edinburgh.

Russell, S. W., Gillespie, G. Y., and McIntosh, A. T., 1977b, Inflammatory cells in solid murine neoplasms. III. Cytotoxicity mediated *in vitro* by macrophages recovered from disaggregated regressing Maloney sarcomas, *J. Immunol.* **118**:1574.

Salmon, S. W., and Hamburger, A. W., 1978, Immunoproliferation and cancer: A common macrophage-derived promoter, *Lancet* **1**:1289.

Snyderman, R., and Pike, M. C., 1976, Defective macrophage migration produced by neoplasms: Identification of an inhibitor of macrophage chemotaxis, in: *The Macrophage in Neoplasia* (M. A. Fink, ed.), p. 49, Academic Press, New York.

Steele, G., and Pierce, G. E., 1974, Effects of cyclophosphamide on immunity against chemically induced syngeneic murine fibrosarcomas, *Int. J. Cancer* **13**:572.

Szymaniec, S., and James, K., 1976, Studies on the Fc receptor bearing cells in a transplanted methylcholanthrene induced mouse fibrosarcoma, *Br. J. Cancer* **33**:36.

Ziegler, J. L., Morrow, R. H., Fass, L., Kyalwali, S. K., and Carbone, P. P., 1970, Treatment of Burkitt's tumor with cyclophosphamide, *Cancer* **26**:474.

Chapter 13

Immunological Stimulation in Situ: The Acute and Chronic Inflammatory Responses in the Induction of Tumor Immunity

M. G. Hanna, Jr., C. D. Bucana, and V. A. Pollack

Cancer Biology Program
NCI Frederick Cancer Research Center
Frederick, Maryland 21701

I. INTRODUCTION

The success of immunotherapy both in experimental animals and in man depends upon the stage of the tumor at the time of treatment. The major potential for immunotherapy is its use as an adjunct to chemotherapy or surgery of the primary tumor when there is only minimal regional lymph node metastasis and micrometastatic disease in the visceral organs. Nonspecific immunomodulation with the aim to enhance immune reactivity against disseminated minimal residual malignancy has been attempted clinically with such microbial vaccines as *Mycobacterium bovis* strain bacillus Calmette–Guérin (BCG), *Corynebacterium parvum*, several polynucleotides, levamisole, and lately interferon. The unsuccessful or equivocal results of these problematic, albeit feasible, clinical protocols may be partly attributable to the low degree of antigenicity of human tumors, while the successful animal models for nonspecific immunotherapy involved relatively antigenic transplantable murine tumors. Although immunopotentiators can enhance immune responses in general, the complicated host–tumor interrelationship indicates that in the immunocompetent host the immune response has a finite capacity to counteract any given antigen. Thus, it is unlikely that generalized immunopotentiation will result in a sufficiently elevated immuno- logical capacity that would significantly alter the growth of a weakly antigenic tumor or affect micrometastases.

There has also been a substantial effort to actively immunize autochthonous or syngeneic hosts with irradiated or chemically modified tumor cells in an attempt to achieve active specific immunotherapy. Inherent in this approach is the assumption that tumor cells express tumor-specific transplantation antigens. Treatment of tumor cells with a variety of unrelated agents such as radiation, mitomycin C, lipophilic agents, neuraminidase, viruses, or admixture of the cells with bacterial adjuvants has yielded nontumorigenic tumor cell preparations that are immunogenic upon injection into syngeneic hosts (Bartlett and Zbar, 1972; Bekesi *et al.*, 1971; Martin *et al.*, 1971; Prager and Baechtel, 1973; Ray *et al.*, 1975). Basically, these results support the concept that antigens not found in normal adult tissues are frequently found in tumors and that the immunogenicity of these tumor cells can be expressed and even enhanced in normal and tumor- bearing hosts. These experimental results have validated the rationale of active specific immunotherapy of neoplasia.

Beginning with the pioneering studies of Mathé *et al.* (1973), who treated acute lymphocytic leukemia with BCG, killed leukemic blasts, or both, similar protocols for treatment of acute or chronic granulocytic leukemia (Powles *et al.*, 1973; Sokal *et al.*, 1973), malignant melanoma (Morton *et al.*, 1976), and lung tumor (Hollingshead, 1978) have produced encouraging results by prolonging disease-free intervals. However, as of now, none of the treatments have signifi- cantly increased patient survival. Not all immunotherapy trials have been suc- cessful, even with respect to maintenance of disease-free intervals, as shown by recent studies of stage IIB malignant melanoma in which allogeneic or autoch- thonous tumor cells were used (Hedley *et al.*, 1978). The approach of active specific immunotherapy, although recognized as biologically sound, has been burdened by technical limitations that must be overcome before being practical in the laboratory or clinic (Prager, 1978).

The weakly immunogenic L10 hepatocarcinoma of strain 2 guinea pigs has proven to be a useful experimental model for examining certain aspects of active specific immunotherapy and has provided a system to evaluate a potent immuno- stimulant, *Mycobacterium bovis* (BCG). Intratumoral injection of viable BCG produced regression of established tumors of limited size growing in the skin and the elimination of regional lymph node metastases (Zbar and Tanaka, 1971; Hanna *et al.*, 1972); it also conferred immunity to a second intradermal (i.d.) challenge with L10 tumor cells (Zbar *et al.*, 1972; Hanna *et al.*, 1973). Also, more recently it has been demonstrated that vaccines composed of viable BCG organisms admixed with metabolically active but nontumorigenic L10 cells were effective in eliminating established visceral micrometastases (Hanna and Peters, 1978*a,b*). These observations imply that mixing the BCG with tumor cells may provide an effective immune stimulus despite the weak antigenicity of the tumor cells. In this guinea pig model the resultant tumor-specific immune response can eliminate established micrometastases. It is important to note that common to both the elimination of localized tumor by BCG alone and the induction of tumor-specific immunity by BCG-tumor cell vaccination is the development of a chronic inflammatory reaction resulting in epithelioid granuloma formation (Hanna and Bucana, 1979). The relationship between the chronic BCG-induced granulomatous inflammation (Adams, 1976; Boros, 1978) and the induction of systemic, tumor-specific immunity in this experimental guinea pig model is unclear.

Of the two therapeutic approaches, intratumoral BCG or BCG plus tumor cell immunization, the latter would appear to be more generally applicable in cancer treatment. Recent investigations have focused on various parameters of the vaccine preparation and administration. The two variables of BCG dose and tumor cell viability were found to profoundly influence the efficacy of the vaccine in the guinea pig immunotherapy model (Hanna *et al.*, 1979; Peters *et al.*, 1979). Significant protection against disseminated tumor required a minimum of two vaccinations administered 1 week apart with the initial immunization containing at least 10^7 viable BCG organisms admixed with 10^7 or more tumor cells. Tumor cell viability above 85% in the *final vaccine preparation* was critical. Thus, any manipulation of the tumor cells such as disaggregation from a solid tumor, cryobiologic preservation, or X irradiation would have to be accomplished while maintaining the prerequisite of cell viability. Also, no protection was achieved when another syngeneic, but antigenically distinct, hepatocarcinoma was used in the vaccine, thus suggesting that this was active specific immunotherapy.

An important feature of the model is its adaptability to studies of active specific immunotherapy as an adjunct to surgery (Hanna and Peters, 1978*a*). This allows the translation of information from this model to cases in which specific immunotherapy is used to treat micrometastasis after surgical excision of the primary tumor.

The reasons for the efficacy of BCG-tumor cell immunization are not understood. Histological and ultrastructural evidence indicates that cells of the macrophage-histiocyte system play a key role in the destruction of tumor cells following intratumoral BCG injection (Hanna *et al.*, 1972; Snodgrass and Hanna, 1973). However, this process must also require the participation of lymphocytes, since intratumoral injection of BCG in antilymphocyte-treated, tumor-bearing animals did not result in tumor destruction (Hanna *et al.*, 1973). Macrophages, and to a lesser extent lymphocytes, from BCG-cured guinea pigs were cytotoxic to tumor cells *in vitro* (Fidler *et al.*, 1976*a,b*).

In this chapter we will review the histology and ultrastructure of the induction site of active specific immunotherapy using BCG plus tumor cell vaccines. The morphology of reactions induced by effective or noneffective vaccines was compared and was correlated with functional tumor immunity as assessed by survival after therapy of established micrometastases in the viscera. Evaluations were made of tumor cell localization and persistence within the skin site, as well as of the composition and interactions of the cellular infiltrate within this microenvironment. The morphological findings at the dermal immunization sites correlated with the efficacy of the BCG–tumor cell vaccines and clarified some of the variables that tip the balance toward success or failure of active specific immunotherapy. Also, studies of the mechanism of action of BCG–tumor cell immunization as it affects tumor-specific immunity will be presented. The approach was to determine the effect of surgical interruption of granulomagenesis. Specifically, guinea pigs were immunized by i.d. vaccination, and the immunization sites and regional lymph nodes were surgically excised at strategic times during the acute and chronic inflammatory responses, prior to and after granuloma formation. The animals were then challenged i.d. with a lethal dose of tumor cells and evaluated for delayed hypersensitivity to tumor challenge and resistance to tumor growth.

II. EFFICACY OF BCG PLUS TUMOR CELL VACCINES FOR THERAPY OF MICROMETASTATIC MALIGNANT DISEASE

The L10 hepatocarcinoma was induced in strain 2 guinea pigs by diethylnitrosamine feeding, as described previously (Rapp *et al.*, 1968). The antigenic and biological properties of the transplantable ascites tumors derived from the primary hepatocarcinomas have also been described (Zbar *et al.*, 1969). To establish disseminated micrometastases in various visceral organs of the experimental animals, freshly harvested ascites cells, washed three times in HBSS, were injected into the dorsal penile vein. Injections of 10^5 or 10^6 cells were routinely fatal in all control animals. The time of death varied with dose. Fatalities occurred from metastases in the lungs, mediastinal and tracheobronchial lymph nodes, and the viscera.

For preparation of the vaccine, ascites cells were removed and washed in HBSS and used either fresh or frozen and thawed. Suspensions of fresh and frozen–thawed L10 cells were X irradiated with a Phillips MG301 X-irradiation unit at 500R/min. A total X-irradiation dose of 20,000 R was attained. Cell viability counts were performed using the trypan blue dye exclusion test or by staining with fluorescein diacetate (Rotman and Papermaster, 1966). Viability after irradiation of either fresh or frozen–thawed cells was generally greater than 80%, with less than 10% variation between the fresh or frozen–thawed cells. Phipps strain BCG (10^9 organisms/ml) was added in equal volume to viable L10 cells (10^8 cells/ml) for a vaccine ratio of 10:1. For ratios of 1:10, BCG (10^9 organisms/ml) was diluted 1:100 in HBSS, and aliquots were admixed with

10^8 viable L10 cells/ml. All immunizations consisted of an i.d. injection of 0.2 ml and were performed less than 1 h after preparation of the BCG–tumor cell mixtures. Immunizations were given i.d. beginning in the right upper dorsal quadrant. Second immunizations were given in the opposite quadrant. Immunizations were performed 1 and 7 days after i.v. L10 injection. Two modes of immunization and three ratios of viable BCG to tumor cells have been tested in guinea pigs injected i.v. with L10 cells. The BCG–tumor cell ratios were 1:10, 1:1, and 10:1, respectively. These doses were administered as either single i.d. injections or two i.d. immunizations separated by 6 days. The survival results are shown in Table I.

Compared to the untreated tumor-bearing guinea pigs, no significant difference in survival was detected in animals treated with two i.d. injections of BCG or tumor cells alone. Single BCG plus tumor cell immunizations at a ratio of 1:10 or 10:1 did not lead to significant protection. In contrast, significant differences in survival were achieved in tumor-bearing guinea pigs when the second vaccination was an identical BCG–L10 mixture. Survival in these treatment groups was a function of the BCG–L10 cell ratio. Without exception, in the guinea pigs given 10^5 or 10^6 cells i.v., a vaccine containing BCG–L10 cells at a ratio of 1:1 or 10:1 resulted in significant protection ($p < 0.01$) whereas a ratio of 1:10 was ineffective. Also, it is apparent at these tumor burdens that

Table I. Survival of Guinea Pigs Given i.v. Injections of 10^5 or 10^6 Syngeneic L10 Hepatocarcinoma[a]

Treatment[b]	No. of survivors/total No. of animals per group at 2 i.v. tumor cell doses	
	10^5	10^6
None	0/10	0/10
(10^8 BCG) (10^8 BCG)	0/10	0/10
(10^7 L10) (10^7 L10)	0/10	0/10
(10^6 BCG + 10^7 L10)[c]	1/10	0/10
(10^8 BCG + 10^7 L10)[c]	2/10	0/10
(10^6 BCG + 10^7 L10) (10^6 BCG + 10^7 L10)	1/10	1/10
(10^7 BCG + 10^7 L10) (10^7 BCG + 10^7 L10)	10/10	3/10
(10^8 BCG + 10^7 L10) (10^8 BCG + 10^7 L10)	10/10	5/10
(10^8 BCG + 10^7 LV[d] L10) (10^8 BCG + 10^7 LV L10)	–	0/10

[a]These experiments were terminated at 240 days after tumor injection. All nontreated controls in the 10^5 group died by 95 days and all nontreated controls in the 10^6 group died by 77 days. Significance of differences in survival was calculated by the Fisher two-tailed exact test.
[b]Vaccinations were administered i.d., 6 days apart on opposite sides.
[c]Vaccination was administered i.d., as a single injection.
[d]Low viability.

a second immunization is mandatory for therapy, although previous studies have shown that BCG is not essential in the second immunization.

III. GROSS MORPHOLOGY AND MEASUREMENT OF DERMAL IMMUNIZATION SITES

Sequential measurements of two perpendicular diameters were made on the primary and secondary immunization sites of guinea pigs immunized with 10^8 BCG, 10^7 L10 cells, 10^8 BCG + 10^7 L10 cells, 10^7 BCG + 10^7 L10 cells, and 10^6 BCG + 10^7 L10 cells. The tumor cells used for these injections were >80% viable at the time of injection. Also, for comparison, immunizations were carried out with suboptimally cryopreserved L10 cells, possessing viability of 30% or less at the time of immunization. These cells were injected alone or admixed with 10^8 BCG. The gross morphology of these sites at various intervals was recorded photographically. The dermal sites of animals immunized with 10^8 BCG + 10^7 L10 cells and 10^7 BCG + 10^7 L10 cells were similar and will be described together.

The primary immunization site for the 10^8 BCG alone underwent a progressive, almost linear swelling to day 13, followed by a reparative phase (Fig. 1a). No ulceration was observed until after 13 days; however, redness of the immunization sites was marked by day 7. Swelling at the secondary immunization site peaked 24 h after injection, then decreased. Two days after the second immunization there was another progressive swelling phase with redness of these immunization sites and ulcerative lesions as early as day 4. This reaction peaked at day 7.

In all treatment groups receiving L10 cells, regardless of the presence or dose of BCG, there was a marked acute swelling without redness 1 day after primary immunization (Fig. 1b–d). In all of these treatment groups there was a 50% or greater reduction in the swelling of these primary immunization sites over the next 5 days. The absence of this 24-h increase in papule size (surface area) in the BCG-only treatment group suggests that this effect is related to the volume of the tumor cell inoculum, not to a cellular infiltrate. A marked and chronic secondary swelling phase with redness was detected in the group treated with 10^8 BCG + 10^7 L10 cells (Fig. 1c). Although a sharp increase in papule size was observed at 24 h with all secondary immunizations, it was most marked and progressive in animals receiving 10^8 BCG + 10^7 L10 cells.

In comparison, guinea pigs receiving a primary immunization of low-viability L10 cells alone showed swelling in the immunization site within 24 h without redness, and there was no measurable papule 3 days after immunization. A secondary immunization with these cells followed a similar pattern. The primary and secondary immunization sites of guinea pigs inoculated with 10^8 BCG + 10^7 low-viability L10 cells had the same gross appearance as guinea pigs receiving primary and secondary immunizations of BCG alone.

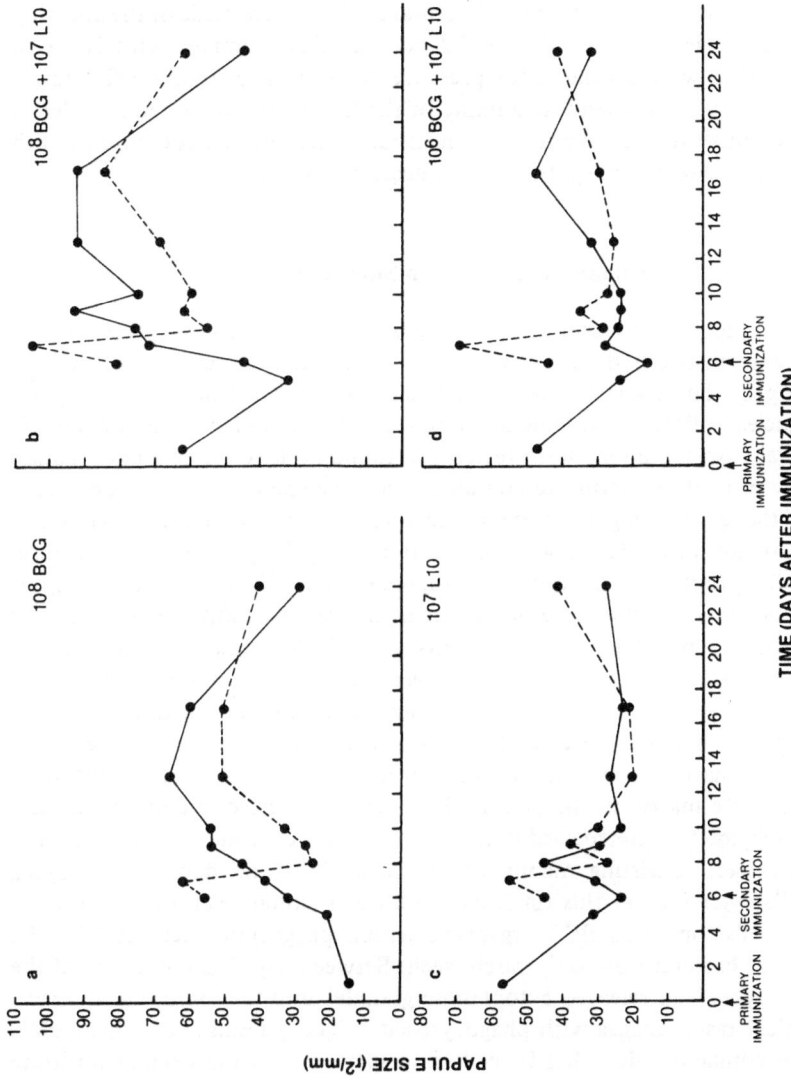

Figure 1. Sequential measurements of the vaccination papules from four treatment groups: (a) 10^8 BCG, (b) 10^8 BCG + 10^7 L10, (c) 10^7 L10, and (d) 10^6 BCG + 10^7 L10. Solid lines indicate primary immunization site, and broken lines indicate secondary immunization site measurements.

IV. MORPHOLOGICAL ANALYSIS OF PRIMARY AND SECONDARY
IMMUNIZATION SITES IN TUMOR-BEARING GUINEA PIGS
TREATED WITH IMMUNOTHERAPEUTIC VACCINES

Sequential histological and ultrastructural analyses were made of the injection sites of guinea pigs immunized with 10^7 or 10^8 BCG admixed with 10^7 L10 cells. These sites were evaluated for presence and survival of tumor cells and for cellular infiltrate. Histochemical staining of the tissue was performed in order to better distinguish the cell types in the infiltrates. Because the response in both treatment groups was similar, they will be described together.

A. Primary Immunization Sites, Days 1 to 7

At day 1, loose aggregates of tumor cells consisting of a few cells to several hundred were distributed throughout the papillary and reticular regions of the dermis (Fig. 2). There was an extensive cellular infiltrate consisting mainly of poly-morphonuclear (PMN) cells, some monocytes, and occasionally lymphocytes. At this interval frozen sections were tested and found positive for acid phosphatase with many cells of the infiltrate containing positive granules. At the edematous border of the reticular region of the dermis there were many tumor cell ghosts or damaged tumor cells. These were characterized by karyorrhexis and diffuse, eosinophilic cytoplasm. PMN cells were still predominant by day 3, but monocytes and lymphocytes became more numerous in the cellular infiltrate. Tumor cells with occasional mitotic figures were established in the loose matrix of the dermis. The mitotic figures of the tumor cells were morphologically disorganized and aberrant, with evidence of X-irradiation-induced chromosome stickiness.

At day 4 a major architectural change occurred at the injection site: there was a transformation from a loosely organized tumor cell–host cellular infiltrate to a more dense matrix in the dermis. The matrix consisted of a proteinaceous, fibrous background, interspersed with nests of tumor cells and cellular infiltrate. Focal abscesses, consisting mainly of pyknotic PMN and damaged or dying tumor cells, were seen at this time. At the ultrastructural level, the majority of the PMN cells contained BCG organisms within phagocytic vacuoles (Fig. 3). Extracellular bacteria were only rarely seen. Between days 2 and 4, many of the PMN cells lysed and released cytoplasmic granules into the extracellular space. Mononuclear macrophages with phagocytosed BCG organisms and/or dead PMN cells were common (Fig. 4). L10 cells interspersed with the cellular infiltrate were highly vacuolated, and while in many cells intact membranes were common, the cytoplasm generally appeared to be degenerating and disorganized. Many L10 cells with blebbing membranes and/or cytoplasmic vesicles were in apposition to mononuclear phagocytes (Fig. 5). This plasma membrane vesiculation on day 4

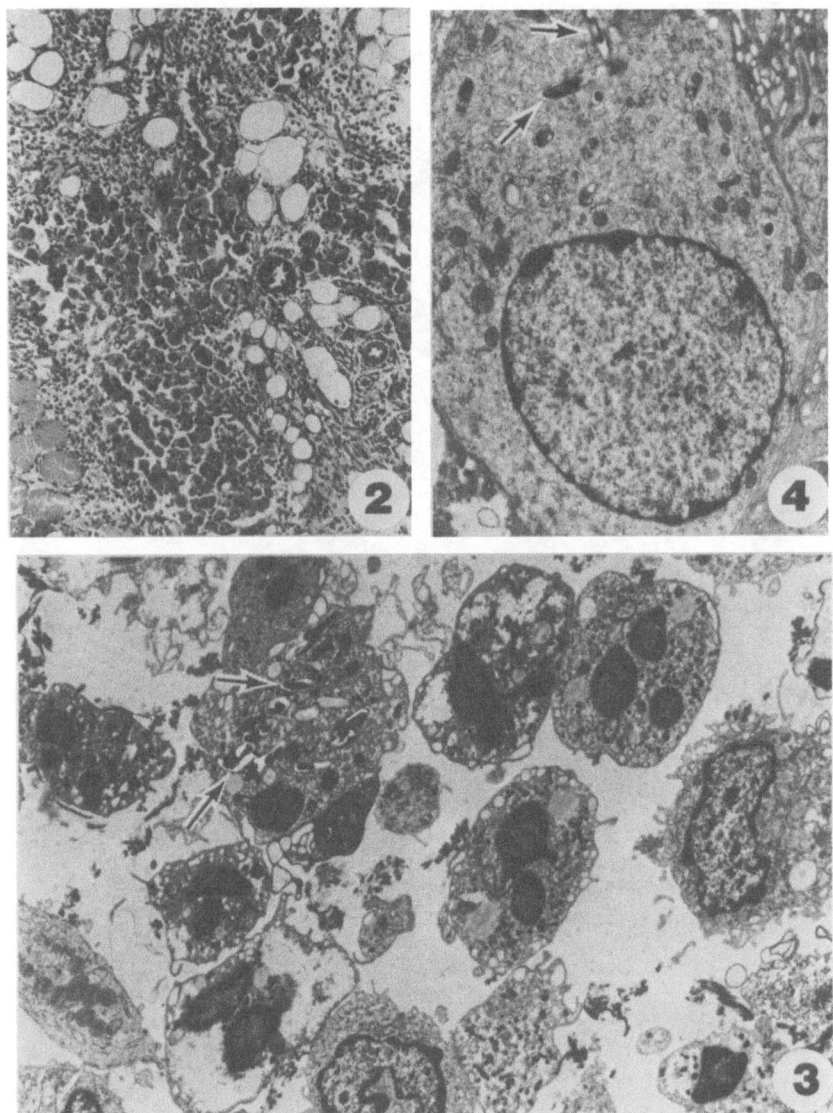

Figure 2. Loose aggregation of L10 tumor cells located throughout the reticular region of the dermis 1 day after injection of 10^8 BCG + 10^7 L10 cells. An intense infiltration of mononuclear and PMN cells surrounds and pervades the nests of tumor cells ($\times$150, reproduced at 65%).

Figure 3. Inflammatory cells seen at the injection site on day 4 consist mainly of PMN cells containing BCG organisms (arrows). Occasional monocytes were also observed ($\times$4200, reproduced at 65%).

Figure 4. Mononuclear macrophage with phagocytosed BCG organisms (arrows) seen at day 7 after primary immunization ($\times$7900, reproduced at 65%).

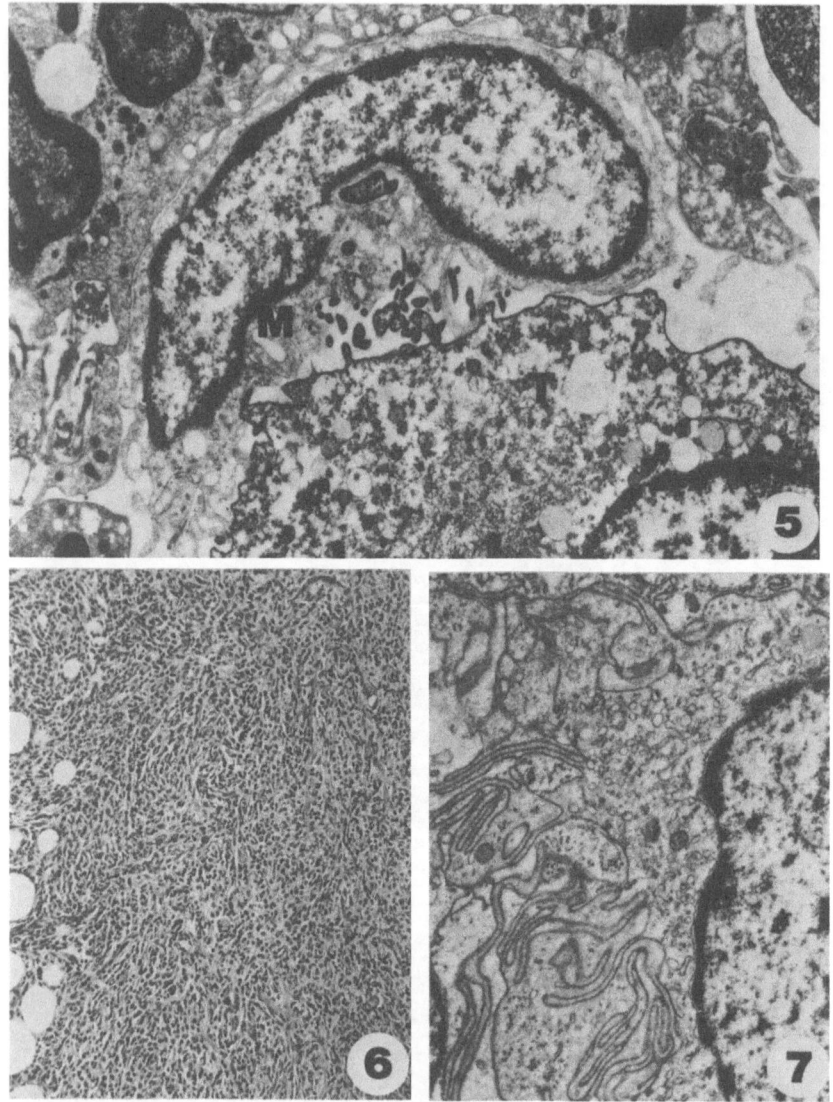

Figure 5. Electron micrograph of tumor cell (T) membrane vesiculation. A mononuclear macrophage (M) appears to be phagocytosing blebs and vesicles released by the tumor cell (×11,200, reproduced at 65%).

Figure 6. Light micrograph of syncytial histiocytosis observed in the injection site at day 7 (×100, reproduced at 65%).

Figure 7. Ultrastructure of a histiocyte showing numerous long cytoplasmic processes forming pronounced interdigitating contacts with neighboring cells (×10,000, reproduced at 65%).

provided morphological support for the metabolic activity of these irradiated L10 tumor cells.

At day 7, the injection site was devoid of tumor cells and consisted of a relatively solid fibrotic matrix interspersed with PMN cells, monocytes, and lymphocytes (Fig. 6). The matrix contained mainly tissue histiocytes that appeared to form a syncytium. At the ultrastructural level, however, it could be seen that these tissue histiocytes possessed numerous long cytoplasmic processes interdigitating with processes from neighboring cells, and thus are not an actual syncytium (Fig. 7). Histochemical preparations of frozen sections revealed a concentration of acid phosphatase-positive cells at the region of marked histiocytosis. This histiocytosis was characteristic of the reaction seen in animals injected with BCG alone and correlated with the hard, nodular gross lesions observed at the skin injection sites in animals receiving BCG alone or 10^8 BCG + 10^7 tumor cells (see Fig. 1).

B. Primary Immunization, Days 8 to 26

During the second to fourth weeks after primary immunization, the histological changes can best be characterized as an epithelioid granulomatous response with intense reactivity for nonspecific esterase stain. This involved a transition from a local histiocytosis to an epithelioid granuloma that was interspersed with focal necrotic abscesses and giant inflammatory cells (Fig. 8). There clearly was a transition from histiocyte and macrophage predominance to epithelioidlike cells and finally to an established epithelioid granuloma (Fig. 9). The prominent large cell, which has been classified by others as an epithelioid cell, had a giant, ovoid nucleus with reticulate chromatin, one or two large nucleoli, and a sharp, delicate nuclear membrane. The abundant cytoplasm was eosinophilic, and finely granular and positive for nonspecific esterase stain. The poorly defined cytoplasmic margins appeared to merge with those of the neighboring cells. On the ultrastructural level there appeared to be a transition between days 13 and 26 from nonphagocytic cells of the histiocyte–macrophage series to epithelioid cells. Most of the nonphagocytic histiocytes had well-developed, dilated, smooth endoplasmic reticulum, Golgi bodies, and some rough-surfaced endoplasmic reticulum (Fig. 10). Between days 17 and 26, epithelioid cells were prominent in the injection site and these cells could be distinguished from the nonphagocytic histiocytes by virtue of a well-developed, rough-surfaced endoplasmic reticulum, arranged in arrays adjacent to the nucleus (Fig. 11). Polysomes were prominent in the cytoplasm, and the morphology was suggestive of an active secretory cell. At day 27 the injection site was composed mainly of epithelioid cells with few phagocytic macrophages and PMN cells (Fig. 12).

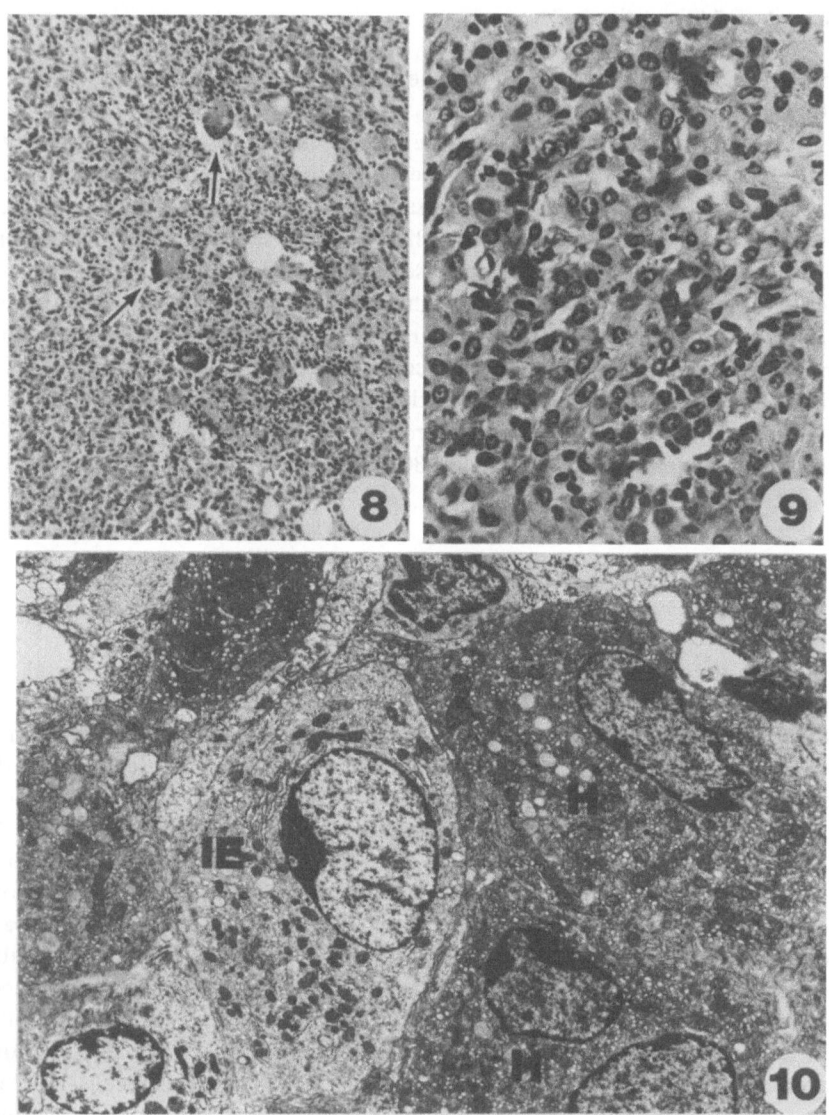

Figure 8. Light micrograph of several giant inflammatory cells in the injection site at day 11. Note the polar accumulation of nuclei in some of these cells (arrows) (×150, reproduced at 65%).

Figure 9. Epithelioid granuloma is established at the injection site by day 26. Note the contrasting ovoid or epithelioid appearance of these cells as opposed to the spindlelike appearance of the histiocytes observed at day 7, shown in Fig. 6 (×450, reproduced at 65%).

Figure 10. Ultrastructure of the transition stage from the histiocytic to epithelioid composition of the injection site. Histiocytes (H) with long cytoplasmic processes are seen, as well as cells that appear to be intermediate between histiocyte and epithelioid cell (IE) (×4950, reproduced at 65%).

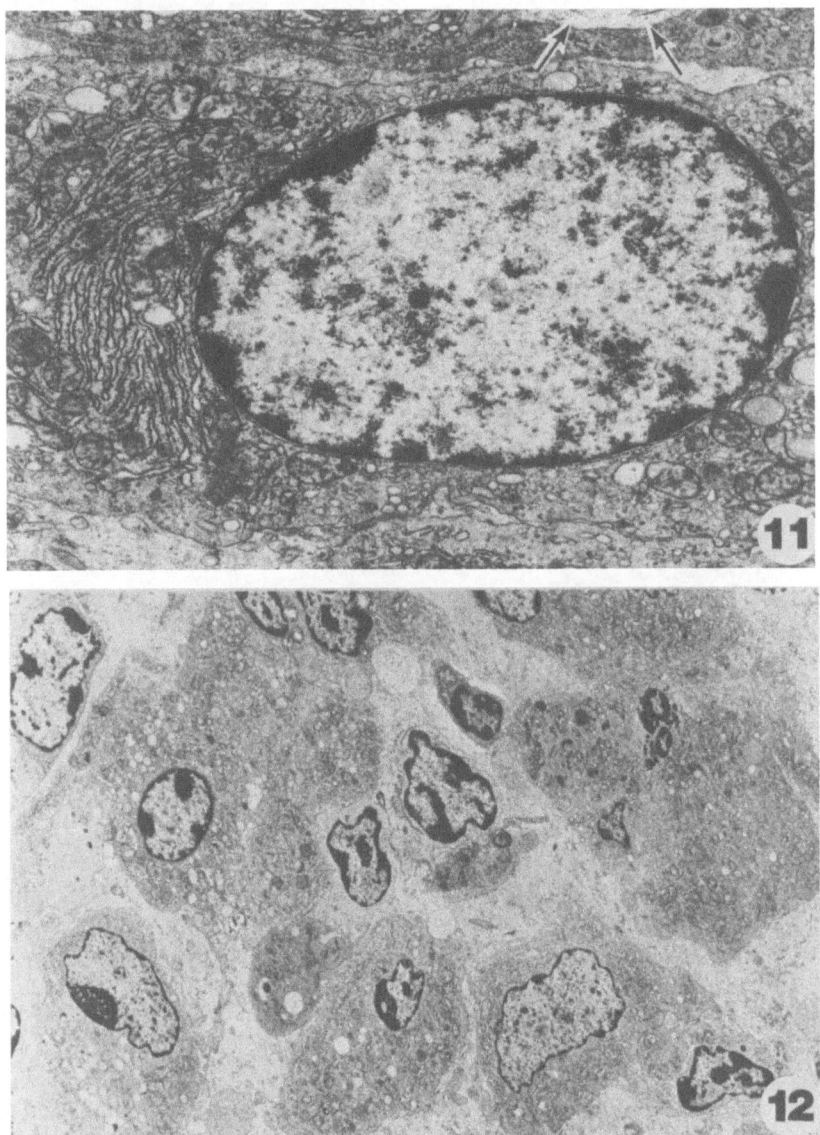

Figure 11. An epithelioid cell showing an array of rough-surface endoplasmic reticulum and prominent polysomes in the cytoplasm. Collagen fibrils are often seen interspersed between the cells (arrows) (×14,800, produced at 65%).

Figure 12. At day 26, the predominant cells in the injection site are the epithelioid cells (×3300, reproduced at 65%).

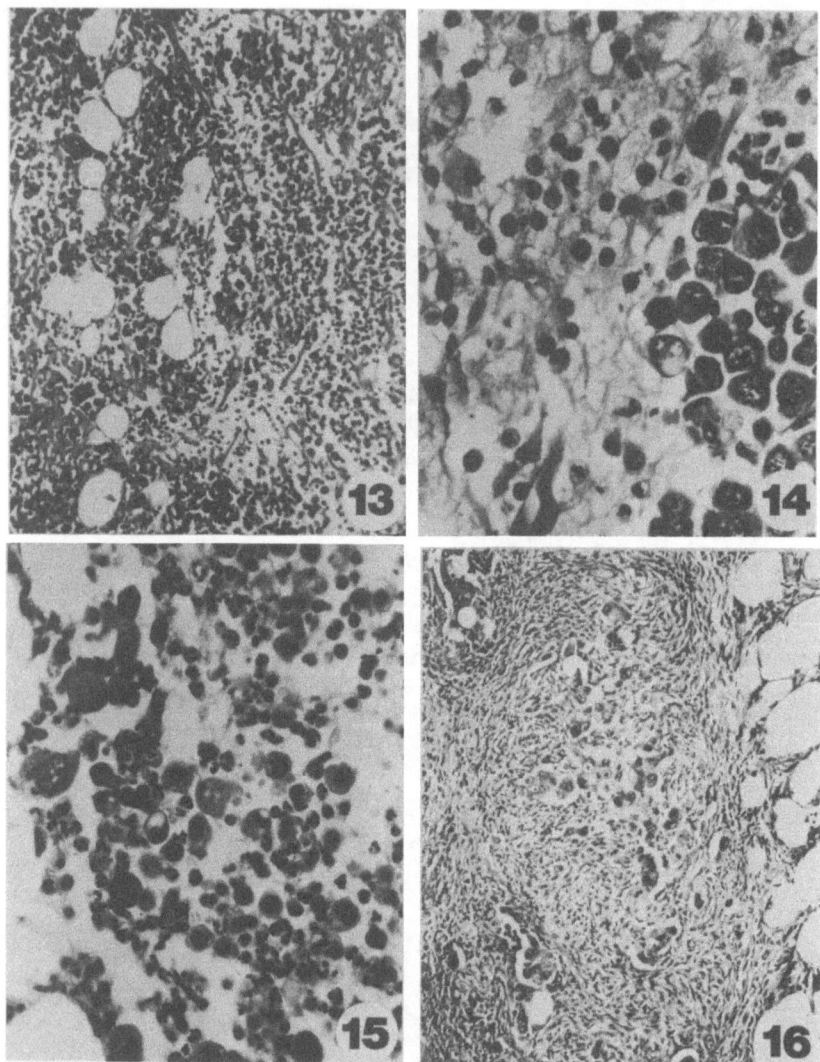

Figure 13. At day 1 after secondary immunization with 10^8 BCG + 10^7 L10 cells, aggregates of tumor cells are seen infiltrated by host inflammatory cells ($\times 150$, reproduced at 65%).

Figure 14. At day 1 after secondary immunization, monocytes and PMN granulocytes are seen in close proximity to tumor cells. The tumor cells are vacuolated at this early time point ($\times 400$, reproduced at 65%).

Figure 15. At day 4 after secondary immunization, numerous inflammatory cells and a few isolated tumor cells are seen at the injection site. The tumor cells have pyknotic nuclei and condensed cytoplasm, indicating early signs of degeneration ($\times 400$, reproduced at 65%).

Figure 16. L10 cells encapsulated in a fibrotic network in the injection site of L10-only vaccine at day 1 after injection. Note absence of the host inflammatory cells that were seen in Fig. 13 ($\times 150$, reproduced at 65%).

C. Secondary Immunization Site, Days 1 to 20

At day 1, aggregations of tumor cells were closely associated with the cellular infiltrate (Fig. 13). While the latter was mostly perivascular, the mononuclear leukocytes and PMN cells appeared to be infiltrating nests of tumor cells as early as 24 h after injection (Fig. 14). The prominent cellular infiltrate consisted of approximately equal numbers of monocytes and PMN cells, while lymphocytes were present in smaller numbers. The monocytes were morphologically of the histiocyte–macrophage series. The abundance of monocytes, along with lymphocytes, distinguishes this reaction from the 24-h response at the primary immunization site. Also, numerous L10 cells in the secondary immunization site between days 1 and 4 were vacuolated and exhibited karyorrhexis, suggesting an early cytolytic response that would be characteristic of hypersensitivity (Fig. 15). L10 cells could not be detected in these sites after day 4. By day 7, the presence of epithelioid cells, phagocytes, and giant cells was apparent. This granulomatous response was established by day 11 and was accompanied by caseating necrosis. Overall, the composition of the cellular infiltrate was comparable in both primary and secondary vaccination sites. However, the secondary vaccination site showed a more rapid evolution of the granulomatous response and an earlier development of focal necrosis.

V. MORPHOLOGICAL ANALYSIS OF PRIMARY AND SECONDARY IMMUNIZATION SITES IN TUMOR-BEARING GUINEA PIGS TREATED WITH NONIMMUNOTHERAPEUTIC VACCINES

Two immunizations of 10^8 BCG, 10^7 L10 cells, or 10^6 BCG admixed with 10^7 L10 cells were ineffective in eliminating established micrometastases. Primary and secondary immunization sites for all three vaccines were studied starting 1 day after the second immunization.

A. BCG Alone

The primary immunization site, in which 10^8 BCG was injected, developed a granulomatous reaction following extensive PMN and mononuclear cell infiltration. This reaction terminated with caseating necrosis that began as early as day 11. While there were similarities between this reaction and the reaction with 10^8 BCG + 10^7 L10 cells, the latter was more extensive as determined by measurement of diameters as well as gross appearance of the papules. The secondary immunization site in which BCG alone was injected had little epithelioid cell response and a more marked caseating necrosis than that seen in animals injected with 10^8 BCG + 10^7 tumor cells.

B. L10 Cells Alone

The primary injection site of irradiated L10 cells of high viability was characterized by nests of tumor cells encapsulated by a fibrotic network. This network was infiltrated with few host leukocytes (Fig. 16). L10 cells could be observed in the primary injection sites as late as 20 days after injection. During this observation period the fibrotic reactivity became more consolidated, and the number of L10 cells diminished. A more prominent perivascular mononuclear cell response was observed during the first week of the secondary immunization with L10 cells alone, and the tumor cells were eliminated by day 11. Thus, grossly (Fig. 1b compared with 1c) and histologically, there appeared to be a delayed-type hypersensitivity response to the L10 cells in animals receiving two injections of tumor cells alone.

Only occasional tumor cells were observed at 1 day, and none were observed 2 days after i.d. injection of 10^7 suboptimally cryopreserved (low viability) L10 cells. This is in marked contrast to the prolonged localization (26 days) of highly viable, nontumorigenic L10 cells. The histologic changes after immunization with 10^8 BCG + 10^7 low-viability L10 cells were identical to the response described after immunization with BCG alone: no intact L10 cells could be detected in the injection sites beyond day 1 after immunization.

C. 10^6 BCG + 10^7 L10 Cells

L10 cells entrapped in a loose fibrotic network, infiltrated with mononuclear and PMN cells, were observed 11 days after the primary immunization. The development of a histiocytosis was apparent at this time, but a distinct epithelioid granulomatous reaction was not observed until day 18. The size and degree of the reaction were diminished compared with that observed when the vaccine contained 10^8 or 10^7 BCG. This was also seen in the measurements of papule diameter (Fig. 1d).

In the secondary vaccination sites a few L10 cells were detected 7 days after injection. The cellular infiltrate consisted predominantly of mononuclear and PMN cells with lymphocytes, indicating a delayed-type hypersensitivity response. By day 11, the local skin sites had a typical granulomatous reaction with epithelioid cells and histiocytes.

VI. HISTOLOGICAL CHANGES IN SUPERFICIAL DISTAL AXILLARY (SDA) LYMPH NODES

The lymph nodes draining the primary injection site in all guinea pigs injected with BCG showed similar architectural changes. The major difference was in the

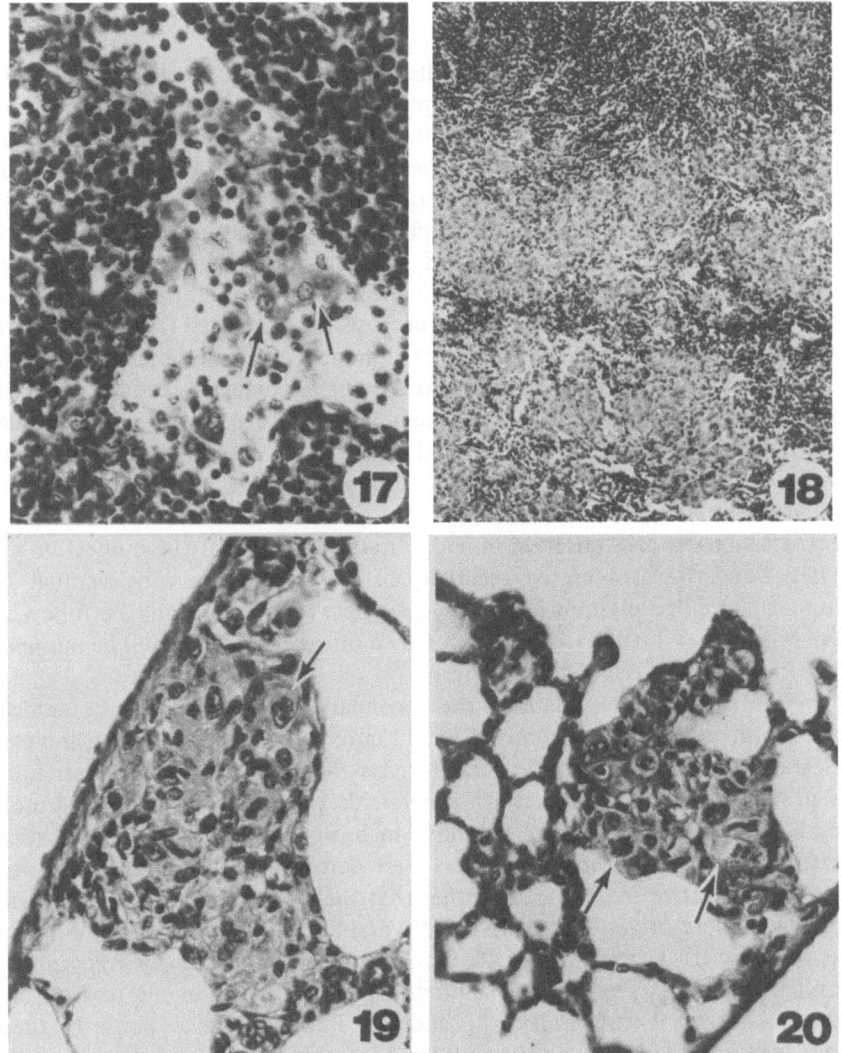

Figure 17. Mononuclear cells (arrows) with large ovoid nuclei and foamy cytoplasm characteristic of phagocytic macrophages, infiltrated medullary sinuses of regional nodes of animals treated with 10^8 BCG alone or admixed with 10^7 L10 cells ($\times 400$, reproduced at 65%).

Figure 18. Large areas of coalesced granulomas are seen in the SDA nodes of 10^8 BCG-treated animals between days 9 and 13 after primary immunization ($\times 150$, reproduced at 65%).

Figure 19. At day 20 after secondary immunization with 10^8 BCG + 10^7 L10 cells, a pulmonary nodule or remnant could be detected that may have been a metastatic foci eliminated by cell-mediated reactivity. One pleomorphic L10 cell (arrow) remains in this remnant ($\times 450$, reproduced at 65%).

Figure 20. At day 20 after secondary immunization with 10^8 BCG + 10^7 L10 cells, a remnant of a metastatic pulmonary nodule can be seen with several pleomorphic L10 cells (arrow) and infiltrating mononuclear cells ($\times 450$, reproduced at 65%).

degree of responsiveness, which was directly proportional to the dose of BCG. For each BCG treatment group, the lymph nodes draining the primary immunization sites underwent three to fourfold increases in size. Eight days after primary immunization with 10^8 BCG either alone or admixed with L10 cells, granulomas were observed in the cortical and paracortical regions of the SDA lymph nodes. Mononuclear cells with large ovoid nuclei and foamy cytoplasm, characteristic of phagocytic macrophages, infiltrated the medullary sinuses of these lymph nodes (Fig. 17). Between days 9 and 13 after primary immunization, the granulomas coalesced and areas of caseating necrosis were observed (Fig. 18). For the remainder of the study, this was the predominant response observed in these lymph nodes. Little or no lymphocyte reactivity was detected, and the syncytial histiocytosis ultimately occluded the medullary sinuses in these nodes. A similar pattern was observed in animals injected with 10^7 or 10^6 BCG + 10^7 L10 cells. However, in both cases granuloma development lagged behind the response observed with 10^8 BCG.

The major response observed in nodes draining the primary immunization site of L10 alone was proliferative reactivity of the cortical area with eventual development of hyperplastic germinal centers between days 13 and 26 following primary injection. Little to no infiltration by mononuclear cells could be observed in the medullary sinuses of these nodes.

In the lymph nodes draining the secondary vaccination sites of animals treated with BCG alone or admixed with tumor cells, the histiocytosis and general granulomatous response was less intense than that seen in nodes draining the primary immunization sites. In general, these nodes showed a much more prominent lymphoproliferative response in both the cortical and paracortical areas. No hyperplastic germinal centers were detected during the course of this lymphoproliferative response, suggesting that the cells may have been primarily of T-lymphocyte origin. The lymph nodes draining the secondary immunization sites of animals treated with L10 alone were distinguished by hyperplastic germinal centers at day 11 and a progressive hyperplasia in the cortical and paracortical areas between days 11 and 20. Basically, the response of these nodes was not markedly different from that seen in the nodes draining the primary vaccination sites.

VII. EFFECT OF SYSTEMIC IMMUNITY ON PULMONARY METASTASES

All guinea pigs that died during the course of the survival study had widespread visceral metastases and tumor foci in the lungs. Examination of the lungs in animals killed for morphological studies at 11 and 20 days after secondary immunization demonstrated that in those animals immunized with 10^8 or 10^7 BCG admixed with L10 cells (eight guinea pigs) no gross pulmonary hepato-

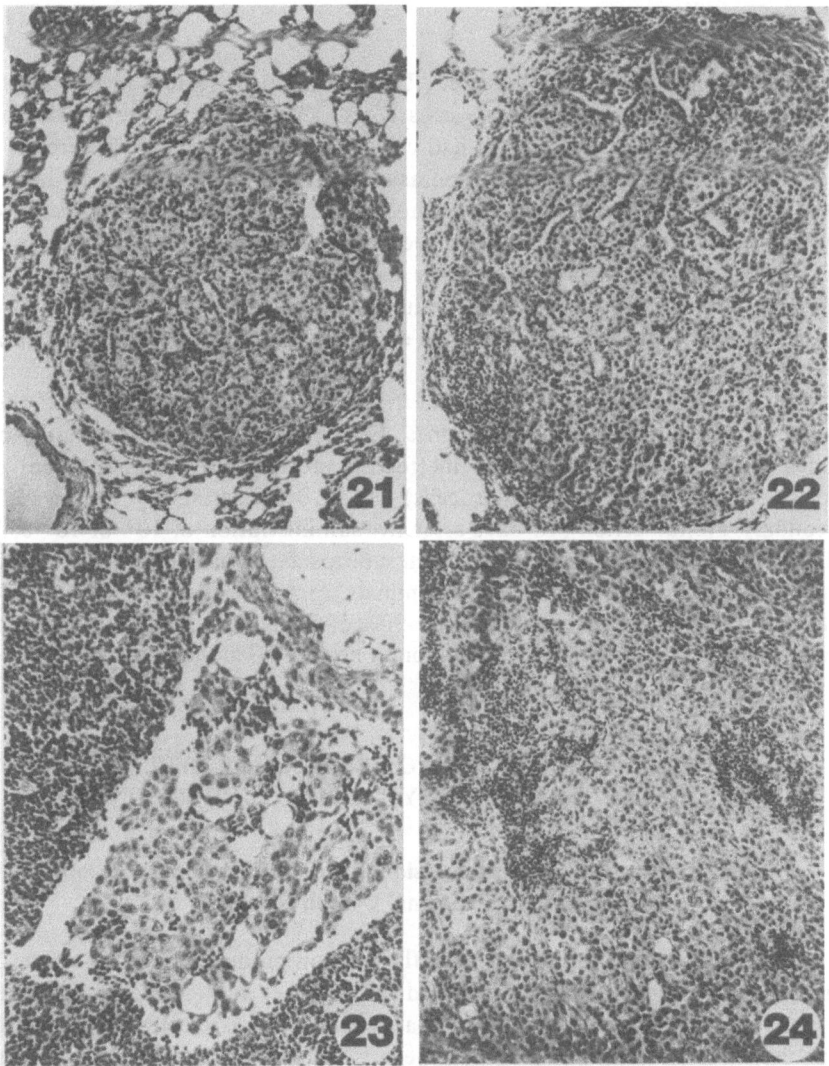

Figure 21. A large metastatic L10 tumor nodule found in the lung of a guinea pig treated with irradiated L10 vaccine at day 20 after secondary treatment ($\times$150, reproduced at 65%).

Figure 22. A tumor nodule in the lung of a guinea pig treated with 10^6 BCG + 10^7 L10 cells. Note the mononuclear cell infiltration at the periphery of the nodule ($\times$150, reproduced at 65%).

Figure 23. Tumor cell metastases to the tracheobronchial nodes of guinea pigs treated with 10^6 BCG + 10^7 L10 vaccine at day 20 after secondary immunization. Note tumor infiltration in the subcapsular medullary sinus of the node ($\times$150, reproduced at 65%).

Figure 24. Massive infiltration of tumor cells in the tracheobronchial node of animals treated with L10 alone obliterated most of the lymphoid tissue in the node at day 20 after secondary immunization ($\times$150, reproduced at 65%).

carcinoma nodules could be detected. The predominant feature in the lungs of these guinea pigs was occasional scars (Figs. 19 and 20). These consisted of fibrotic areas, some of which still had cells that morphologically appeared to be pleomorphic L10 tumor cells with occasional mitotic figures. Many of the scars were infiltrated with PMN and mononuclear leukocytes. Thus, these scars were suggestive of metastatic foci that had been eliminated by a cell-mediated reaction. In contrast, the animals treated with ineffective vaccines showed gross and microscopic metastatic nodules in the lungs by day 11. These were large, vascularized tumor nodules, with little or no evidence of mononuclear cell infiltration (Figs. 21 and 22).

No L10 cells were observed in the tracheobronchial lymph nodes of those animals treated with optimum vaccines. However, the tracheobronchial lymph nodes of all animals treated with ineffective vaccines (BCG alone, tumor cell alone, or 10^6 BCG + 10^7 tumor cells) had L10 metastases by 11 days after secondary immunization (18 days after i.v. administration of 10^5 or 10^6 cells). The extent of the metastasis ranged from subcapsular medullary sinus infiltration and paracortical L10 infiltration in animals immunized with 10^6 BCG + 10^7 L10 cells (Fig. 23) to approximately 80–90% of the nodes infiltrated with metastases in those animals treated with tumor alone or BCG alone (Fig. 24).

VIII. MECHANISMS OF ACTION OF BCG–TUMOR CELL VACCINES IN THE GENERATION OF SYSTEMIC TUMOR IMMUNITY

A. The Effect of Surgical Excision of the Dermal Immunization Site and Regional Lymph Node

As discussed, the granulomatous inflammation produced by BCG–tumor cell vaccines administered i.d. is associated with potent tumor-specific immunity. Mycobacteria and tumor cells injected at separate sites are ineffectual immunostimulants, suggesting that granulomagenesis, and immune induction are synergistically interrelated. In order to identify those stages of immunization that are requisite for systemic tumor immunity, we examined the effect of interrupting granulomagenesis on the induction of immunity. The vaccination site (groups A–F) or both the vaccination site and regional SDA lymph nodes (groups G–L) were surgically excised at various times (i.e., 1, 4, 7, 11, 15, and 22 days) after vaccination with 10^8 BCG organisms admixed with 10^7 X-irradiated L10 cells (Table II). An i.d. challenge of 10^6 viable L10 cells was consistently fatal to unvaccinated animals, whereas vaccinated, but surgically untreated, animals (group M) were almost completely protected when challenged 37 days after vaccination (100% and 19% mortality, respectively). Excision of vaccination sites at 4–22 days after immunization had no discernible effect on the induction of

Table II. Effect of Surgical Excision of Vaccination Site and Superficial Distal Axillary Lymph Nodes on the Development of Systemic Tumor Immunity after BCG–Tumor Cell Vaccination

Treatment group	Vaccinate 10^8 BCG, 10^7 L10 i.d.	Surgery					Tumor challenge 10^6 L10 i.d.	Progressors/ total	%
	0[a]	5	10	15	20	22	37		
Excise vaccination site									
A	+ +						+	8/16	50
B	+	+					+	1/16	6
C	+		+				+	0/16	0
D	+			+			+	0/16	0
E	+				+		+	0/16	0
F	+					+	+	2/16	13
Excise vaccination site + SDA nodes									
G	+ +						+	5/5	100
H	+	+					+	6/6	100
I	+		+				+	5/6	83
J	+			+			+	4/6	67
K	+				+		+	2/6	33
L	+					+	+	2/5	40
No surgery									
M	+						+	3/16	19
N	−						+	15/15	100

[a]Numbers indicate days after vaccination with 10^8 BCG organisms admixed with 10^7 X-irradiated L10 cells.

tumor immunity, since the incidence of progressive tumor growth did not differ from that of animals not subjected to surgery (M), as determined by the Fisher exact probability test ($p > 0.05$). Though it may appear that excision of immunization sites 1 day after vaccination blocked the development of immunity in group B (50% progressors) as opposed to the untreated controls (19%), this difference was not statistically significant.

Excision of the vaccination site and the regional lymph nodes, however, resulted in a severe impairment in the generation of systemic antitumor immunity. Progressive tumor growth occurred in 100% of animals surgically treated 1 and 4 days after vaccination (G and H); only partial protection was conferred to animals surgically treated 7 or more days after vaccination (I-L).

The length of time that the vaccination sites and regional lymph nodes remained intact was critical to the development of antitumor immunity. The incidence of progressive tumor growth steadily declined as the time increased between vaccination and surgical excision. For groups A-G and H-L, this trend was highly significant, using the Cochran-Armitage test for analysis of trends (one-tailed test, $p < 0.005$ and 0.001, respectively.) The data suggest that early stages of the inflammatory response prior to granulomagenesis are associated with maximal induction of antitumor immunity and that the involvement of the vaccination site and the regional lymph nodes is minimal after 4 and 15 days, respectively.

IX. DELAYED HYPERSENSITIVITY RESPONSE TO L10 TUMOR CHALLENGE

Immunization with BCG-tumor cell vaccines affected sensitization to tumor antigens. This was detectable by the delayed hypersensitivity response, and was independent of the timing or the extent of surgical intervention (Fig. 25). The responses of all immunized groups were significantly greater than those of the unimmunized controls ($p < 0.001$). Surgical excision of the vaccination site or both the vaccination site and the regional lymph nodes as soon as 1 day after injection did not prevent sensitization, although the magnitude of the response was clearly less than that of the vaccinated, but surgically untreated, control group ($p < 0.01$). Excision of the immunization site at 4 days had no effect on the delayed hypersensitivity response after challenge compared with the control group ($p < 0.05$), whereas excision at 7, 15, or 22 days enhanced the delayed hypersensitivity response ($p < 0.01$). Removal of both the vaccination site and regional lymph nodes, however, impaired the development of delayed hypersensitivity. The responses of these groups did not equal those of animals in the control group ($p < 0.05$), demonstrating that the intact regional lymph nodes

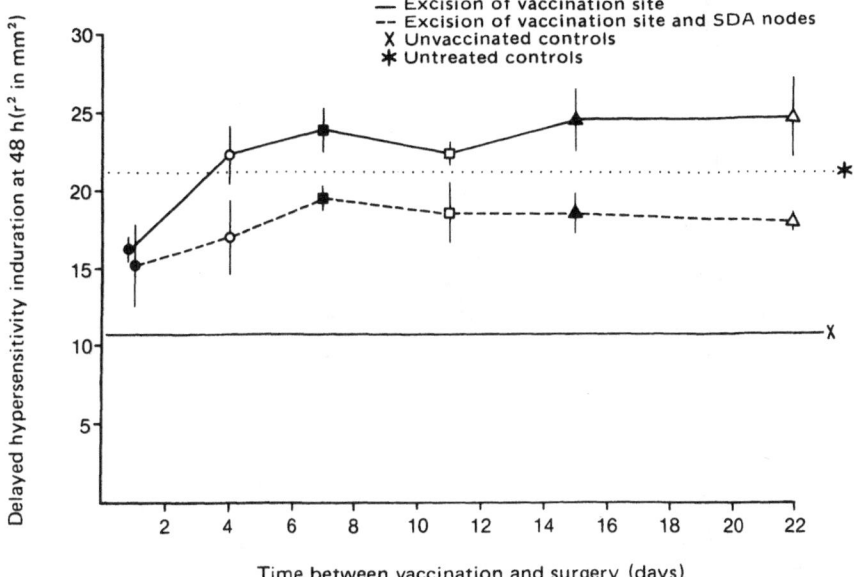

Figure 25. Effect of surgical excision of the immunization site (solid line) or immunization site and SDA lymph node (dashed line) on sensitization to tumor antigens detectable by the delayed hypersensitivity response, measured 48 h after i.d. tumor challenge with 10^6 L10 tumor cells 37 days after vaccination. Surgical interruption of granulomagenesis was performed 1 (●), 4 (○), 7 (■), 11 (□), 15 (▲), and 22 (△) days after i.d. vaccination with 10^8 BCG admixed with 10^7 L10 tumor cells. The delayed hypersensitivity responses of normal, unvaccinated animals (X) and vaccinated, but surgically untreated, controls (∗) are also shown.

were essential for delayed hypersensitivity and contribute to the response for as long as 22 days after immunization.

The relationship between the delayed hypersensitivity response to tumor challenge and the course of subsequent tumorigenesis (i.e., tumor growth rate) is depicted in Fig. 26. The minimal delayed hypersensitivity response of unvaccinated animals to tumor challenge was associated with rapid tumor progression, whereas the response of vaccinated animals was characterized by elevated delayed hypersensitivity associated with either slower tumor growth or tumor regression. The chi square test was applied to these data, and the results indicate that the point distribution is not random: $\chi^2 = 84.182$, where the minimum expected value is 0.258. The data are consistent with a polynomial regression of the third degree (i.e., a sigmoidal curve or threshold effect) rather than with a linear regression model. The distribution of points suggests that, under defined conditions of animal strain—vaccination methods, tumor challenge dose, etc.— there exists a threshold delayed hypersensitivity response compatible with tumor

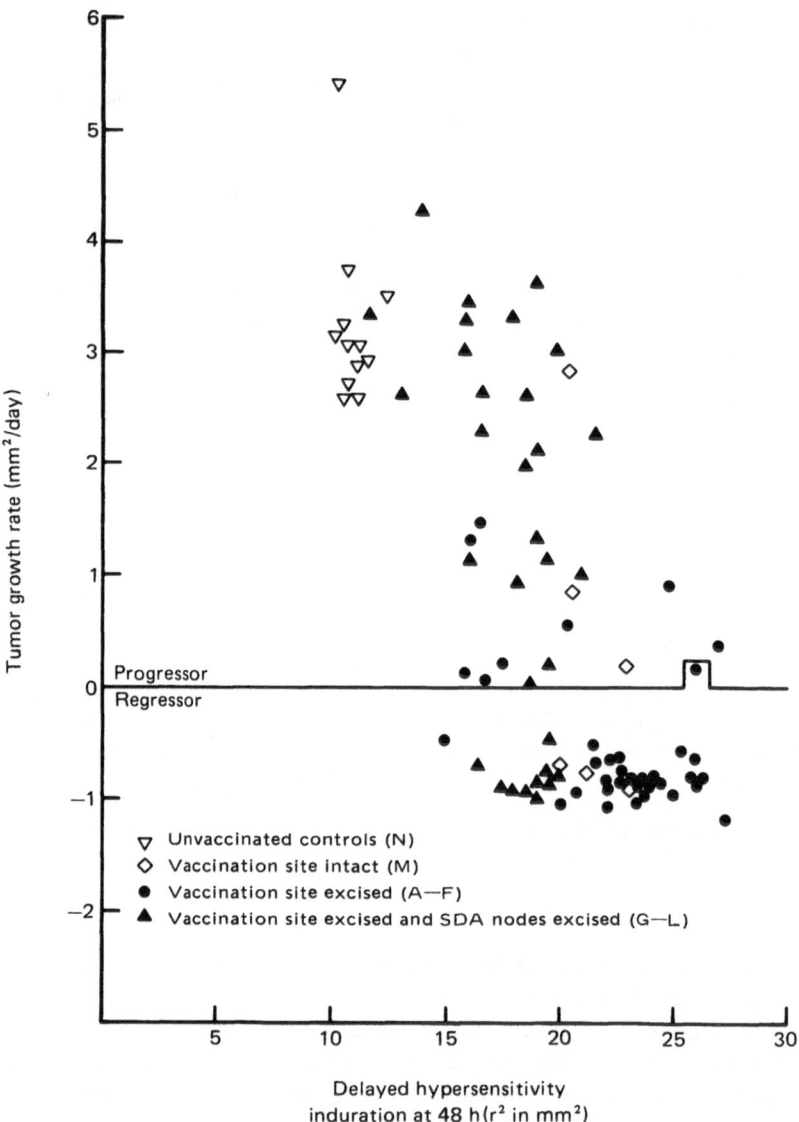

Figure 26. Relationship between the delayed hypersensitivity response to tumor challenge and subsequent tumor growth rates. Guinea pigs were vaccinated i.d. with 10^8 BCG admixed with 10^7 L10 tumor cells on day 0; and at various times thereafter, either the immunization site (groups A–F, ●) or the immunization site and SDA node (groups G–L, ▲) were surgically excised. The responses of normal, unvaccinated animals (▽) and vaccinated, but surgically untreated, controls (◇) are also shown. All animals received an i.d. tumor challenge of 10^6 L10 cells 37 days after vaccination and the delayed hypersensitivity response (induration at the challenge site) was measured 48 h after challenge; tumor growth rates (mm^2/day) were calculated from measurements of tumor papule size (mm^2) made on alternate days for 3 weeks after challenge.

regression. We estimate that the threshold may be contained within the interval 20–25 mm^2.

X. CONCLUSION

The major histopathologic alterations in BCG and/or L10 cell immunization sites can be used to examine the variables in different vaccine preparations and to analyze the host responses that contribute to the efficacy of treatment and control of minimal residual malignancy (Table III). It is interesting to note that nontumorigenic, viable L10 tumor cell suspensions (attenuated), when injected alone at a dose of 10^7 cells, can be histologically observed in the skin site up to 26 days after injection. These cells indeed do elicit a weak inflammatory response manifested by a fibrotic encapsulation, often characteristic of foreign-body reactions. L10 cell suspensions that are suboptimally cryopreserved and have low viability are totally destroyed by 48 h after i.d. injection and elicit a minimal host response. The host responses elicited by optimal doses of BCG (10^8 or 10^7) are qualitatively the same in the presence or absence of high viability L10 cells. In fact, the BCG-induced inflammatory response contributes to the destruction of tumor cells during the first week after a primary immunization.

A fundamental observation of this study regarding induction sites of specific tumor immunity using BCG–tumor cell vaccines is that there is a requirement for persistence of intact tumor cells and thus, presumably, tumor antigen(s), during a critical phase of the development of a chronic inflammatory response. This chronic inflammatory response is characterized by a reaction in which the end point is an epithelioid granuloma. In this experimental immunotherapy model of guinea pigs in which the effectiveness of the induced tumor immunity was assayed by the elimination of disseminated visceral micrometastasis, it was clear that the persistence of intact tumor cells in the dermal injection site, while necessary, was not entirely sufficient for induction of effective tumor immunity. Also, the chronic inflammatory response with development of epithelioid granuloma, as elicited by i.d. injection of an optimal dose of viable BCG, in itself was not immunotherapeutic in this experimental model. It becomes obvious then that the conversion of the BCG-induced acute inflammatory reaction to a chronic inflammatory reaction between days 4 and 7, and the destruction and immunologic processing of tumor antigen(s) during this time period by the infiltrating blood-borne monocytes, lymphocytes, and PMN cells are all essential factors that contribute to effective induction of specific cell-mediated tumor immunity.

Several conclusions can now be developed from these observations. The failure of some previous experimental and clinical attempts at active specific immunotherapy using BCG and autologous tumor cell vaccines are probably

Table III. Synopsis of Major Histological Alterations in BCG and/or L10 Cell Immunization Sites

Treatment	Vaccine	Days after immunization				
		1	4	7	17	26
Primary immunization	10^8 BCG + 10^7 HV[a] L10 10^7 BCG + 10^7 HV L10	+++ Tumor cells	++ Tumor cells	– Tumor cells→		
		+++ Acid phosphatase————————→			+++ Nonspecific esterase————————→	+++ Epithelioid cells
						++ Nonphagocytic histiocytes
						++ Lymphocytes
		Host cellular infiltrate				
		+++ PMN[b] cells	+++ MN[c] cells	+++ Nonphagocytic histiocytes	+++ Nonphagocytic histiocytes	
		++ MN cells	++ PMN cells	++ MN cells	++ MN cells	
		± Lymphocytes	± Lymphocytes	++ PMN cells	++ Epithelioid cells	
				+ Lymphocytes	+ Giant inflammatory cells———→	+ Macrophages
					± Plasma cells	
					± PMN cells	
			Loose proteinaceous stroma————→	"Syncytial" histiocytosis————→		Epithelioid granuloma
				Focal abscesses containing PMN cells	Focal necrotic areas	Collagenous stroma
Primary immunization	10^7 HV L10	+++ Tumor cells————————→		++ Tumor cells	+ Tumor cells	± Tumor cells
				Host cellular infiltrate		
				+ MN cells		
				+ PMN cells		
				± Lymphocytes		
				Fibrotic stroma————————————————————→		
Primary immunization	10^7 LV[d] L10	± Tumor cells	– Tumor cells————→			

[a] HV, high viability.   [b] PMN, polymorphonuclear.   [c] MN, mononuclear macrophages.   [d] LV, low viability.

attributable to the use of tumor cell suspensions of low viability. An acute antigenic exposure instead of a prolonged tumor cell challenge during the development of a chronic inflammatory response could be at fault. One technical problem with some of these past studies has been suboptimal cryobiologic preservation. Also, prior to the present studies, it had been assumed that nontumorigenic preparations required nonviable and metabolically inactive cells. In the present study the cells were metabolically active and underwent a limited number of mitotic divisions. It can be assumed that with 20,000 R X-irradiation, many of the cells were blocked in the G_1 phase of cell division and the cells were destined to die during the subsequent mitosis. Possibly, the interruption of cell division in G_1 preserved the cells and their metabolic activity. The ultrastructurally observed plasma membrane vesiculation could represent a persisting source of tumor antigen that provided chronic immunogenic exposure for optimum induction of cell-mediated immunity.

We have now demonstrated that a nontumorigenic vaccine can affect immunotherapy. Past results in this experimental model demonstrated that there is a critical dose for BCG in the initial vaccination, but that BCG is not essential in the subsequent vaccination. Thus, the BCG-induced chronic inflammatory response that is essential in the primary immunization for the afferent recognition and elicitation of immunological memory to the tumor antigen is not required for the enhancement of memory to the tumor antigen. Based on this observation, one can speculate about the relationship of cellular immunity to granulomatous inflammation. Although the basic morphology of chronic inflammatory responses and epithelioid granuloma development is well known, little is known about the relationship of the apparently secretory epithelioid cells to the development of systemic cellular immunity.

Surgical excision of the immunization sites and regional lymph nodes at strategic points in the development and maturation of the acute and chronic inflammatory reaction was expected to block critical events in immune induction. This process is known to involve antigen recognition and processing at the injection site, followed by emigration (or transport) to and proliferation in the regional lymph nodes by specifically sensitized, immunocompetent lymphoid cells (Hanna and Peters, 1978 b). Excision of the vaccination sites as early as 4 days after vaccination did not prevent sensitization to tumor antigens or inhibit the generation of antitumor immunity. This indicates that antigen processing at the injection site occurs maximally during the acute inflammatory response and between the transformation of the acute inflammatory response to a chronic inflammatory reaction. These results clearly indicate that antigen processing is minimal during the chronic inflammatory response and the formation of the mature epithelioid granuloma.

Since tumor cells are not observable in histologic sections of the dermal immunization sites taken 7 days after vaccination, it may be argued that the vaccination site is functional only as long as metabolically active tumor cells persist in the tissue; later stages in granulomagenesis may be fully competent but lacking in tumor antigens. However, we have recently found that reinjection of developing BCG–tumor cell-induced granulomas with 10^7 metabolically active L10 cells at 4 or 13 days after vaccination did not improve the efficacy of the vaccine (unpublished data). This suggests that immune induction may be restricted to discrete stages of granulomagenesis, and that later stages may be irrelevant or even inhibitory to the generation of antitumor immunity.

Excision of both the vaccination site and the regional lymph nodes inhibited sensitization to tumor antigens and blocked the development of antitumor immunity, as evidenced by depressed delayed hypersensitivity responses and decreased resistance to tumor challenge, respectively. The role of the regional lymph nodes, therefore, in immune induction is crucial, since the lymph nodes were shown to contribute to the delayed hypersensitivity response for at least 22 days after immunization. The lymph nodes probably function as a site of clonal proliferation of tumor antigen-sensitive immunocytes, although their function in antigen processing cannot be excluded by these experiments.

Thus, in this immunotherapy model of guinea pigs some critical parameters in the induction of functional tumor-specific immunity are (1) persistence of intact and metabolically active tumor cells, (2) BCG-mediated recruitment of a host cellular infiltrate at the immunization site (acute inflammatory response), (3) antigen processing at the immunization site during the period of transformation from an acute to chronic inflammatory response, and (4) the resultant sensitization and induction of tumor specific immunity in the intact regional lymph node. This experimental guinea pig model supports the concept of active specific immunotherapy when proper consideration is given to the technical details of vaccine preparation and parameters of host responses. The findings reported in this study clarify some possible reasons for past failures and provide a useful model for further examination of the variables of active specific immunotherapy with respect to vaccine preparation, regimen, and host response. Continued studies in this experimental model could lead to a better understanding of the mechanisms that contribute to the effective induction of specific cell-mediated tumor immunity for treatment and control of minimal residual malignancy.

ACKNOWLEDGMENTS

Research sponsored by the National Cancer Institute under Contract N01-CO-75380 with Litton Bionetics, Inc. V. A. Pollack is a postdoctoral fellow supported by a grant made possible by United Order True Sisters, Inc.

We are grateful for the invaluable help given by Drs. L. C. Hoyer and H. C. Hoover, and the excellent technical assistance of Diane Plentovich, Leona Peters, and Jane Brandhorst.

XI. REFERENCES

Adams, D. O., 1976, The granulomatous inflammatory response: A review, *Am. J. Pathol.* 84:164-191.

Bartlett, G. L., and Zbar, B., 1972, Tumor-specific vaccine containing *Mycobacterium bovis* and tumor cells: Safety and efficacy, *J. Natl. Cancer Inst.* 49:1709-1726.

Bekesi, J. G., St-Arneault, G., and Holland, J. F., 1971, Increase of leukemia L1210 immunogenicity by *Vibrio cholerae* neuraminidase treatment, *Cancer Res.* 31:2130-2132.

Boros, D. L., 1978, Granulomatous inflammations, *Progr. Allergy* 24:183-267.

Fidler, I. J., Budmen, M. B., and Hanna, M. G., Jr., 1976a, Characterization of *in vitro* reactivity by BCG-treated guinea pigs to syngeneic line-10 hepatocarcinoma, *Cancer Immunol. Immunother.* 1:179-186.

Fidler, I. J., Kataoka, T., and Hanna, M. G., Jr., 1976b, A comparison of *in vitro* cell-mediated reactivity against syngeneic tumor cells by various lymphoid cell populations from *Bacillus Calmette-Guérin*-tumor-cured, tumor-sensitized, tumor-bearing, and normal inbred guinea pigs, *Cancer Res.* 36:4459-4466.

Hanna, M. G., Jr., and Bucana, C., 1979, Active specific immunotherapy of residual micrometastasis: The acute and chronic inflammatory response in induction of tumor immunity by BCG-tumor cell immunization, *J. Reticuloendothel. Soc.* 26:439-452.

Hanna, M. G., Jr., and Peters, L. C., 1978a, Specific immunotherapy of established visceral micrometastases by BCG-tumor cell vaccine alone or as an adjunct to surgery, *Cancer* 42:2613-2625.

Hanna, M. G., Jr., and Peters, L. C., 1978b, Immunotherapy of established micrometastases with *Bacillus Calmette-Guérin* tumor cell vaccine, *Cancer Res.* 38:204-209.

Hanna, M. G., Jr., Zbar, B., and Rapp, H. J., 1972, Histopathology of tumor regression and intralesional injection of *Mycobacterium bovis*. I. Tumor growth and metastasis, *J. Natl. Cancer Inst.* 48:1441-1455.

Hanna, M. G., Jr., Snodgrass, M. J., Zbar, B., and Rapp, H. J., 1973, Histopathology of tumor regression after intralesional injection of *Mycobacterium bovis*. IV. Development of immunity to tumor cells and BCG, *J. Natl. Cancer Inst.* 51:1897-1908.

Hanna, M. G., Jr., Brandhorst, J. S., and Peters, L. C., 1979, Active specific immunotherapy of residual micrometastasis: An evaluation of sources doses and ratios of BCG with tumor cells, *Cancer Immunol. Immunother.* 7:165-173.

Hedley, D. W., McElwain, T. J., and Currie, G. A., 1978, Specific active immunotherapy does not prolong survival in surgically treated patients with stage IIB malignant melanoma and may promote early recurrence, *Br. J. Cancer* 37:491-496.

Hollingshead, A. C., 1978, Active-specific immunotherapy, in: *Immunotherapy of Human Cancer* (E. Hersh, ed.), pp. 213-233, Raven Press, New York.

Martin, W. J., Wunderlich, J. R., Fletcher, F., and Inman, J. K., 1971, Enhanced immunogenicity of chemically-coated syngeneic tumor cells, *Proc. Natl. Acad. Sci. USA* 68:469-472.

Mathé, G., Weiner, R., Pouillart, P., Schwarzenberg, L., Jasmin, C., Schneider, M., Hrynt, M., Amiel, J. L., DeVassal, F., and Rosenfeld, C., 1973, BCG in cancer immunotherapy. I. Experimental and clinical trials of its use in the treatment of leukemia minimal and/or residual disease, *Natl. Cancer Inst. Monogr.* 39:165-175.

Morton, D. L., Eilber, F. R., Holmes, E. C., Sparks, F. C., and Ramming, K. P., 1976 Present status of BCG immunotherapy of malignant melanoma, *Cancer Immunol. Immunother.* 1:93-98.

Peters, L. C., Brandhorst, J. S., and Hanna, M. G., Jr., 1979, Preparation of immunotherapeutic autologous tumor cell vaccines from solid tumors, *Cancer Res.* 39:1353-1360.

Powles, R. L., Crowther, D., Bateman, C. J. T., Beard, M. E. J., McElwain, T. J., Russel, J., Lister, T. A., Whitehouse, J. M. A., Wrigley, P. F. M., Pike, M., Alexander, P., and Fairley, G. H., 1973, Immunotherapy for acute myelogenous leukaemia, *Br. J. Cancer* 28:365–376.

Prager, M. D., 1978, Specific cancer immunotherapy, *Cancer Immunol. Immunother.* 3: 157–161.

Prager, M. D., and Baechtel, F. S., 1973, Methods for modification of cancer cells to enhance their antigenicity, in: *Methods in Cancer Research*, Vol. 9 (H. Busch, ed.), pp. 339–400, Academic Press, New York.

Rapp, H. J., Churchill, W. H., Jr., Kronman, B. S., Rolley, R. T., Hammond, W. G., and Borsos, T., 1968, Antigenicity of a new diethylnitrosamine-induced transplantable guinea pig hepatoma: Pathology and formation of ascites variant, *J. Natl. Cancer Inst.* 41:1–11.

Ray, P. K., Tahkur, V. S., and Sundaram, K., 1975, Antitumor immunity. I. Differential response of neuraminidase-treated and X-irradiated tumor vaccine, *Eur. J. Cancer* 11: 1–8.

Rotman, B., and Papermaster, B. W., 1966, Membrane properties of living mammalian cells as studied by enzymatic hydrolysis of fluorogenic esters, *Proc. Natl. Acad. Sci. USA* 55: 134–141.

Snodgrass, M. J., and Hanna, M. G., Jr., 1973, Histopathology of tumor regression after intralesional injection of *Mycobacterium bovis*. Ultrastructural studies of histiocyte-tumor cell interactions, *Cancer Res.* 33:701–716.

Sokal, J. E., Aungst, C. W., and Grace, J. T., Jr., 1973, Immunotherapy of chronic myelocytic leukemia, *Natl. Cancer Inst. Monogr.* 39:195–198.

Zbar, B., and Tanaka, T., 1971, Immunotherapy of cancer: Regression of tumors after intralesional injection of living *Mycobacterium bovis*, *Science* 172:271–273.

Zbar, B., Wepsic, H. P., Rapp, H. J., Borsos, T., Kronman, B. S., and Churchill, W. H. J., 1969, Antigenic specificity of hepatomas induced in strain 2 guinea pigs by diethylnitrosamine, *J. Natl. Cancer Inst.* 43:833–841.

Zbar, B., Bernstein, I. D., Bartlett, G. L., Hanna, M. G., Jr., and Rapp, H. J., 1972, Immunotherapy of cancer: Regression of intradermal tumors and prevention of growth of lymph node metastases after intralesional injection of living *Mycobacterium bovis* (*bacillus Calmette-Guérin*), *J. Natl. Cancer Inst.* 49:119–130.

Chapter 14

Tumor Immunity in the Peritoneal Cavity

Gideon Berke and Barbara Schick

Department of Cell Biology
The Weizmann Institute of Science
Rehovot, Israel

I. INTRODUCTION

Multicellular organisms are equipped with an intricate system to recognize and neutralize foreign and potentially dangerous components such as parasites, microorganisms, and neoplastic cells. However, many neoplastic tissues are capable of proliferative growth eventually leading to the death of the host, despite potential host antitumor cellular and humoral immunity. Inefficient antitumor activity is probably due to a complex series of events and factors that may include malfunction or suppression of host cells involved in antitumor responses and/or modification of tumor cells, for example, nonexpression or modification of antigenic determinants, inhibition of potential antitumor responses by antigen, sera, and/or tumor cell membrane complexes, accessibility of the tumor to components of the immune system, and a rate of tumor growth that outstrips the responses generated against it. An understanding of the characteristics, functions, and interactions of humoral and cellular host components involved in such responses might enable manipulation to benefit the individual.

II. STUDIES OF *IN SITU* VERSUS PERIPHERAL IMMUNITY

Studies of tumor- or graft-associated cells are important because the induction and execution of cell-mediated immune responses depend on events that occur at the site (Haskill *et al.*, 1978; Cohen and Livnat, 1976; Cerottini and Brunner,

1974; Hellström and Hellström, 1974; Herberman, 1974; Canty and Wunderlich, 1971; Wilson and Billingham, 1967; Amos, 1962b). Since intensive circulation occurs in the lymphatic system, it is possible to obtain immunopotent cells by tapping peripheral lymph organs or vessels far from the allograft or tumor site (Ford, 1975; Pederson and Morris, 1970). Since the isolation of immune cells from solid tissues is difficult, most studies on immune responses have been performed with cells from peripheral lymph organs or vessels. Using such an approach it has been shown that immune T cells, B cells, and macrophages, as well as nonimmune lymphocytes, exhibit antitumor or allograft immunity by themselves or in cooperation with humoral components (Cerottini and Brunner, 1974; Hellström and Hellström, 1974; Herberman, 1974; Levy and Wheelock, 1974). Although such studies have yielded valuable information about effector populations, their precursors, and induction, differentiation, and effector mechanisms, the findings may not be representative of those responsible for rejection *in situ*. Therefore, attention has recently focused on the host cells anatomically associated with tumors and allografts (Strom *et al.*, 1977, see Haskill *et al.*, 1978, for overall review). The cell types that infiltrated the area were first determined by microscopic observation. Infiltration of graft parenchyma by mononuclear cells is common in allograft rejection and delayed hypersensitivity reactions (Waksman, 1970, 1974). Macrophage infiltration of tumor sites is also common (Evan, 1972).

Presence of cells at the tumor or allograft site does not establish their involvement in immune responses. Therefore, cells from such sites have been isolated and their immunological functions studied. Since most immunological reactions occur within solid masses of tissue, drastic procedures, either chemical or physical, are necessary to isolate host cells from the area in question. Enzymatic digestion can be used to obtain single-cell suspensions from which host cells can then be separated on density gradients (Russell *et al.*, 1976; Zettergren *et al.*, 1973). Variations in the size and density of cells hamper isolation of homogenous subpopulations with gradients, and the enzymatic or physical separation techniques may damage cells and their surface markers. These difficulties have been overcome by implanting fibroblast-infiltrated sponge matrices in allogeneic rats and removing the infiltrating host cells by simply squeezing the sponge (Roberts and Häyry, 1977). However, the implantation of sponge matrices induces nonspecific histiocyte infiltration.

III. TUMOR AND ALLOGRAFT IMMUNITY IN THE PERITONEAL CAVITY

A. The Peritoneal Cavity

The wealth of lymphatic tissues and connections contained within the peritoneal cavity, such as lymphoid patches, mesenteric nodes, retroperitoneal nodes, and the spleen, probably facilitate the migration of immunocompetent host cells to and from the peritoneal cavity (Straube *et al.*, 1955). This migration may promote infiltration of peritoneal tumors by immunocompetent cells, migration of triggered cells to a milieu conducive to effector cell differentiation, and migration of mature effector cells to the tumor site. The variety of lymphocytes trapped in the peritoneal cavity, in conjunction with the lymphatic plexi, may create an environment conducive to a reaction similar to *in vitro* mixed lymphocyte reactions *in vivo*, thus allowing effector differentiation in the peritoneal cavity. Tumors capable of multiplying as single cells within the peritoneal or pleural cavity are referred to as ascitic tumors. During advanced stages of syngeneic ascites tumor growth, tumor membrane fragments and vesicles are detected in the ascitic fluid (Nowotny *et al.*, 1974; Van Blitterswijk *et al.*, 1977, 1979; Raz *et al.*, 1978). Immunization of nonimmune syngeneic hosts with these tumor membrane fragments and vesicles can induce immunity to the tumor. Furthermore, these preparations can inhibit the adhesion of tumor cells to nonimmune peritoneal macrophages *in vitro* (Raz *et al.*, 1978). Since the tumor cell vesicles and membrane fragments express tumor antigens, it has been postulated that the vesicles may compete with the ascitic cells in host antitumor responses and facilitate tumor escape from host immune responses (Nowotny *et al.*, 1974; Raz *et al.*, 1978; Van Blitterswijk *et al.*, 1979).

B. Early Studies on Syngeneic and Allogeneic Systems

Since established ascites tumors grow as single cells and are not subject to intense vascularization and necrosis as is the case with solid tumors (Gorer, 1956), their use as models to examine antitumor and allograft responses has been widespread. Pioneering studies of the immune responses within the peritoneal cavity relied mainly upon visual observations. Upon intraperitoneal (i.p.) injection into syngeneic hosts, ascitic tumors multiply rapidly (Patt and Straube, 1956). Sometimes a slight lag period is observed after injection, and a decrease in the number of tumor cells may occur prior to host death. Initially the growth of ascitic tumors in the peritoneal cavities of allogeneic hosts is similar to that observed in syngeneic ones; however, after about 5 days a dramatic decrease in the number of tumor cells occurs (Amos, 1960, 1962b; Amos and Wakefield, 1959; Baker *et al.*, 1962; Berke and Amos, 1973a). In syngeneic ascites systems, only slight changes in the host cell populations are visually observed (Baker *et al.*, 1962). This is not the case with the majority of allogeneic tumor systems examined, where dramatic variations in the number of peritoneal macrophages are observed that correspond to the changes in the tumor cell population, suggesting that macrophages are responsible for the tumor rejection (Amos, 1960, 1962a,b; Baker *et al.*, 1962). At the peak of ascitic tumor growth, peritoneal macrophages have been reported to consist primarily of small cells with compact cytoplasm and rounded nucleus and to exhibit little phagocytic activity for the tumor cells

(Amos, 1960). Upon decline of the tumor population, larger macrophages, which contain irregular lipid granules and tumor cell fragments (Amos, 1960) and which adhere to the tumor cells *in vivo* (Baker *et al.*, 1962) are observed. In the allogeneic Sarcoma I system employed by Baker and co-workers, no other host cell type was observed that exhibited affinity for the tumor cells. Furthermore, the injection of Sarcoma I cells into the peritoneal cavity of alloimmune mice led to the formation of tumor cell–macrophage clusters within 30 min and the generation of cellular debris and large macrophage–tumor cell clumps within several hours. Immunity to the Sarcoma I was adoptively transferred by immune spleens and macrophage-rich immune peritoneal exudates, but not by sera, cell-free ascites, or sonic extracts of alloimmune cells (Baker *et al.*, 1962). Alloimmune peritoneal cells that could phagocytose iron prevented the growth of the DBA/2 lymphoma L1210 in allogeneic C3H mice (Amos, 1962*a*). These findings further suggested that macrophages are involved in the i.p. rejection of allogeneic tumors. Although tumor cell fragments are observed within many macrophages during the decline in the tumor population, it did not appear that the macrophages act as scavengers, since few free-floating dead (trypan blue including) tumor cells were detected in the peritoneal exudates (Amos, 1960). At various stages after the injection of allogeneic ascites tumors, tumor cells and/or host cells in the presence of complement are lysed *in vitro*. Furthermore, alloimmune peritoneal macrophages can be lysed upon exposure to antitumor or antihost antibodies and complement (Amos, 1960, 1962*a*). These findings suggested that host cells can become coated with tumor antigens and antigen–antibody complexes. It was further suggested that the lysis of such cells in the presence of complement causes the release of factors that can lyse both host and tumor cells nondiscriminately. This could explain the almost simultaneous decrease in tumor and host macrophage populations during advanced stages of the allogeneic ascites tumor growth. However, when one compatible and one incompatible ascites tumor are co-injected i.p., only the incompatible one is rejected (G. Klein and Klein, 1956; E. Klein and Klein, 1972), thus discounting the possibility of nonspecific immune lysis of cells in the peritoneal cavity.

Even when grafts are not administered i.p., an immunopotent population of cells can be obtained from the cavity (Old *et al.*, 1963; Zbar *et al.*, 1970). After s.c. injection of the methylcholanthrene-induced sarcoma (Meth A) to syngeneic BALB/c mice, the macrophage-rich peritoneal exudates obtained specifically suppressed the s.c. growth of Meth A cells in nonimmune mice (Old *et al.*, 1963). Co-injection of Meth A cells with peritoneal cells obtained from nonimmune mice or mice immunized with other tumors did not affect Meth A growth. These findings prompted an investigation of the mechanism by which peritoneal exudate cells (PEC) inhibit tumor growth. In the presence of relevant alloantisera that can opsonize cells, normal or immune peritoneal macrophage monolayers are capable of phagocytosing tumor cells. Although leukemia cells are the most susceptible to phagocytosis, sarcoma and normal lymphocytes are also susceptible in the presence of relevant antisera. The peritoneal macrophages obtained from immunized mice do not require the addition of antisera in order to phagocytose cells. However, they lose this capacity when washed, suggesting that it is due to antibodies adsorbed on the macrophages. Although a correlation between *in vitro* and *in vivo* mechanisms of tumor destruction is expected, three points suggest that a mechanism other than opsonization and total ingestion by macrophages can account for immune PEC inhibition of tumor growth: (1) peritoneal cells and not sera of hyperimmune mice can transfer immunity; (2) when the phagocytosing ability of peritoneal cells from isoimmune donors is abolished by washing, which removes the adsorbed antisera, they still inhibit tumor growth *in vivo;* and (3) co-inoculation of excess nonimmune PEC and tumor cells in the presence of immune sera does not suppress tumor growth (Old *et al.*, 1963). In fact, antisera and cell-free peritoneal exudates of immune mice that contain antibodies can enhance tumor growth.

Three different mechanisms of immune destruction of a DBA/2 thymoma by C57BL/6 mice were reported on by Weaver (1958). After a single i.p. injection of the tumor, most of the tumor cells were phagocytosed and destroyed by host peritoneal macrophages. Others were lysed after adhering to host peritoneal lymphocytes. This second type of immune response was observed *in vitro* with alloimmune peritoneal lymphocytes and tumor cells. The lymphocyte-dependent destruction of the tumor cells became more pronounced upon reimmunization of the allogeneic mice. Thirdly, tumor cell death observed independent of interaction with host cells was attributed to interaction with cell-free antibodies.

Precise elucidation of the host cells and components involved in the response to ascites tumors required the fractionation of PEC and testing *in vitro* of the cells and components present therein. Peritoneal exudates of Donryu rats primed s.c. with nitrogen-mustard-treated Yoshida sarcoma and challenged i.p. with Yoshida cells exhibited antitumor activity, as determined by adoptive transfer, tumor neutralization, and diffusion chamber experiments (Hashimoto *et al.*, 1965). That the antitumor effect was due to intact cells of the alloimmune exudates was demonstrated by the fact that lysed exudate preparations displayed no antitumor activity and that sarcoma cells inside diffusion chambers in the peritoneal cavities of alloimmune mice were not lysed, although when alloimmune PEC were present within the chamber lysis occurred. Adherent cells were removed from the alloimmune exudates to obtain lymphocyte-enriched fractions whose cytolytic activities *in vitro* were examined (Hashimoto *et al.*, 1968). When these peritoneal exudate lymphocyte (PEL) preparations were incubated with tumor cells at ratios of 30 : 1, more than 90% of the tumor cells were destroyed within 7 h. Adherence of the alloimmune PEL to Yoshida cells was observed *in vitro* within 1 h. Also a correlation between the number of bound lymphocytes and the antitumor activity was noticed. Yoshida cells to which two or more lymphocytes bound were lysed within several hours, and after incubation for 24–48 h even one adherent PEL could cause tumor cell destruction.

Several groups have demonstrated that PEC populations exhibit more potent antitumor activity than spleen, thymus, lymph node or peripheral blood lymphocytes after i.p. injection of tumors (Fig. 1) (Berke et al., 1972; Cerottini and Brunner, 1971; Takasugi and Klein, 1970). Upon removal of macrophages from the PEC of immunized mice and rats, a cell population demonstrating increased antitumor activity is obtained (Berke et al., 1972; Hashimoto et al., 1968). This population, referred to as nonadherent PEL, is capable of adoptive transferring immunity and of tumor neutralization. Studies in vitro have demonstrated that the major effector cells in ascites allograft systems are nonadherent, nonphagocytic, small- to medium-sized T lymphocytes that must come into physical contact with the target cells to cause lysis (Berke and Amos, 1973a; Berke, 1980). When the leukemia EL4 of C57BL/6 (H-2^b) mice was injected i.p. into the C57BL/6 mutant strain B6.C-H-2^{ba}, a large percentage of the recipients (20/26 males and 23/38 females) rejected the tumor (Berke and Amos, 1973b). The PEL of these immunized mice lysed ^{51}Cr-labeled EL4 in vitro and exhibited

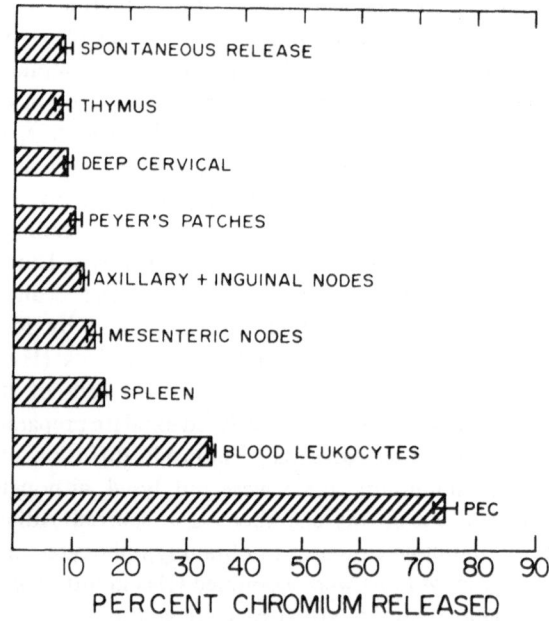

Figure 1. ^{51}Cr release from labeled C57BL/6 EL4 leukemia cells in the presence of cells obtained from BALB/c mice immunized i.p. with EL4. Triplicates of BALB/c cells and ^{51}Cr-labeled EL4 at a 10:1 ratio were incubated at 37°C for 2.5 h with rocking. (Modified from Berke et al., 1973.)

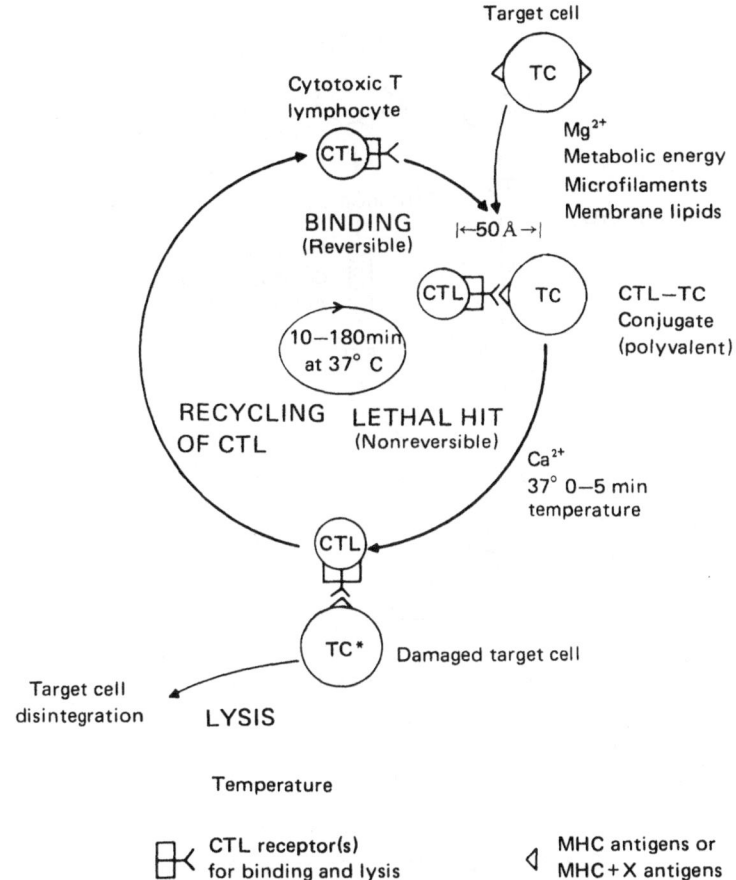

Figure 2. The cytotoxic T lymphocyte (CTL) lytic cycle. (Modified from Berke and Amos, 1973a.)

higher antitumor activity than spleen preparations. No evidence of antibody activity was detected in the immunized mice even after six injections, thus confirming that antibody production is not essential for allograft rejection.

PEL have been used to investigate the mechanism by which cytotoxic T lymphocytes (CTL), specifically bind to and lyse target cells (TC) (Berke and Amos, 1973a; Berke, 1980). A scheme summarizing current knowledge of the mechanism of specific CTL interaction with TC leading to TC lysis, compiled from work done with PEL and other types of CTL, is presented in Fig. 2 (Berke, 1979; Golstein and Smith, 1977; Henney, 1977; Martz, 1977; Berke and Amos, 1973a). Figure 3 depicts the procedures by which PEL are prepared and their functional activities tested. Two assays are routinely used: (1) release of ^{51}Cr

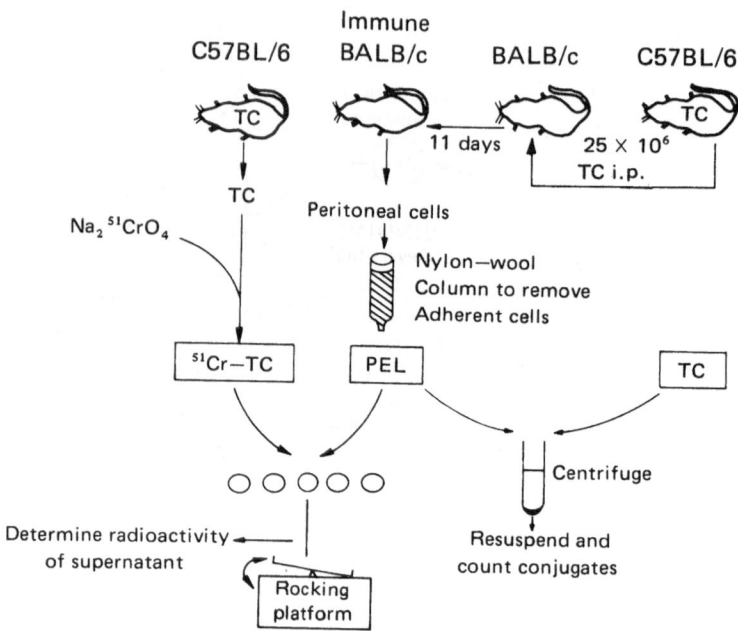

Figure 3. Preparation and functional monitoring of immune peritoneal exudate cytotoxic T lymphocytes (PEL). (For details see Berke *et al.*, 1972, 1975.)

from labeled TC to monitor lytic activity, and (2) conjugation (formation of CTL–TC clusters, Fig. 4) to monitor specific binding activity.

C. Contemporary Studies on Syngeneic Systems

In syngeneic hosts, ascites tumors continuously multiply in the peritoneal cavity and eventually lead to host death. Several groups have investigated the possibility that PEC associated with the tumor possess cytostatic or cytolytic activities. Allison (1972) has reported the presence of cells that exhibit antibody-dependent cell-mediated cytotoxicity (ADCC) in the peritoneal cavity of normal mice. Tracey *et al.* (1975) tested whether ADCC activity was associated with murine ascites tumors. In eight syngeneic ascites tumors they detected ADCC activity against mouse antibody-coated chicken red blood cells, which was removed when adherent cells or cells displaying 19 S Fc receptors were absorbed out. The ADCC activity was probably not due to the tumors, since tumor lines *in vitro* did not exhibit ADCC activity. The ADCC activity associated with the ascitic tumors may be due to a host cell population similar to the major nonphagocytic ADCC effectors found in the peritoneal cavities of normal mice. There are several explanations as to why these cells, which exhibit ADCC activity

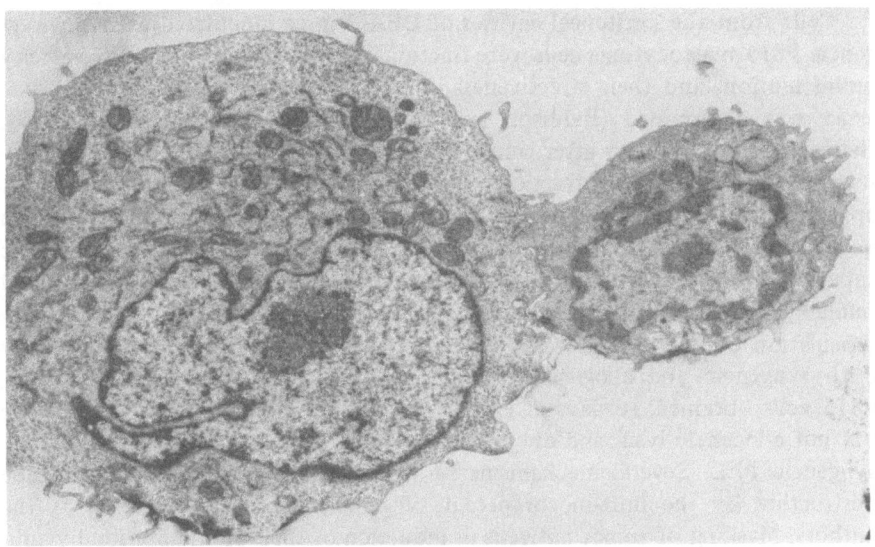

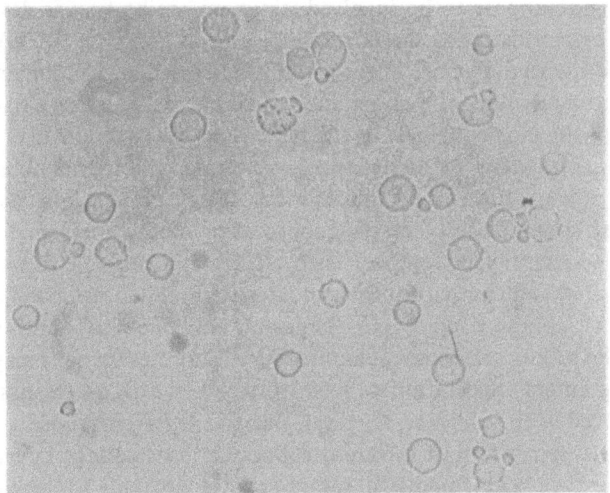

Figure 4. Light and electron micrographs of conjugates formed between peritoneal exudate lymphocytes (PEL) and tumor cells. The small cells are PEL from BALB/c mice immunized against the C57BL/6 leukemia EL4 (the large cells). [The electron micrograph ($\times$10,000, reproduced at 70%) is courtesy of Dr. Dalia Rosen of this laboratory.]

against chicken red blood cells *in vitro*, do not counter the tumor growth *in vivo* (Tracey *et al.*, 1975). First, the tumor targets would have to be coated with an appropriate type and amount of antibody; second, tumor cells might not be appropriate targets for this type of ADCC activity; and third, there is an overwhelming excess of tumor cells.

Cells from the peritoneal cavities of DBA/2 mice inoculated with 10^3 syngeneic P815 mastocytoma cells were fractionated on the basis of size by velocity sedimentation, and their effectiveness in a cell-mediated ^{51}Cr release cytotoxic assay was determined (Biddison and Palmer, 1977; Biddison et al., 1977). Between 8 and 16 days after tumor injection, cell-mediated cytotoxic activity was observed in the PEC fractions that sedimented between 2 and 6 mm/h. It appears that this cytolytic activity present within the growing tumor is due to T cells, since incubation with anti-Thy-1.2 and complement reduced the lytic capacity, whereas anti-immunoglobulin sera plus complement or heat-aggregated human gamma globulin had no effect. P815 cells obtained 10 days after the i.p. inoculation of 10^3 cells were as susceptible as in vitro-grown P815 to lysis by both syngeneic and allogeneic effector cell-mediated cytotoxicity. However, P815 cells obtained 16 days after the inoculation were resistant to syngeneic but not allogeneic lysis, and did not inhibit the lysis of in vitro-grown P815 by syngeneic PEL. Several mechanisms by which the day 16 P815 may escape destruction by the immunocompetent syngeneic PEC were discussed by the authors. Masking of tumor antigens or induction of their internalization by antibodies does not appear to be involved, since no antibody was detected on the tumor cells or circulating in the host (Biddison and Palmer, 1977). Whether host cells that sedimented at more than 6 mm/h possessed antitumor activities could not be determined, since the abundance of tumor cells in these fractions would compete with the labeled targets in the lytic assay used (Biddison et al., 1977).

The major drawback of ascites tumor systems is the tremendous tumor overgrowth that occurs and hampers study of host cell populations associated with the tumor, although upon successful mobilization of the host's immune response the number of tumor cells declines. Theoretically it is possible to specifically lyse allogeneic tumor cells in peritoneal exudates with alloantisera and complement. However, such an approach requires large amounts of specific antisera, complete removal of the tumor cells is not guaranteed and nonrelevant cells may be affected by the complement. Separation of host from tumor cells on the basis of size can also be achieved with gradients; however, due to the heterogeneity of cell populations, absolute separation of different subpopulations cannot be ensured. Alternatively, one can inject modified tumors whose capacity to replicate has been inhibited.

Resistance of DBA mice to the syngeneic lymphoma L518Y was conferred by a single i.p. injection of irradiated (irr) L518Y cells (Evans and Alexander, 1970). This immunity can be transferred to other DBA mice by spleen or lymph node cells of the immunized mice, but neither immune spleen nor lymph node cells of the immunized mice exhibit cytotoxic or cytostatic activity in vitro. The mechanism of this tumor immunity was examined in vitro. Monolayers of peritoneal macrophages from the immunized mice or of nonimmune peritoneal macrophages incubated with immune spleen cells inhibited L518Y growth in vitro. Sera from immunized mice and supernates from cultures of immune spleen cells did not render macrophages cytotoxic. The inhibition of the tumor growth *in vitro* was immunologically specific, did not require the addition of complement, and was dependent upon direct contact with the macrophages and not to some factor in the medium. Thus, the antitumor response observed *in vitro*, which might reflect the mechanism of immunity *in vivo* appears to be due to cooperation between immune lymphocytes and macrophages. The authors suggested that in allogeneic systems in which immune lymphocytes alone are cytoxic, such cooperation might occur but would be hard to detect. After a single i.p. injection of irr-L518Y cells, peritoneal macrophages exhibiting cytostatic effects were observed on day 11 but not on days 7 or 14.

Multiple i.p. injections of irr-EL4 into syngeneic C57BL/6 mice protected the mice against subsequent challenges with nonirradiated EL4 (Johnson *et al.*, 1975). Low levels of cytotoxic lymphoid activity were also detected in the PEC of syngeneic and allogeneic mice after multiple injections of the irr-tumor cells. A single i.p. injection of leukemia EL4 cells, exposed to ^{60}Co irradiation, induced resistance to non-irr-EL4 in syngeneic C57BL/6 and allogeneic BALB/c mice (Schick and Berke 1977*a*). Tumor resistance was demonstrated at both the tumor inoculation (Fig. 5) and peripheral sites (Table I). Tumor-associated PEC lysed

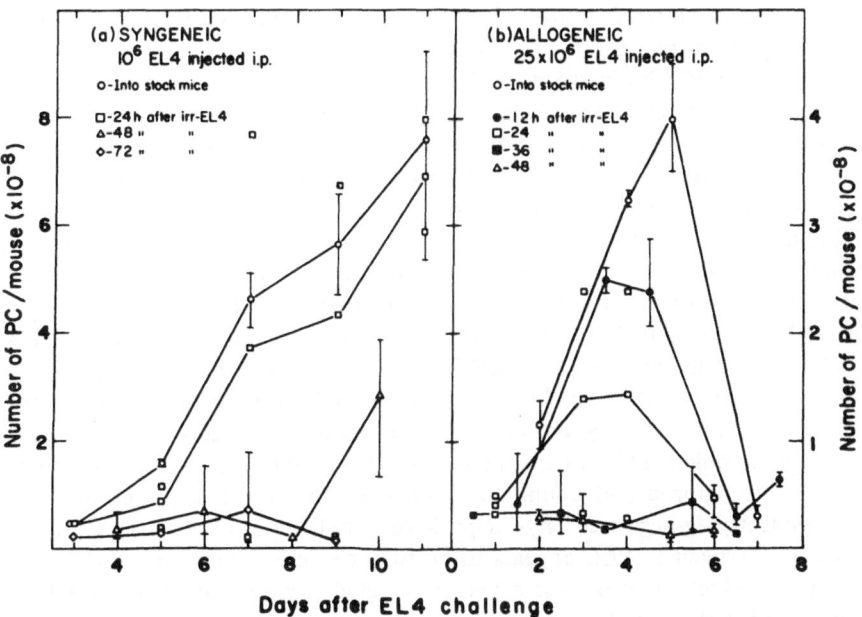

Figure 5. Inhibition of EL4 growth in the peritoneal cavities of C57BL/6 (a) and BALB/c (b) mice primed with 150 and 25 × 10⁶ irr-EL4, respectively. The average number of cells present in the peritoneal cavities from three mice and the spread, if any, are shown. (Reproduced with permission from *Schick and Berke*, 1977*a*.).

Table I. Resistance of Stock and Primed[a] C57BL/6 Mice to s.c. Challenge of Nonirradiated EL4

Exp.	No. of i.p. primings	s.c. challenge with EL4[b]	Average lifespan	Survivors/ total	Mouse lifespan (days)
1	0	5×10^3	21.5	0/5	18, 18, 25, 25
	1		37.2	0/5[c]	10, 33, 37, 49, 57
	0	5×10^4	23.0	0/5	20, 22, 22, 25, 26
	1		25.3	0/5	22, 22, 25, 32
	0	5×10^5	15.2	0/5	12, 15, 15, 17, 17
	1		19.4	0/5	17, 18, 19, 19, 24
2	0	5×10^3	22.3	0/6	16, 17, 25, 25, 25, 26
	1		33	1/5	29, 34, 40
	3		–	5/6	29
	0	5×10^4	30.6	1/6	25, 26, 34, 34, 34
	1		30.5	3/5	26, 35
	3		–	6/6	–

[a] 150×10^6 irr-EL4/0.5 ml phosphate buffered saline, i.p.
[b] Challenged 5 days after the last priming.
[c] Died from ascitic not s.c. growth.

EL4 in cytolytic assay *in vitro* (Schick and Berke, 1977a) as early as 3 days after irr-EL4 injection, peaking on days 5–6 (Fig. 6). Adoptive immunity was exhibited by syngeneic PEC obtained 5 days after priming. Therefore a single i.p. injection of irr-tumor cells can induce a cell-mediated immune respose at the tumor inoculation site, which can be measured *in vivo* and *in vitro*, in addition to conferring resistance *in vivo* against the nonirradiated tumor. A more potent immune response can be generated by repeated i.p. injections of irr-tumor cells (Table I and unpublished results). Fractionation of immune allogeneic and syngeneic PEC induced by irr-tumors, on nylon–wool columns, yielded a nonadherent, Ig-negative, Thy-1.2-positive PEL fraction with increased anti-EL4 activity *in vitro* (Table II; Schick and Berke, 1977b). The cytolytic and conjugating capacity of the PEL paralleled the cytolytic activity of unfractionated PEC peaking on days 5–6 (Schick and Berke, 1977b). That thymus-derived lymphocytes in the PEL exhibit antitumor activity was demonstrated by immunofluorescence and antibody-plus-complement lysis experiments (Tables II and III). The tumor-associated PEL that recognized and bound to tumor cells, thus forming conjugates, were predominantly Ig-negative, Thy-1.2-positive lymphocytes (Table III). Cytolytic activity of syngeneic PEL appears to be tumor-specific, since only C57BL/6 T leukemias, which may possess a yet undetected common antigen, were lysed (Schick and Berke, 1977a).

The cytolytic capacity of effector PEL induced by irr-EL4 is lower than that induced by non-irr-EL4 (Schick and Berke, 1977a). Since the irradiation (5000 R, ^{60}Co) of EL4 seems not to affect their cellular antigenicity *in vitro* (Schick and Berke, 1977a), the weaker response elicited by irr-EL4 cannot be explained by gross antigenic changes due to irradiation (see also Herberman *et al.*, 1976). The difference may be due to the amount of cellular antigen available for sensitization, since the prolific multiplication of non-irr-EL4 in the peritoneal cavity (Berke and Amos, 1973a) provides more cellular antigen than the irr-EL4, which do not multiply. The early decline in anti-irr-EL4 PEL activity may be caused by migration of immune PEC from the peritoneal cavity once the sensitizing cellular antigen is no longer present. Thus, the response induced by irr-EL4 may parallel early events in immunity against nonirradiated EL4 that are usually masked by

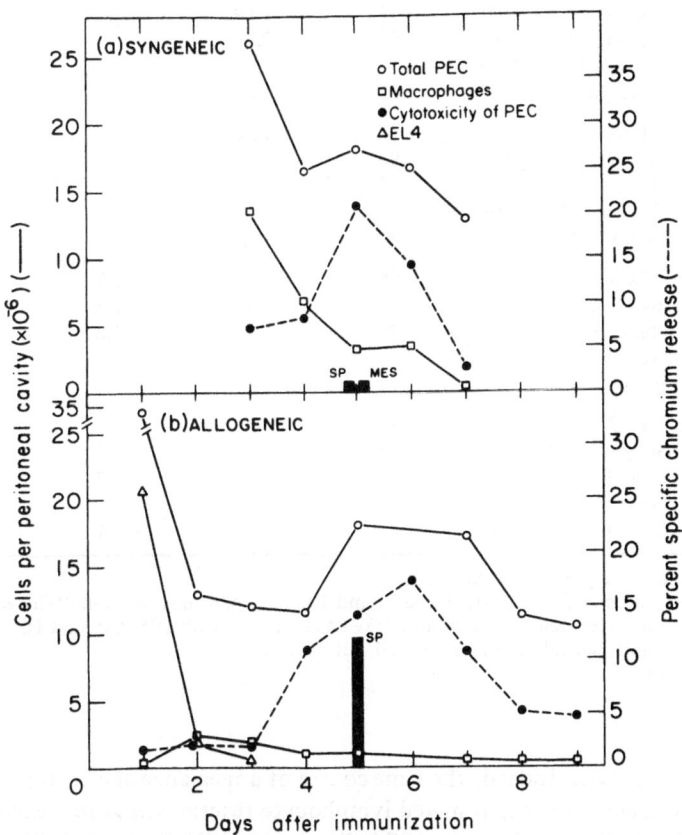

Figure 6. Cell populations and cytolytic activity of PEC from C57BL/6 (a) and BALB/c (b) mice inoculated i.p. with 150 and 25 × 10⁶ irr-EL4, respectively. Effector: ^{51}Cr–EL4 ratios of 20:1 (syngeneic PEC), 4:1 (allogeneic PEC), 100:1 (spleen–SP), and 50:1 (mesenteric node lymphocytes–MES) were employed in a 2-h ^{51}Cr-release cytotoxic assay. Heavily granulated cells were considered to be macrophages. (Reproduced with permission from Schick and Berke, 1977a.)

Table II. Involvement of Theta-Positive C57BL/6 Anti-irr-EL4 PEL in the Conjugation and Cytolysis of EL4

Exp.	Treatment	% Viability[a]	% Specific lysis[b]	No. conjugates $(\times 10^4)^c$	% Of control
1	PBS–FCS[d]	99	14.3	–	100
	AKRα(θ)C3H (1:10)[e]	98	17.9	–	125
	Guinea pig C' (1:10)[f]	95	7.3	–	51
	AKRα(θ)C3H (1:10)+				
	guinea pig C' (1:10)	53	0.7	–	5
2	PBS–FCS	98	38.5	–	100
	AKRα(θ)C3H (1:10)	97	48.4	–	126
	Guinea pig C' (1:10)	92	23.6	–	61
	AKRα(θ)C3H (1:10)+				
	guinea pig C' (1:10)	31	4.8	–	12
3	PBS–FCS	95	12.6	–	100
	AKRα(θ)C3H (1:10)	95	21.5	–	170
	Rabbit C' (1:16)	72	9.8	–	78
	AKRα(θ)C3H (1:10)+				
	rabbit C' (1:16)	32	2.5	–	20
4	PBS–FCS	86	–	3.7	100
	AKRα(θ)C3H (1:5)	86	–	2.8	75
	Rabbit C' (1:8)	70	–	2.8	75
	AKRα(θ)C3H+				
	rabbit C' (1:8)	<18	–	0.7	19
5	PSB–FCS	88	–	3.7	100
	AKRα(θ)C3H (1:5)	83	–	3.9	105
	Guinea pig C' (1:20)	87	–	3.2	86
	AKRα(θ)C3H+				
	guinea pig C' (1:20)	8	–	1.1	30

[a] Determined by trypan blue exclusion.
[b] PEL:EL4 ratios of 20:1 (exps. 1 and 2) and 14:1 (exp. 3) during a 2-h ^{51}Cr release assay.
[c] Conjugation performed according to Berke et al. (1975) with 10^6 PEL and 10^6 EL4.
[d] Phosphate buffered saline plus 10% fetal calf serum.
[e] 30 min on ice.
[f] 45 min at 37°C.

tumor overgrowth. Indeed, the time course of appearance of effector cell activity in this system parallels that mixed lymphocyte reactions *in vitro* (Andersson and Häyry, 1975; Cerottini et al., 1974; Wagner and Röllinghoff, 1973), while no effector cells were detected in peripheral lymph of syngeneic hosts on day 5 (Fig. 6). Thus, in this system as in several others, it appears that cytolytic effectors may differentiate at the tumor site. No differences in the characteristics of the PEL induced by irr-tumor cells as compared to allogeneic tumor cells have been observed.

Table III. Test for θ, Ig, and Fc-Positive Cells in PEL and PEL–EL4 Conjugates[a]

PEL donor	Serum[b,c]	PEL		Conjugated PEL	
		Stained/ total	% Positive	Stained/ total	% Positive
C57BL/6	GAMG-F1	16/400	4	–	–
(syngeneic)	GAMM-F1	1/100	1	–	–
	GAMA-F1	2/200	1	–	–
	AggHγG-F1 [d]	17/533	3	2/50	4
	AKRα(θ)C3H +GAMG-F1	416/440	94	95/100	95
BALB/c	GAMG-F1	7/219	3	–	–
(allogeneic)	AKRα(θ)C3H[e] +GAMG-F1	186/195	95	67/69	97

[a] Reproduced with permission from Schick and Berke, 1977b.
[b] Fluoresceinated goat antisera to mouse 7 S globulin (GAMG-F1), IgA (GAMA-F1), and IgM (GAMM-F1). Fluoresceinated aggregated human gamma globulin (AggHγG-F1). Incubations 30 min on ice unless indicated.
[c] Diluted 1:10. In control experiments, 30–40% normal spleen cells were stained by GAMG-F1, 30% by GAMM-F1, 20% GAMA-F1, and 40% by AggHγG-F1. Less than 0.5% of thymocytes were strained by GAMG-F1, GAMM-F1, and GAMA-F1. Five percent of thymocytes were stained by AggHγG-F1.
[d] Diluted 1:4, 50λ, 30 min at room temperature.
[e] Diluted 1:2.

IV. SUMMARY

This review has summarized the major contributions of studies using ascites tumors to our understanding of cell-mediated responses *in situ* to syngeneic and allogeneic tumors. Tapping of the peritoneal cavity during an ongoing antitumor response yields single-cell suspensions, from which host cells can easily be obtained and their functional activities monitored *in vivo* and *in vitro*. Although pioneering studies suggested that macrophages were the predominant host cell type responsible for elimination of certain ascites tumors, more recent studies have indicated that cytotoxic T lymphocytes play a major role in this response. An assessment *in vitro* of the development of a cell-mediated immune response *in vivo* directed against irradiated ascites leukemias at the tumor site in syngeneic and allogenic mice was described. This tumor–host system allowed the continuous monitoring of cell populations present at the tumor site that can bind to and lyse tumor target cells and that are probably directly involved in the immune response against tumors. Peritoneal exudate cells that lysed tumor cells *in vitro* were detected as early as three days after irr-tumor administration and were capable of adoptively transferring immunity. Incubation of the immunized peritoneal exudate cells on nylon–wool columns yielded a macrophage-free, nonadherent lymphocyte fraction with enhanced cytolytic activity *in vitro*. This cytolytic capacity was T-cell-associated and specific and paralleled the ability of nonadherent immune lymphocytes to bind (conjugate) to tumor cells. The individual host cells that bound to the tumor cells *in vitro* were Ig-negative, Thy-1.2-positive lymphocytes. The induction, development, and characteristics of this cell-mediated immune response will further our understanding of an organism's defense mechanisms against neoplastic tissues.

ACKNOWLEDGMENTS

We wish to express our gratitude to Z. Fishelson, D. Gabison, and M. (Weinstein) Sela, who performed some of the experiments; and to S. Gohali, P. Reitman, D. Rosen, B. Tannenbaum, and R. (Tzur) Wolfson for excellent assistance. Part of the work mentioned in this review was supported by NIH Contract CB-74183.

V. REFERENCES

Allison, A. C., 1972, Immunity and immunopathology in virus infections, *Ann. Inst. Pasteur, Paris* 123:585.
Amos, D. B., 1960, Possible relations between the cytotoxic effects of isoantibody and host cell function, *Ann. N. Y. Acad. Sci.* 87:273.
Amos, D. B., 1962*a*, Host response to ascites tumors, in: *Mechanism of Cell and Tissue Damage Produced by Immune Reactions*, p. 210, Benno Schwabe and Co., Basel, Switzerland.
Amos, D. B., 1962*b*, The use of simplified systems as an aid to the interpretation of mechanisms of graft rejection, *Prog. Allergy* 6:468.
Amos, D. B., and Wakefield, J. D., 1959, Growth of ascites tumor cells in diffusion chambers. II. Lysis and growth inhibition by diffusible isoantibody, *J. Natl. Cancer Inst.* 22:1077.
Andersson, L. C., and Häyry, P., 1975, Clonal isolation of alloantigen-reactive T Cells and characterization of their memory, *Transplant. Rev.* 25:121.
Baker, P., Weiser, R. S., Jutila, J., Evans, C. A., and Blandau, R. J., 1962, Mechanisms of tumor homograft rejection: The behavior of Sarcoma I ascites tumor in the A/Jax and C57BL/6K mouse, *Ann. N. Y. Acad. Sci.* 101:46.
Berke, G., 1980, Interaction of cytotoxic T lymphocytes and target cells, *Prog. Allergy* 27:69–133.
Berke, G., and Amos, D. B., 1973*a*, Mechanism of lymphocyte-mediated cytolysis: The LMC cycle and its role in transplantation, *Transplant. Rev.* 17:71.
Berke, G., and Amos, D. B., 1973*b*, Cytotoxic lymphocytes in the absence of detectable antibody, *Nature (London) New Biol.* 242:237.
Berke, G., Sullivan, K., and Amos, D. B., 1972, Rejection of ascites tumor allografts. I. Isolation, characterization, and *in vitro* reactivity of peritoneal lymphoid effector cells from BALB/c mice immune to EL4 leukosis, *J. Exp. Med.* 135:1334.
Berke, G., Gabison, D., and Feldman, M., 1975, The frequency of effector cells in populations containing cytotoxic T lymphocytes, *Eur. J. Immunol.* 5:813.

Biddison, W. E., and Palmer, J. C., 1977, Development of tumor cell resistance to syngeneic cell-mediated cytotoxicity during growth of ascitic mastocytoma P815, *Proc. Nat. Acad. Sci. USA* **74**:329.

Biddison, W. E., Palmer, J. C., Alexander, M. A., Cowan, E. P., and Manson, L. A., 1977, Characterization and specificity of murine anti-tumor cytotoxic effector cells within an ascitic tumor, *J. Immunol.* **118**:2243.

Canty, T. G., and Wunderlich, J. R., 1971, Quantitative assessment of cellular and humoral responses to skin and tumor allografts, *Transplantation* **11**:111.

Cerottini, J. C., and Brunner, K. T., 1971, Cytotoxic lymphocytes as effector cells of cell-mediated immunity, in: *Progress in Immunology*, Vol. 1 (D. B. Amos, ed.), p. 385, Academic Press, New York.

Cerottini, J. C., and Brunner, K. T., 1974, Cell-mediated cytotoxicity, allograft rejection and tumor immunity, *Adv. Immunol.* **18**:67.

Cerottini, J. C., Engers, H. D., MacDonald, H. R., and Brunner, K. T., 1974, Generation of cytotoxic T lymphocytes in vitro. I. Response of normal and immune mouse spleen cells in mixed leukocyte cultures, *J. Exp. Med.* **140**:703.

Cohen, I. R., and Livnat, S., 1976, The cell-mediated immune response: Interactions of initiator and recruited T lymphocytes, *Transplant. Rev.* **29**:24.

Evans, R., 1972, Macrophages in syngeneic animal tumors, *Transplantation* **14**:468.

Evans, R., and Alexander, P., 1970, Cooperation of immune cells with macrophages in tumor immunity, *Nature (London)* **228**:620.

Ford, W. L.. 1975, Lymphocyte migration and immune responses, *Prog. Allergy* **19**:1.

Golstein, P., and Smith, E. T., 1977, Mechanism of T-cell-mediated cytolysis: The lethal hit stage, in: *Contemporary Topics in Immunobiology*, Vol. 7 (O. Stutman, ed.), pp. 273–300, Plenum Press, New York.

Gorer, D., 1956, Some recent work on tumor immunity, *Adv. Cancer Res.* **4**:149.

Hashimoto, Y., and Sudo, H., 1968, Studies on acquired transplantation resistance. III. Cytocidal effect of sensitized peritoneal lymphocytic cells of Donryu rats against the target Yoshida sarcoma cells in vitro, *Gann* **59**:7.

Hashimoto, Y., Ishidate, M., and Takaku, M., 1965, Studies on acquired transplantation resistance. II. Action of peritoneal exudate cells of Donryu rats immune to the tumor against Yoshida sarcoma, *Gann* **56**:23.

Haskill, J. S., Häyry, P., and Radov, L. A., 1978, Systemic and local immunity in allograft and cancer rejection, in: *Contemporary Topics in Immunobiology*, Vol. 8 (N. L. Warner and M. D. Cooper, eds.), pp. 107–170, Plenum Press, New York.

Hellström, K. E., and Hellström, I., 1974, Lymphocyte-mediated cytotoxicity and blocking serum activity to tumor antigens, *Adv. Immunol.* **18**:209.

Henney, C. S., 1977, T-cell-mediated cytolysis: An overview of some current issues, in: *Contemporary Topics in Immunobiology*, Vol. 7 (O. Stutman, ed.), pp. 245–272, Plenum Press, New York.

Herberman, R. B., 1974, Cell-mediated immunity to tumor cells, *Adv. Cancer Res.* **19**:207.

Herberman, R. B., Campbell, D. A., Oldham, R. K., Bonnard, G. D., Ting, C. C., Holden, H. T., Glaser, M., Djeu, J., and Oehler, R., 1976, Immunogenicity of tumor antigens, *Ann. N.Y. Acad. Sci.* **276**:26.

Johnson, T. S., Hudson, J. L., Feldman, M. E., and Irvin, G. L., 1975, Innumoprophylaxis and cytotoxic effector cells against EL4 leukemia induced in syngeneic C57BL/6J mice by use of irradiated EL4 cells, *J. Natl. Cancer Inst.* **55**:561.

Klein, E., and Klein, G., 1972, Specificity of homograft rejection in vivo, assessed by inoculation of artificially mixed compatible and incompatible tumor cells, *Cell. Immunol.* **5**:201.

Klein, G., and Klein, E., 1956, Conversion of solid neoplasms into ascites tumors, *Ann. N.Y. Acad. Sci.* **63**:640.

Levy, M. H., Wheelock, E. F., 1974, The role of macrophages in defense against neoplastic diseases, *Adv. Cancer Res.* **20**:133.

Martz, E., 1977, Mechanism of specific tumor cell lysis by alloimmune T lymphocytes: Resolution and characterization of discrete steps in the cellular interaction, in: *Contemporary Topics in Immunobiology*, Vol. 7 (O. Stutman, ed.), pp. 301–361, Plenum Press, New York.

Nowotny, A., Groshsman, J., Abdelnoor, A., Rote, N., Yang, C., and Waltersdorff, R., 1974, Escape of TA3 tumors from allogeneic immune rejection: Theory and experiments, *Eur. J. Immunol.* **4**:73.

Old, L. J., Boyse, E. A., Bennet, B., and Lilly, F., 1963, Peritoneal cells as an immune population in transplantation studies, in: *Cell-Bound Antibodies* (B. Amos and H. Koprovski, eds.), p. 89, Wistar Press, Philadelphia.

Patt, H. M., and Straube, R. L., 1956, Measurement and nature of ascites tumor growth, *Ann. N.Y. Acad. Sci.* **63**:728.

Pedersen, N. C., and Morris, B., 1970, The role of the lymphatic system in the rejection of homografts: A study of lymph from renal transplants, *J. Exp. Med.* **131**:936.

Raz, A., Goldman, R., Yuli, I., and Inbar, M., 1978, Isolation of plasma membrane fragments and vesicles from ascites fluid of lymphoma-bearing mice and their possible role in the escape mechanism of tumors from host immune rejection, *Cancer Immunol. Immunother.* **4**:53.

Roberts, P. J., and Häyry, P., 1977, Effector mechanism in allograft rejection. II. Density, electrophoresis, and size fractionation of allograft-infiltrating cells demonstrating several classes of killer cells, *Cell. Immunol.* **30**:326.

Russell, S. W., Doe, W. F., Hoskins, R. G., and Cochrane, C. G., 1976, Inflammatory cells in solid murine neoplasms. I. Tumor disaggregation and identification of constituent inflammatory cells, *Int. J. Cancer* **18**:322.

Schick, B., and Berke, G., 1977a, Activity of tumor-associated lymphoid cells at short intervals after administration of irradiated syngeneic and allogeneic tumor cells, *J. Immunol.* **118**:986.

Schick, B., and Berke, G., 1977b, Tumor-associated lymphoid cells: Analysis of host cells that bind to syngeneic and allogeneic tumor cells shortly after tumor administration, *Transplant. Proc.* **9**:1157.

Straube, R. L., Hill, M. S., and Patt, H. M., 1955, Vascular permeability and ascites tumor growth, *Proc. Am. Assoc. Cancer Res.* **2**:49.

Strom, T. B., Tilney, N. L., Paradysz, J. M., Bancewicz, J., and Carpenter, C. B., 1977, Cellular components of allograft rejection: Identity, specificity, and cytotoxic function of cells infiltrating acutely rejecting allografts, *J. Immunol.* **118**:2020.

Takasugi, M., and Klein, E., 1970, A microassay for cell-mediated immunity, *Transplantation* **9**:219.

Tracey, D. E., Pross, H. F., Jondal, M., and Witz, I. P., 1975, Antibody-dependent cell-mediated cytotoxic activity in syngeneic mouse ascites tumors, *Int. J. Cancer* **16**:870.

Van Blitterswijk, W. J., Emmelot, P., Hilkmann, H. A. M., Oomen-Meulemans, E. P. M., and Inbar, M., 1977, Differences in lipid fluidity among isolated plasma membranes of normal and leukemic lymphocytes and membranes exfoliated from their cell surface, *Biochim. Biophys. Acta* **467**:309.

Van Blitterswijk, W. J., Emmelot, P., Hilkmann, H. A., Hilgers, J., and Feltkamp, C. A., 1979, Rigid plasma-membrane-derived vesicles enriched in tumor associated surface antigens (MLr) occurring in the ascites-fluid of a murine leukemia (GRSL), *Int. J. Cancer* **23**:62.

Wagner, H., and Röllinghoff, M., 1973, *In vitro* induction of tumor-specific immunity. Parameters of activation and cytotoxic reactivity of mouse lymphoid cells immunized *in vitro* against syngeneic and allogeneic plasma cell tumors, *J. Exp. Med.* **138**:1.

Waksman, B. H., 1970, *Atlas of Experimental Immunobiology and Immunopathology*, Yale University Press, New Haven and London.

Waksman, B. H., 1974, The antiallograft response effector mechanism, in: *Progress in Immunology*, Vol. 5 (L. Brent and E. J. Holbrow, eds.), p. 127, North-Holland, Amsterdam.

Weaver, J. M., 1958, Destruction of mouse ascites tumor cells *in vivo* and *in vitro* by homologous macrophages, lymphocytes, and cell-free antibodies, *Proc. Am. Assoc. Cancer Res.* **2**:354.

Wilson, D. B., and Billingham, R. E., 1967, Lymphocytes and transplantation immunity, *Adv. Immunol.* **7**:189.

Zbar, B., Wepsic, H. T., Borsos, T., and Rapp, H. J., 1970, Tumor-graft rejection in syngeneic guinea pigs, Evidence for a two-step mechanism, *J. Natl. Cancer Inst.* **44**:473.

Zettergren, J. G., Luberoff, D. E., and Pretlow, T. G., 1973, Separation of lymphocytes from disaggregated mouse malignant neoplasms by sedimentation in gradients of Ficoll in tissue culture medium, *J. Immunol.* **111**:836.

Chapter 15

The Multicellular Tumor Spheroid: A Quantitative Model for Studies of in Situ Immunity

H. Robson MacDonald and Bernard Sordat

Unit of Human Cancer Immunology
Lausanne Branch
Ludwig Institute for Cancer Research
and Department of Immunology
Swiss Institute for Experimental Cancer Research
1066 Epalinges-sur-Lausanne, Switzerland

I. INTRODUCTION

Current knowledge of the basic cellular events associated with the immune response to solid tumors is severely limited by the lack of availability of model systems that adequately reflect the complexity of the environment *in situ*. Thus, while a number of investigators have isolated and partially purified cells and immunoglobulins from tumors for the purpose of testing their effector functions *in vitro* (this volume), such studies do not directly pertain to the question of whether or not such mechanisms may be operative within the tumor itself. Indeed it is clear from a number of studies that solid tumors differ from dissociated suspensions of tumor cells in a variety of ways apart from obvious differences in geometry. For example, the concentration of critical metabolites such as oxygen and glucose (as well as toxic waste products) is diffusion-limited in solid tumors, resulting in necrotic areas at distances sufficiently removed from the vascular supply (Thomlinson and Gray, 1955; Tannock, 1968). Similar considerations may account for the fact that solid neoplasms have been found to contain an appreciable fraction of tumor cells that progress through the cell cycle either very slowly or not at all (reviewed in Baserga, 1971). These and other factors have been shown to give rise to heterogeneity in the response of solid tumors to experimental radiotherapy and chemotherapy (Gray *et al.*, 1953; Kaplan,

1974), and similar effects of microenvironment on immune responses might be anticipated.

Several experimental approaches to the study of tumor microenvironment have been put forward in recent years. A major goal of such studies has been the reproducible establishment of three-dimensional colonies (or aggregates) of tumor cells *in vitro* (McAllister *et al.*, 1967; Dalen and Burki, 1971; Folkman and Hochberg, 1973; Carlsson and Brunk, 1977). A particularly interesting model system of this type involves the growth of sarcoma or carcinoma cells *in vitro* in the geometrical configuration of multicellular tumor spheroids (MTS) (Sutherland *et al.*, 1971). This system, which will be described in more detail in Section II, has a number of features in common with solid tumors, including considerable heterogeneity in the nutritional and cell cycle status of the constituent tumor cells (reviewed in Sutherland and Durand, 1976). As such, it is obvious that the microenvironment of spheroids simulates in many ways that of certain solid tumors *in vivo*. MTS thus provide a particularly useful experimental model for studies of the possible effect of microenvironment on the response of solid tumors to radiation, drugs, and immune mechanisms.

In the present article, we will restrict ourselves to a brief general description of MTS and a discussion of some immunological aspects of spheroid destruction *in vivo*. For interested readers, a comprehensive review of the possible applications of the MTS model to radiobiology and chemotherapy has been published recently by Sutherland and Durand (1976).

II. THE MTS AS A MICROTUMOR

A. Description of Spheroids

1. General

MTS can be initiated and grown *in vitro* either in spinner flasks (Sutherland *et al.*, 1971), in semisolid agar (Folkman and Hochberg, 1973), or, as described more recently, in liquid medium over a base layer of agar or agarose (Yuhas *et al.*, 1977; Haji-Karim and Carlsson, 1978). All three methods have been shown to provide adequate conditions for a variety of tumor and transformed cell lines to grow as spheroids: they include carcinomas and gliomas of human origin (Haji-Karim and Carlsson, 1978; Yuhas *et al.*, 1977; Lees *et al.*, 1979) (Fig. 1A,B), melanoma and sarcoma from the mouse (Sutherland and Durand, 1976; Folkman and Hochberg, 1973; Yuhas *et al.*, 1977), and lung cell lines originating from the Chinese hamster (Sutherland *et al.*, 1971). Optimal conditions for MTS formation in spinner flasks, as analyzed in detail elsewhere (Sutherland and Durand, 1976), is dependent on the type of cells cultured and on several other factors

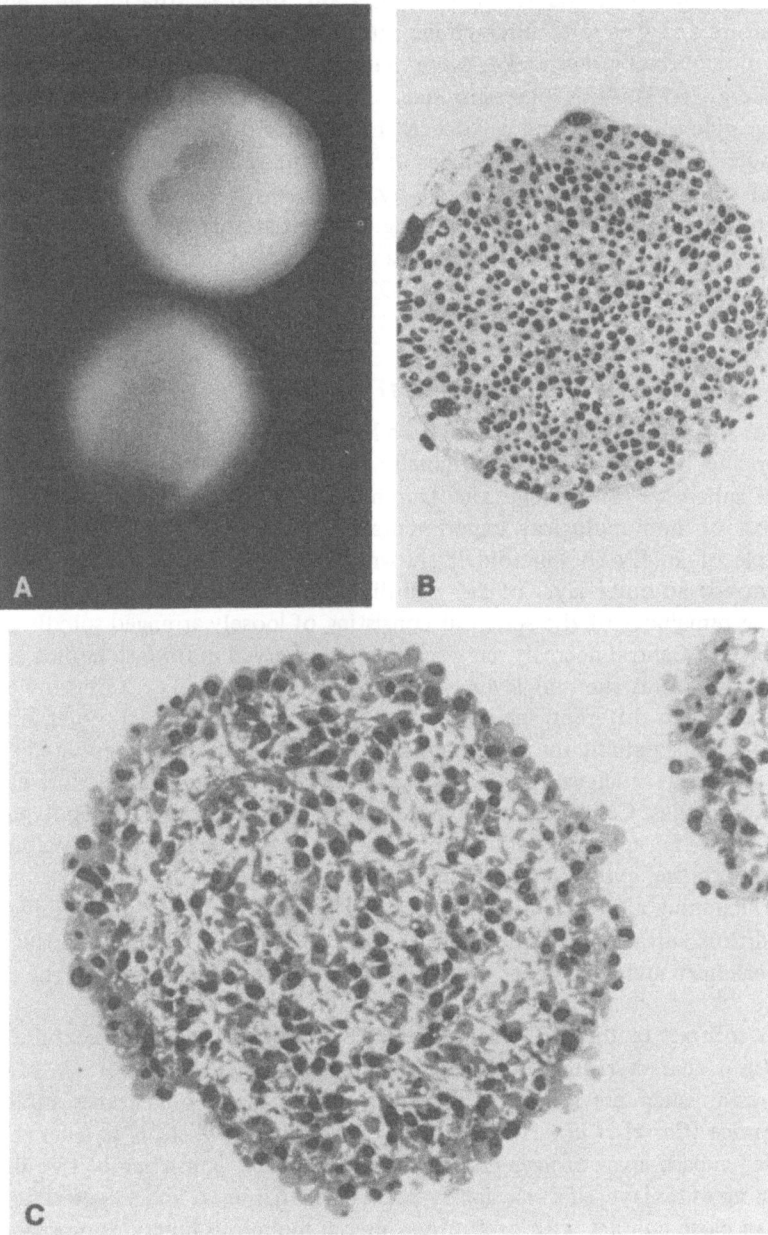

Figure 1. Examples of human and murine MTS. (A) Spheroids of human choriocarcinoma cell line (CCL98) seen under dissecting microscope (actual diameter 1.5 mm). (B) Photomicrograph of CCL98 spheroid (actual diameter 300 μm). (C) Photomicrograph of murine EMT6 spheroid (actual diameter 250 μm).

including initial cell and serum concentration, speed of rotation, and possibly the nature and degree of intercellular attachment. Under appropriate conditions three-dimensional growth takes place that is generally self-limiting (Folkman and Hochberg, 1973). With increasing size, MTS usually develop a necrotic core containing pyknotic nuclei and cell debris. The nonnecrotic part, which is composed of viable tumor cells, can be further divided into two regions: an outer layer of several cell diameters characterized by a high proportion of cycling cells (as detected by mitotic index and labeling with tritiated thymidine), and an inner part that has been shown to contain a large fraction of slowly cycling or noncycling cells (Sutherland and Durand, 1976).

2. The EMT6 Spheroid

For the studies described below, we have utilized the EMT6 mouse mammary tumor line of BALB/c origin originally established by Rockwell et al. (1972). EMT6 spheroids (Sutherland and Durand, 1976) are particularly useful in the context of immunological experiments (Sutherland et al., 1977). A typical example of an EMT6 spheroid is shown in Fig. 1C. Two major zones can be recognized: an outer layer of 2–3 cell diameters that is epithelial in appearance, and the remainder of the spheroid consisting of loosely arranged spindle-shaped EMT6 cells. Central necrosis was occasionally observed in large spheroids.

At the ultrastructural level, variations in intercellular organization can be observed when different spheroid types are compared (Fig. 2). For the EMT6 spheroid, cells exhibit the morphological features of an undifferentiated tumor, such as a large nucleus and a cytoplasm rich in polysomes with some ergastoplasmic profiles. Cells located in the outer part are generally more polygonal in shape than the central sarcomalike elements. In places they display abundant interpenetrating cytoplasmic projections together with point contacts consisting of a thickening along a limited area of cell membrane appositions (see Fig. 2A). In addition, surface microvillous projections are generally numerous at the spheroid periphery and, to a lesser degree, in the free intercellular space of the central zone.

In contrast to the EMT6 spheroid, MTS of human Co-115 cells exhibit ultrastructural characteristics of a more differentiated type of tumor. Co-115 cells were established previously from a human colon carcinoma transplanted into nude mice (Carrel et al., 1976). Co-115 spheroids grown either in spinner flasks or over a base layer of agar resemble hollow spheres consisting of two distinct zones: an outer layer of 8–12 tightly packed cell diameters and a central necrosis. Cells in close contact with each other present numerous junctions mostly of the desmosome type (Fig. 2B). Surface microvilli with cytoplasmic rootlets can be observed. The fine structure of Co-115 cells within spheroids appears to be similar to that of the tumor cells described in culture (Carrel et al., 1976).

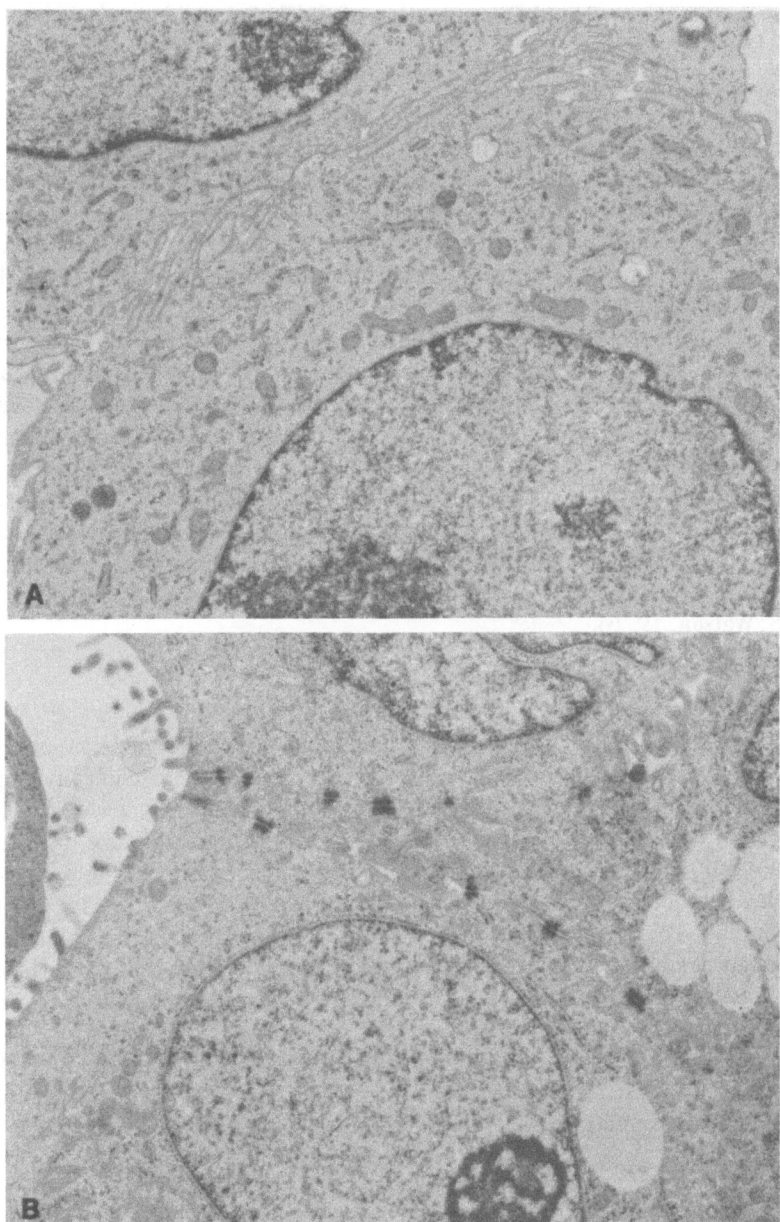

Figure 2. Electron micrographs illustrating two types of intercellular attachment in MTS. (A) EMT6 spheroid. Note interdigitating penetrations and areas of close membrane apposition (×14,500, reproduced at 90%). (B) Co-115 spheroid (human colon carcinoma). Note numerous desmosomes and microvilli (×13,000, reproduced at 90%).

B. Growth and Dissemination of EMT6 Spheroids *in Vivo*

1. Tumor Growth Studies

Comparative studies of the growth of EMT6 solid tumors starting either from cell suspensions or from single spheroids have been carried out. Both sources of EMT6 cells have been inoculated subcutaneously and intraperitoneally to groups of BALB/c or C57BL/6 nude mice. Following subcutaneous inoculation, tumor volume as a function of time was assessed assuming that progressively growing tumors tend to be hemiellipsoids (Dethlefsen *et al.*, 1968). From these data, which are summarized in Fig. 3, it can be seen that a sigmoid growth curve was obtained when single EMT6 spheroids were implanted. There was no evidence of strain- or sex-related differences in the growth of EMT6 tumors under these conditions. The growth curve is characteristically triphasic, with an initial lag period corresponding to local implantation and invasion of the micro-tumor, followed by exponential growth and finally by a late period of growth retardation. At a volume of 0.1 cm^3, the slope of the tangent to the growth curve indicates a doubling time *in vivo* of approximately 43 h, which is in the range of values reported by other authors (Watson, 1976; Twentyman, 1978). Mechanisms to account for this pattern of growth are discussed elsewhere (Dethlefsen *et al.*, 1968; Watson, 1976).

2. Behavior in Situ

Single EMT6 spheroids implanted subcutaneously into nude mice rapidly induced a vascular reaction that can be readily observed macroscopically (Fig. 4). The pattern of EMT6-induced vasculature is characterized by a well-developed peripheral vascularization and a central necrosis. With increasing size, the necrosis develops at multiple central sites, resulting in a polynodular growing tumor edge. At the light-microscopy level, the vasculature of implanted EMT6 spheroids appears mainly peripheral (Fig. 5A). Dilated veins as well as a fine capillary network can be observed. It has been repeatedly suggested that a factor released by tumor cells could be responsible for the proliferative response of the local venous host system (Folkman, 1974).

Local tumors obtained from individual EMT6 spheroids are sarcomalike in appearance, consisting of spindle-shaped cells arranged in bundles. This tumor architecture is similar to that described for earlier passages of the EMT6 line

→

Figure 3. Growth of EMT6 solid tumors in nude mice from cell suspensions or individual spheroids. Tumor volume was monitored at various times after implantation of 10^6 EMT6 cells in suspension (dotted lines) or one EMT6 spheroid (solid line) into groups of C57BL nude (□) or BALB/c nude (■, ●) mice. Confidence limits represent two standard errors of the mean.

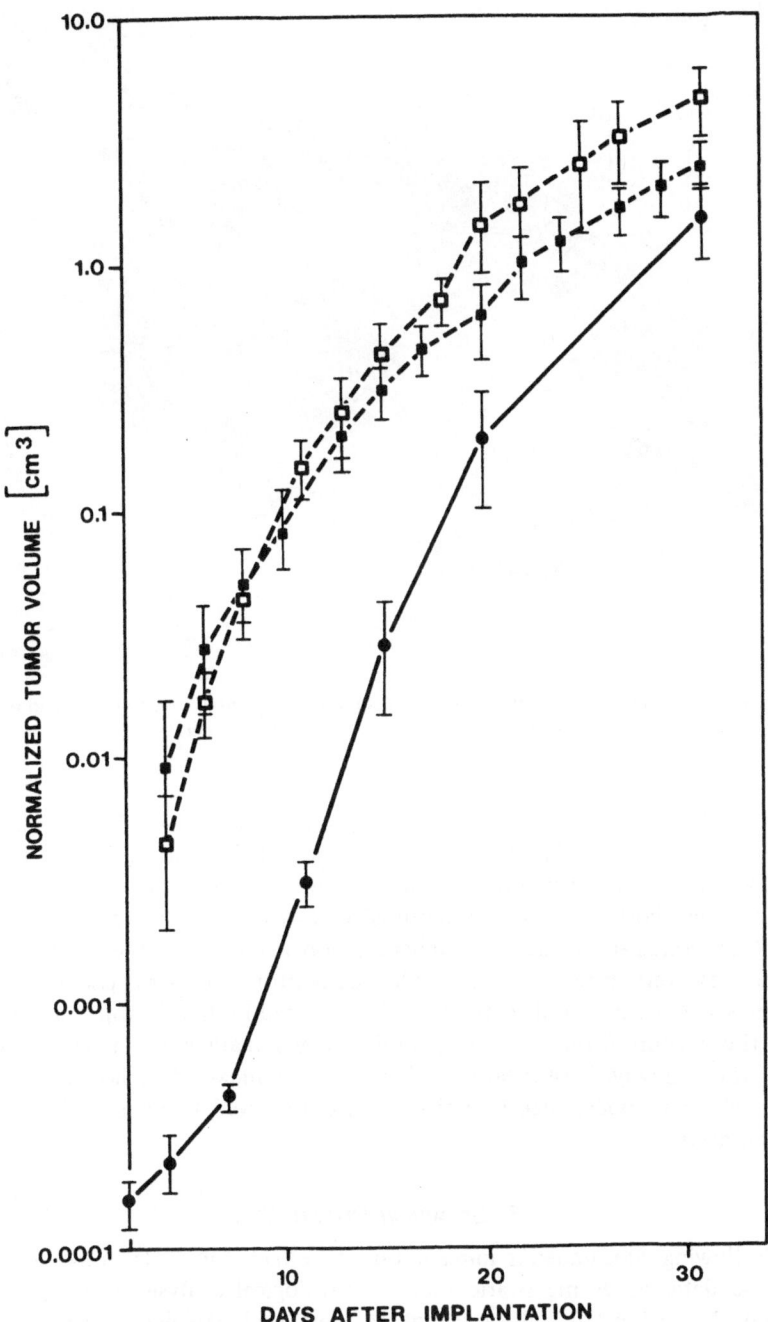

NORMALIZED TUMOR VOLUME [cm³]

DAYS AFTER IMPLANTATION

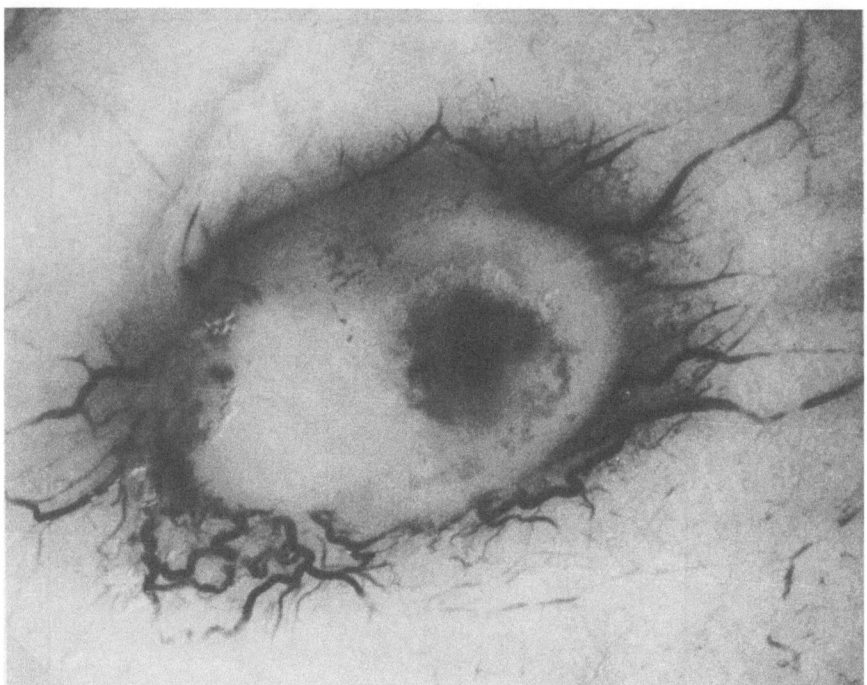

Figure 4. Vascular reaction induced by EMT6 spheroid implanted subcutaneously in BALB/c
nude mouse (day 13). Actual size, 1.2 cm.

(Rockwell *et al.*, 1972). Multinucleated giant cells may be seen both in the solid
tumor *in vivo* and within the EMT6 spheroid. EMT6 cells are highly invasive
locally and penetrate surrounding muscle layers and fat tissue. Neutrophils and
mononuclear host cells may be identified mainly at the tumor periphery. When
EMT6 spheroids are inoculated intraperitoneally in nude mice, they usually attach
to the mesenterium and grow as vascularized peritoneal tumor masses (peritoneal
carcinosis) (Fig. 5B). EMT6 tumor cells may readily detach from these masses
into the peritoneal fluid. Some spheroids may remain loose in the cavity and
grow there slowly. Peritoneal growth is also accompanied by host cell infiltration, which in nude mice is similar to that observed following subcutaneous
implantation.

3. Growth at Distant Sites

Following subcutaneous implantation of EMT6 spheroids, tumor cells can
also be detected as metastatic foci by histological analysis. They frequently
invade the regional lymph nodes where they produce solid masses extending

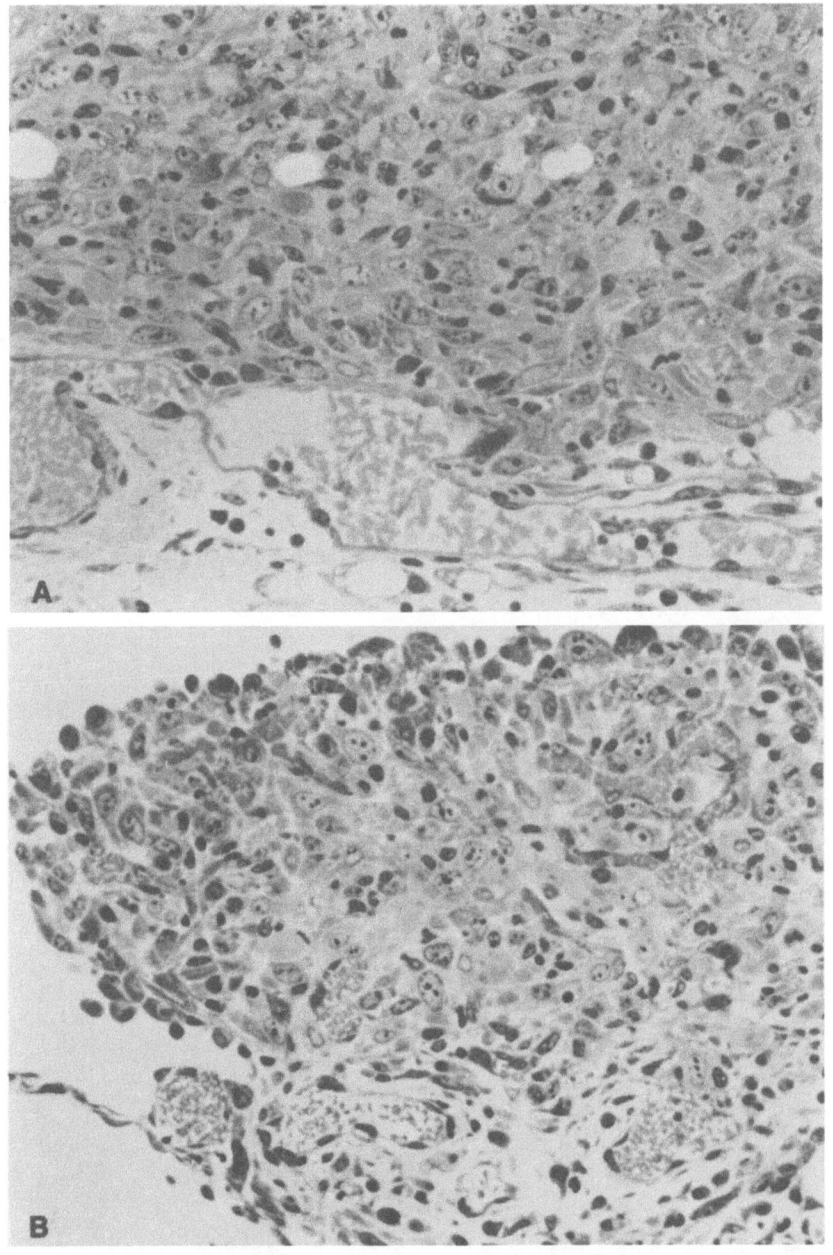

Figure 5. Photomicrographs of local tumors resulting from implantation of EMT6 spheroids at different sites. (A) Subcutaneous implantation (day 31). Tumor of undifferentiated type with peripheral vasculature (× 800, reproduced at 95%). (B) Intraperitoneal implantation (day 17). Tumor appended to mesenterium and well vascularized (× 800, reproduced at 95%).

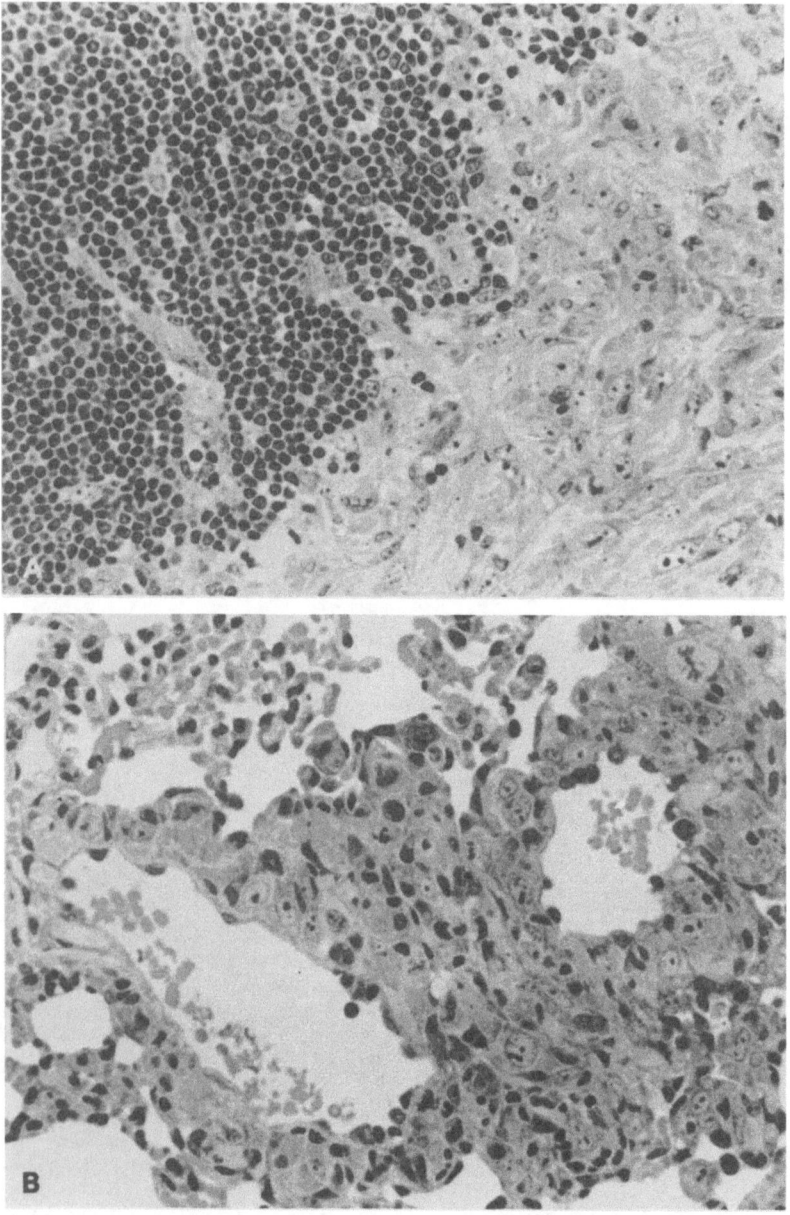

Figure 6. Metastatic behavior of subcutaneous tumors established from EMT6 spheroids. (A) Axillary lymph node metastasis (day 31). Note invasion of marginal sinus (×800, reproduced at 90%). (B) Perivascular lung metastasis, same conditions (×800, reproduced at 90%).

from the marginal sinus into the lymphoid parenchyma (Fig. 6A). With increasing tumor size, mediastinal lymph nodes may also be involved. Furthermore, all animals with very large tumors (inoculated either with cell suspensions or with a single spheroid) have concomitant lung metastases. These may occur as isolated intraseptal aggregates of several tumor cells or as large perivascular foci (Fig. 6B). Artificial metastases of EMT6 tumors have also been observed in the lungs of BALB/c mice following intravenous inoculation of tumor cell suspensions (Twentyman, 1978).

In conclusion, it is clear that growth and dissemination *in vivo* may be obtained from individual EMT6 spheroids. As such, MTS provide a model for microtumors that can be implanted at various sites and that are capable of multiphasic growth, invasiveness, and metastasis.

III. THE MTS AS AN EXPERIMENTAL ALLOGRAFT

A. Destruction of Spheroids Implanted in Normal or Immune Allogeneic Mice

1. Quantitation and Specificity

A major practical advantage of the MTS model system is that the tumor cells forming spheroids are clonogenic in most instances. Thus, immunologically mediated damage to spheroids can be quantitatively assessed by dissociating the spheroids and plating appropriate dilutions of the resulting single-cell suspension in a cloning assay (Sutherland *et al.*, 1977; MacDonald and Howell, 1978). A representative example of the results of such an approach is shown in Table I, in which EMT6 spheroids (of BALB/c origin) were dissociated and plated 48 h after implantation in the peritoneal cavity of either normal or specifically alloimmune C57BL/6 mice. It can be seen that the plating efficiency of the recovered cells was reduced by about 100-fold in the alloimmune group, and the absolute number of clonogenic cells per spheroid (i.e., the product of the plating efficiency times total cell number) was correspondingly reduced. This latter cal-

Table I. Quantitation of EMT6 Spheroid Destruction 48 h after Implantation in the Peritoneal Cavity of Normal or Specifically Alloimmune C57BL/6 Mice

Status of mice	Plating efficiency (%)[a]	Clonogenic EMT6 cells per spheroid
Normal	41 ± 5	8200
Immune	0.04 ± 0.03	70

[a]Mean ± 1 SD of five determinations.

culation is important because implanted spheroids contain a variable (and often large) number of host cells, which complicates any determination of plating efficiency (see Section III.B). Similar reductions in clonogenic tumor cells following implantation of EMT6 spheroids in alloimmune mice have been reported recently by Lord *et al.* (1979).

The immunological specificity of spheroid destruction *in vivo* has also been investigated (MacDonald and Howell, 1978). When strain A mice that had been immunized with either relevant ($H-2^d$) or third-party ($H-2^k$) alloantigens were implanted with EMT6 ($H-2^d$) spheroids for a period of 48 h, a 50-fold-greater reduction in surviving clonogenic tumor cells was observed in the specifically immunized mice. It should be noted, however, that no spheroids bearing $H-2^k$ alloantigens were available as a positive control for these experiments. In the latter context, the recent availability of a wider range of MTS (Section II.A) should facilitate future studies of the immunological specificity of spheroid destruction.

2. Kinetics

A kinetic study of spheroid destruction using the cloning assay has recently been performed (Sordat *et al.*, 1980). A summary of these results for EMT6 spheroids implanted intraperitoneally in specifically alloimmune or normal C57BL/6 mice as well as in athymic C57BL/6 mice is shown in Figure 7. It is clear that the destruction of spheroids proceeds much more quickly in alloimmune than in normal mice, with an initial reduction in clonogenic cells being detectable at 6 h versus 4 days, and 99% reduction occurring at 48 h versus 7 days. No significant reduction was observed in allogeneic athymic mice 7 days after spheroid implantation. In the latter context, it is noteworthy that growth and ultimate dissemination of EMT6 spheroids was observed following implantation in athymic mice (Section II.B).

3. Histopathology and Ultrastructure

A further advantage of the MTS model is that spheroid destruction *in situ* can be directly visualized by conventional histological and ultrastructural techniques. For EMT6 spheroids implanted in normal or alloimmune mice, clear differences in histopathology are apparent within 24–48 h (MacDonald and Howell, 1978; Lord *et al.*, 1979). In agreement with the results of clonogenic studies (Section III.A.), destruction of tumor cells *in situ* is extensive within 48 h in alloimmune mice, whereas many intact tumor cells can be seen following implantation for the same time period in normal allogeneic mice (Fig. 8). In addition, it is clear that numerous infiltrating cells of host origin are present within spheroids in both situations (Fig. 8). Further characterization of these cells will be presented in Section III.B.

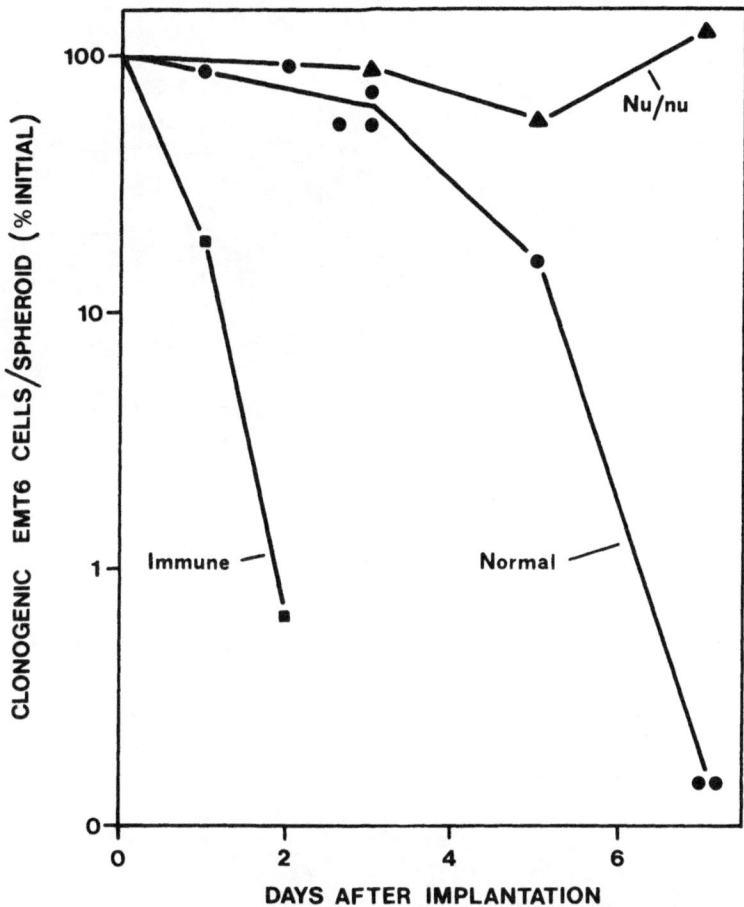

Figure 7. Kinetic analysis of the destruction of EMT6 spheroids implanted intraperitoneally in normal, alloimmune, or athymic (nu/nu) C57BL/6 mice. At the times indicated, spheroids were dissociated and the number of viable (clonogenic) EMT6 cells was determined in a colony formation assay. Normalized results from several experiments are presented.

More recently, we have investigated the kinetics of spheroid infiltration and destruction in greater detail (Sordat *et al.*, 1980). As can be seen in Fig. 9, infiltration of spheroids by host cells occurs very rapidly in specifically alloimmune mice. Within minutes, attachment of some cells to the outer surface of spheroids can be detected (Fig. 9A), and progressive infiltration occurs in a matter of hours (Fig. 9B,C). The heterogeneous nature of this spheroid infiltrate, which is apparent from Figs. 8 and 9, will be analyzed quantitatively in a subsequent section. It is interesting to note, however, that a massive influx of host cells occurs before any significant damage to the tumor cells is apparent.

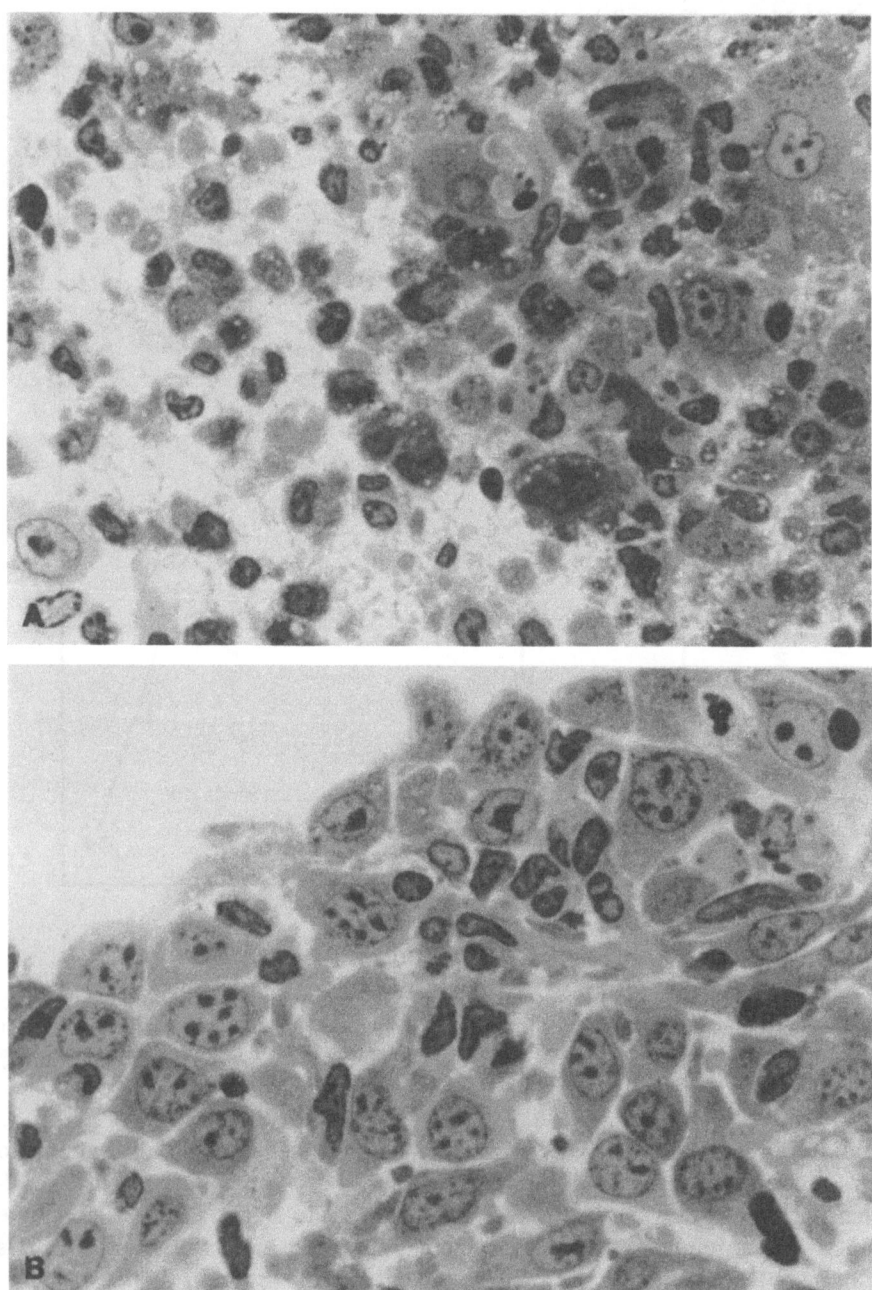

Figure 8. Photomicrographs of EMT6 spheroids implanted intraperitoneally for 48 h in specifically alloimmune (A) or normal (B) C57BL/6 mice. Note tumor cell destruction (A) and prominent host cell infiltration (A, B) (×1800).

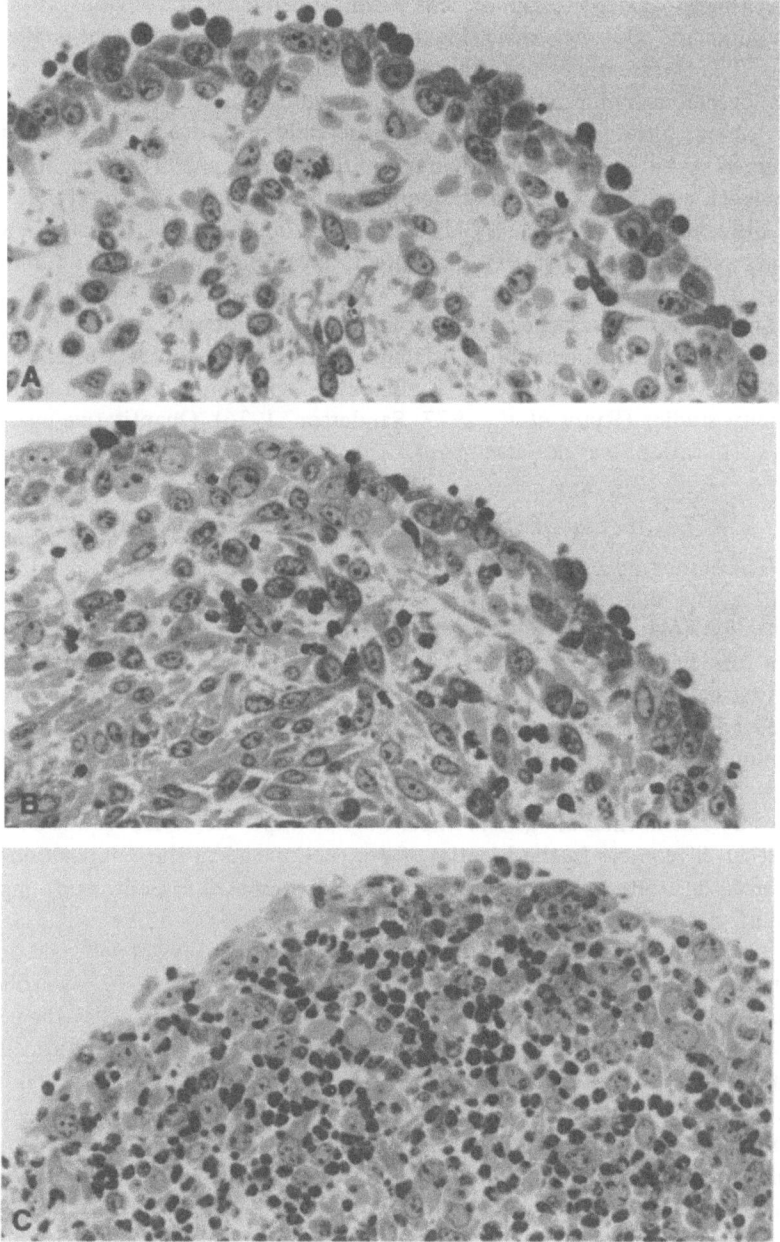

Figure 9. Photomicrographs illustrating progressive infiltration of EMT6 spheroids implanted intraperitoneally in alloimmune C57BL/6 mice for 10 min (A), 1.5 h (B), or 4 h (C) (×1000, reproduced at 90%).

Although damage to tumor cells within spheroids is not obvious within 48 h in nonimmune allogeneic mice (Fig. 8B), such damage does eventually take place. After 7 days, essentially no viable tumor cells can be seen in spheroid sections. In allogeneic athymic mice, damage to spheroids is not observed within this 7-day period, although infiltration by host cells does occur. Thus, the results obtained by histology, while not quantitative, are in general agreement with the clonogenic studies insofar as assessment of spheroid damage is concerned.

Ultrastructural studies of EMT6 spheroids implanted in normal or alloimmune mice indicate a variety of contacts between lymphoid and tumor cells (Lord *et al.*, 1979; Sordat *et al.*, 1980). As can be seen in Fig. 10, contacts between tumor cells and either macrophages, lymphocytes, or neutrophils were regularly observed in spheroids. In general terms, these contacts often resemble those seen between sensitized T lymphocytes and tumor cells in *in vitro* cytotoxicity studies (Ryser *et al.*, 1977; Sanderson, 1976). Quantitative analysis of these associations was not attempted.

4. Destruction of Spheroids Implanted at Other Sites or in Vitro

The limited number of studies of the immunological destruction of spheroids to date have concentrated on the peritoneal cavity as the site of spheroid implantation (MacDonald and Howell, 1978; Lord *et al.*, 1979). Recently, we have also begun to assess the effect of subcutaneous spheroid implantation (Sordat *et al.*, unpublished data). In preliminary studies, we have been able to recover EMT6 spheroids 48 h after subcutaneous implantation in normal or alloimmune C57BL/6 mice. Clonogenic assays have shown that spheroid destruction is essentially complete in alloimmune mice at this time, whereas little damage is detectable in normal allogeneic mice. Further experiments are required to assess whether differences in the kinetics of destruction and/or the composition of the spheroid infiltrate exist when subcutaneous (as opposed to peritoneal) implantation of spheroids is carried out.

Little work has likewise been done using *in vitro* assays of spheroid destruction. In a preliminary communication (Sutherland *et al.*, 1977), we observed a significant but incomplete reduction in clonogenic tumor cells when EMT6 spheroids were exposed *in vitro* to specifically alloimmune lymphoid cells generated in mixed leukocyte cultures. Further experimentation in this model system failed to increase the proportion of tumor cells killed *in vitro*, even when alloimmune peritoneal exudate cells (PEC) were used as a source of effector cells under a variety of assay conditions (MacDonald and Howell, unpublished data). Thus, it is not clear at the present time whether the rapid (and essentially complete) destruction of spheroids observed *in vivo* reflects a real difference between the two experimental systems (such as cell recruitment *in vivo*, for example) or simply a technical artifact of the *in vitro* assay.

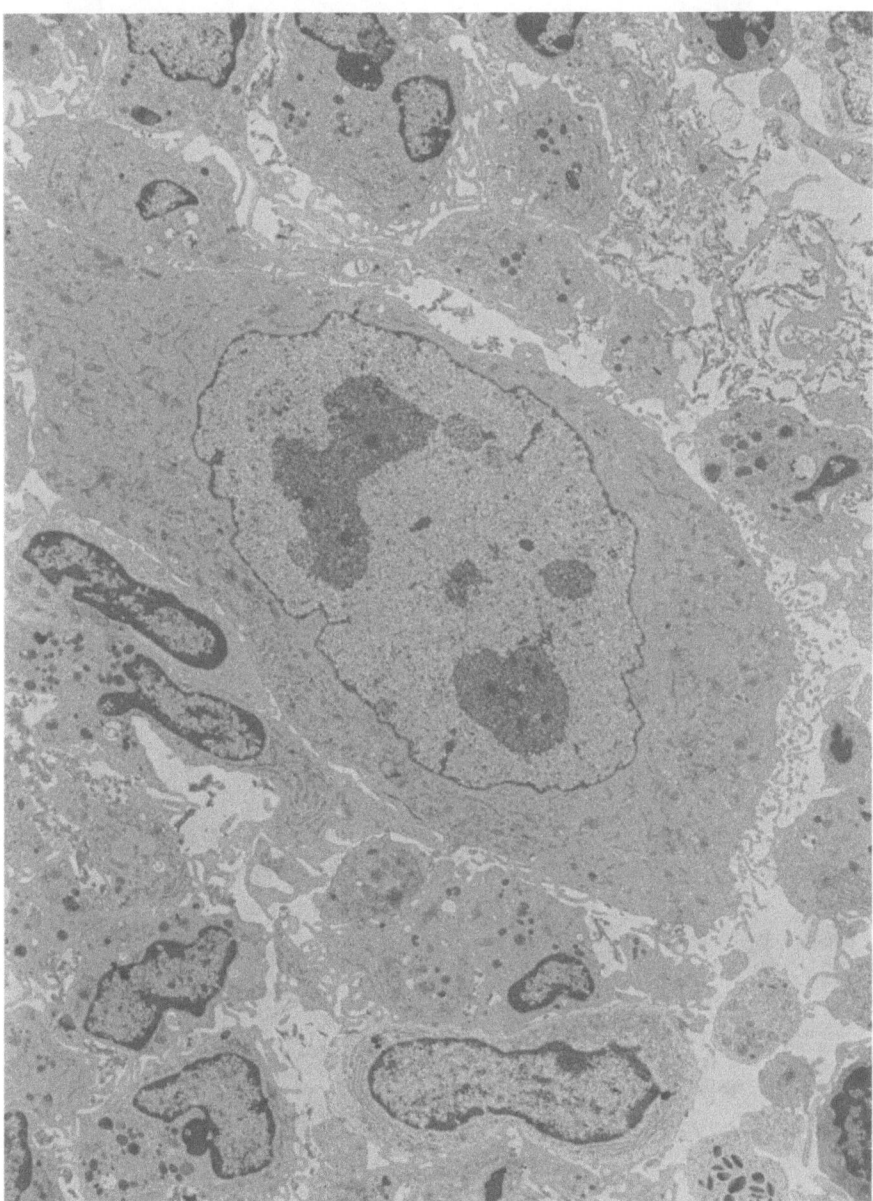

Figure 10. Electron micrograph of EMT6 spheroid implanted intraperitoneally for 48 h in normal C57BL/6 mouse. Note contacts between numerous host cells and central tumor cell (×5500).

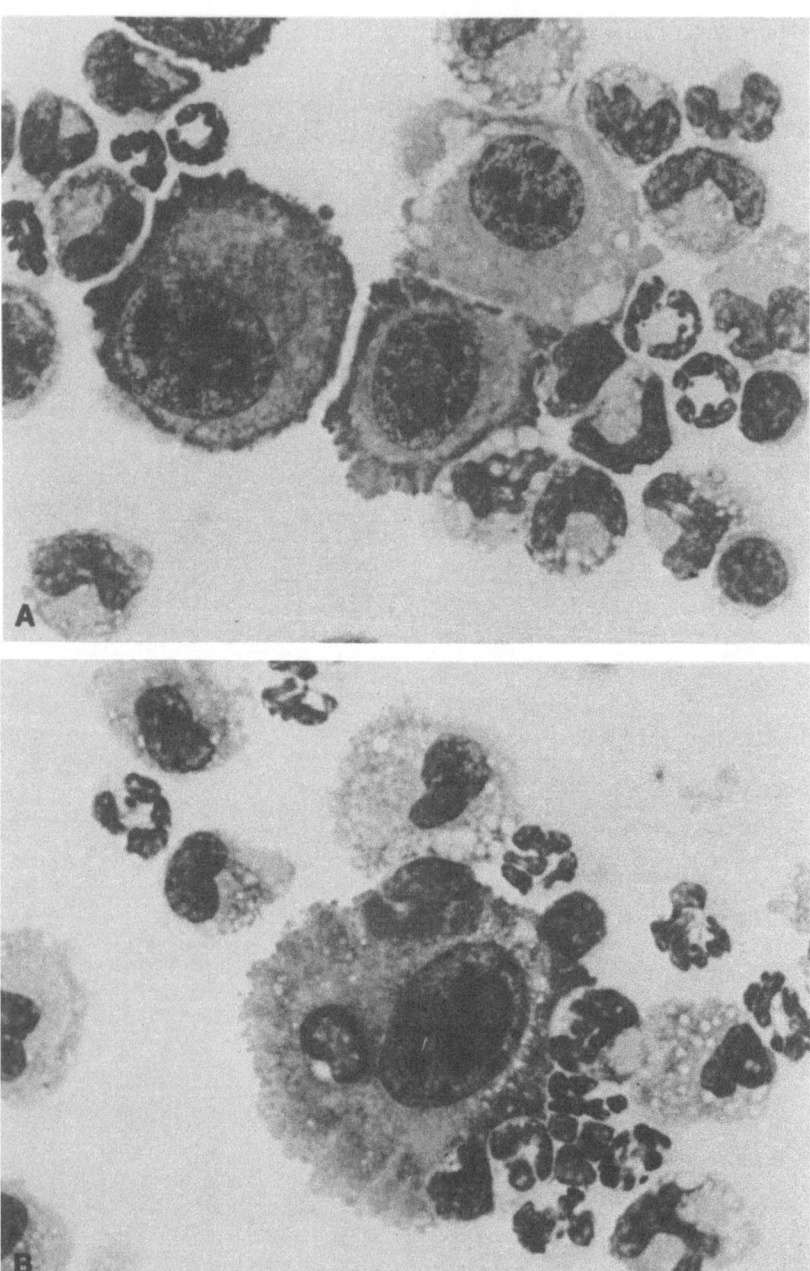

Figure 11. Cytocentrifuge preparations of cell suspensions from EMT6 spheroids obtained 48 h after implantation in normal (A) or specifically alloimmune (B) C57BL/6 mice. Note heterogeneous nature of infiltrating host cells (×1800, reproduced at 95%).

B. Characterization of Spheroid-Infiltrating Cells

1. Morphological

The facility with which spheroids can be dissociated by mild enzymatic treatment allows detailed quantitative studies of the morphological and functional properties of the infiltrating population to be carried out. We have chosen to study the morphology of spheroid-associated cells (SAC) on cytocentrifuge preparations because of the ease of identification of the cell types under these conditions. A typical example of a population of SAC isolated 48 h after implantation of EMT6 spheroids in normal or alloimmune C57BL/6 mice is shown in Fig. 11. It can be seen that SAC are heterogeneous, with tumor cells, neutrophils, macrophages, and lymphocytes all present in detectable numbers. By carrying out differential counts of SAC in normal and alloimmune mice at various times after spheroid implantation, it is thus possible to analyze the kinetics of cellular infiltration in a quantitative fashion (Sordat *et al.*, 1980). A summary of such an analysis for EMT6 spheroids implanted in normal C57BL/6 mice is presented in Table II. As suggested by the histological studies presented earlier (Section III.A. 3), a rapid influx of neutrophils into spheroids can be detected within hours of implantation. Monocytes accumulate within spheroids at later times, reaching a peak at about 2 days. Interestingly, only relatively small numbers of lymphocytes are detectable within spheroids at any time after implantation. Other cell types detectable in the peritoneal cavity surrounding the spheroids (such as eosinophils and, more rarely, mast cells) are never found in significant numbers within spheroids. As far as tumor cells are concerned, it should be noted that a drastic reduction in their number occurs between 4 and 7 days, corresponding to the time when the number of clonogenic cells per spheroid is likewise decreasing (Section III.A.2). Similar results were obtained when spheroids were implanted

Table II. Morphological Classification of SAC at Various Times after Implantation of EMT6 Spheroids in the Peritoneal Cavity of Normal C57BL/6 Mice

Time after implantation (days)	SAC ($\times 10^3$)	Differential count (% total)[a]			
		Tumor cells	Neutrophils	Monocytes	Lymphocytes
0.25	63	65	32	1.5	1.8
1	96	25	51	20	2.8
2	82	28	27	40	3.2
4	96	29	26	39	6.6
7	48	1.5	6.7	78	14

[a]Assessed on cytocentrifuge preparations.

in alloimmune mice, except that the kinetics of infiltration of host cells (and corresponding decrease in the number of tumor cells) was considerably more rapid.

It is clear from such quantitative morphological analysis that the infiltration of spheroid allografts is a dynamic process, with different cell types being present in different quantities at different times. In this context, it is interesting to compare the relative efficiency of infiltration of each cell type as a function of time. We have performed such a calculation for each morphological cell type mentioned above by dividing the differential count within spheroids (exclusive of tumor cells) by the corresponding differential count in the peritoneal cavity (Sordat *et al.*, 1980). The parameter so determined can be operationally defined as a penetration index and is illustrated for the case of nonimmune allogeneic mice in Table III (using data from Table II). Clear differences in the penetration index of different morphological cell types are apparent from such an analysis, and kinetic variations can also be documented. The high propensity of neutrophils to infiltrate spheroids is particularly evident, as is the relatively low penetration index of lymphocytes and eosinophils under all conditions tested. The marked increase in monocyte penetration as a function of time after spheroid implantation is likewise striking.

2. Functional

Functional analysis of SAC has also recently been carried out (MacDonald *et al.*, 1978; Lord *et al.*, 1979). In particular, SAC recovered 48 h after implantation of EMT6 spheroids in alloimmune C57BL/6 mice have been shown to function as effector cells in a short-term (3 h) ^{51}Cr-release assay using labeled target cells of the same genotype (H-2^d) as the spheroids. SAC recovered from

Table III. Differential Penetration of Various Cell Types into EMT6 Spheroids as a Function of Time after Implantation in Normal C57BL/6 Mice

Cell type	Penetration index[a]			
	6 h	24 h	48 h	96 h
Neutrophils	1.5	2.7	2.9	12.2[b]
Monocytes	0.3	0.9	1.2	1.1
Lymphocytes	0.23	0.10	0.14	0.22
Eosinophils	<0.1	<0.1	0.13	<0.1

[a] Defined as differential count (SAC)/differential count (PEC) after discounting tumor cells. In this way, an index of >1 indicates selective infiltration.
[b] High value resulting from very small number of neutrophils remaining in PEC at this time.

Table IV. Characteristics of Cytolytic SAC Detected
in a Short-Term [51]Cr Release Assay

SAC population[a]	Relative cytolytic activity
Untreated	100
Nonphagocytic[b]	200
Nonadherent[c]	300
T-cell depleted[d]	<3
Large (>6 mm/h)[e]	<10
Small (3 < s < 4 mm/h)[e]	300

[a] SAC recovered 48 h after implantation of spheroids in alloimmune C57BL/6 mice were treated as indicated and subsequently tested for cytotoxicity on ^{51}Cr-labeled DBA/2 mastocytoma cells at various lymphocyte:target cell ratios. Results are expressed as relative lytic units (normalized to the value of the untreated control).
[b] Following exposure to carbonyl iron plus magnet.
[c] Following 60 min incubation on plastic petri dishes.
[d] Following treatment with rabbit antimouse T-cell serum plus complement.
[e] Following separation by 1g velocity sedimentation.

normal or athymic mice were inactive under comparable experimental conditions. Further characterization of the cytotoxic cells (Table IV) indicated that they were nonadherent and nonphagocytic and that they were eliminated by treatment with a heterologous rabbit antimouse T-cell serum (MacDonald *et al.*, 1978). Velocity sedimentation cell separation further identified the cytotoxic cells as small lymphocytes. These experiments thus provide unequivocal evidence that cytotoxic T lymphocytes can be found within spheroids. The possibility that other cell types found within spheroids may also be cytotoxic under different experimental conditions has not yet been investigated.

C. Attempts to Identify the Mechanism of Spheroid Destruction *in Situ*

An obvious question arising from the MTS model system is the question of how spheroid damage may be effected *in situ*. In this context, it is important to bear in mind that the isolation of any particular effector function (be it cellular or humoral) from the spheroid infiltrate is necessary but certainly not sufficient evidence to conclude that such a mechanism is decisive (or even operative) *in situ*. The question of identification of effector mechanisms *in situ* is therefore a complex one encompassing the problem of tumor microenvironment as well as the utilization of suitable functional assays. Indeed it is possible to approach the question of the effect of certain tumor microenvironmental factors on effector functions as a separate issue (Harris, 1976; MacDonald *et al.*, 1976); however,

Table V. Effect of Transferred Alloimmune Cells
and/or Antiserum on the Survival of EMT6 Spheroids
Implanted in Irradiated Normal C57BL/6 Mice

Material transferred	Plating efficiency (%)	Clonogenic EMT6 cells per spheroid
None	54	13,700
PEC[a]	17	2,500
Antiserum[b]	41	13,300
PEC + antiserum	5.3	1,100

[a] 10×10^6 peritoneal cells from C57BL/6 mice immunized
19 days previously with P-815 tumor cells.
[b] 0.25 ml of hyperimmune C57BL/6 anti-DBA/2 antiserum.

since the precise nature of microenvironmental factors in any particular tumor
system is very difficult to evaluate directly, such studies cannot be definitively
interpreted.

In view of the complexity of this problem, we have taken an operational
approach to the identification of spheroid-damaging effector mechanisms *in situ*.
In particular, we have attempted to transfer spheroids to immunoincompetent
(lethally irradiated) C57BL/6 hosts together with various specific alloimmune
components (i.e., cells and/or antibodies) and evaluate spheroid destruction
under such conditions. Our results to date are still somewhat preliminary, but we
have succeeded in demonstrating significant spheroid destruction within 48 h
when EMT6 spheroids were transferred together with alloimmune C57BL/6
peritoneal exudate cells (Table V). In similar experiments, transfer of hyperimmune serum directed against spheroid alloantigens did not in itself induce
detectable damage to spheroids, and a combination of immune cells and serum
was only slightly more cytotoxic than immune cells alone (Table V). Destruction
of EMT6 spheroids in athymic C57BL/6 mice was also observed following
transfer of alloimmune PEC. These results are certainly encouraging, and further
experiments are currently in progress to evaluate the effect of transferring more-
defined cell subpopulations on spheroid survival. In the meantime, no definite
conclusion as to the mechanism(s) of spheroid damage *in situ* can be made.

IV. CONCLUSIONS AND PROSPECTS

Identification and quantitative evaluation of immunological parameters
affecting the growth of solid tumors *in vivo* is an extremely complex problem in
immunobiology. One aspect of this problem that has been extensively investigated
by a few workers in recent years is the isolation and *in vitro* characterization of

immune components from solid tumors, as is discussed in detail in this volume. Another nonexclusive question that has received somewhat less attention is the degree to which immune responses may be influenced by the unique micro-environment of the tumors themselves. In the latter context, the MTS model described in this communication is particularly attractive in the sense that it is characterized by similar variations in metabolite concentration and cell-cycle status as have been observed for a number of solid tumors (Sutherland and Durand, 1976).

For practical reasons, our initial studies have concentrated on applying the MTS model to the problem of allograft rejection in the mouse. In this system, considerable progress has been made in recent years in the domain of identification and quantitation of effector mechanisms both *in vivo* and *in vitro* (see Cerottini and Brunner, 1974; Häyry, 1976). Despite these advances, however, the actual means whereby solid tissue and tumor grafts are damaged *in situ* remain elusive. Data concerning the accumulation of host cells within allografts have been available for some time (Medawar, 1944; Simonsen *et al.*, 1953); however, attempts to investigate the functional properties of such cells have only recently been carried out. From such studies, it has become clear that a heterogeneous mixture of potential effector populations can be isolated from murine sponge matrix allografts (Roberts and Häyry, 1977; Wiktorowicz *et al.*, 1978) and from rat cardiac allografts (Strom *et al.*, 1977). A crucial question in these and other, similar studies is how to relate the isolated effector phenomena with graft damage *in situ*, particularly in situations where the latter parameter cannot be quantitatively assessed.

We have attempted to apply similar methodology to the study of tumor spheroid allografts. A principal advantage of the system over other published work is that the survival of the grafts can be quantitatively assessed at any given time by a simple clonogenic assay (Sutherland *et al.*, 1977; MacDonald and Howell, 1978). Using such analysis, we have shown that spheroids are destroyed within 48 h in specifically alloimmune mice and after 5–7 days in normal allogeneic mice. Spheroid damage is not apparent in athymic (nu/nu) mice. Destruction is immunologically specific and is accompanied by progressive infiltration of neutrophils, monocytes, and some lymphocytes. The proportion of these cell types present within spheroids varies with time after implantation; generally neutrophil influx is extremely rapid, whereas maximum monocyte infiltration does not occur for several days (at least in nonimmune mice). Functional analysis of the spheroid infiltrate using a short-term ^{51}Cr-release assay has revealed the presence of cytotoxic cells that have the properties of small T lymphocytes. The presence of other cells with cytotoxic potential cannot be excluded.

Although it is not yet possible to identify effector cells *in situ* on the basis of these data, certain comparisons between spheroids and other model systems can be made. For example, the presence of directly cytotoxic T cells *in situ* has also been demonstrated at early times after implantation of sponge matrix allografts in mice (Wiktorowicz *et al.*, 1978), as well as in acutely rejecting rat cardiac allografts (Strom *et al.*, 1977). A rapid accumulation of neutrophils and more delayed appearance of monocytes and lymphocytes has likewise been observed in a number of tissue allografts (reviewed in Häyry, 1976), although the functional significance of these cells remains to be determined. With the availability of a transfer system in which the effect of defined alloimmune cell subpopulations can be directly assessed on spheroids (Section III.C), we are hopeful that more definitive answers to these questions will be available in the near future.

Aside from their utility as an allograft model, multicellular tumor spheroids would seem to be ideally suited for quantitative studies of immunity to syngeneic tumors. With this in mind, we are currently growing spheroids of highly immuno-genic oncornavirus-induced sarcoma cells derived from several strains of mice as well as several human MTS (see Section II.A). Along similar lines, Lord (1979) has recently demonstrated destruction of EMT6 spheroids in syngeneic BALB/c mice that had been immunized previously with irradiated EMT6 tumor cells. Since it is also feasible to study dissemination (and metastasis) of tumor cells derived from individual spheroids (see Section II.B), it is clear that MTS may prove to be an extremely useful tool for unraveling the complex series of im-munological (and other) events associated with the growth and dissemination of solid tumors *in vivo*.

ACKNOWLEDGMENTS

We are especially endebted to Rosemary Lees, Robert Howell, and Emil Bogenmann, who collaborated in the experiments described in this chapter. We also wish to thank Drs. Edith Lord and Robert Sutherland for making available their unpublished data. The expert technical assistance of Jeanine Bamat and Lene Kolly as well as the secretarial assistance of Brigitte Favre, Josiane Duc, and Silvia Saulle is gratefully acknowledged. This work was supported in part by Grant 3-136-077 from the Swiss National Foundation for Scientific Research.

V. REFERENCES

Baserga, R., 1971, *The Cell Cycle and Cancer*, Marcel Dekker, New York.

Carlsson, J., and Brunk, U., 1977, The fine structure of three-dimensional colonies of hu-man glioma cells in agarose culture, *Acta Pathol. Microbiol. Scand. Sect. A* 85:183.

Carrel, S., Sordat, B., and Merenda, C., 1976, Establishment of a cell line (Co-115) from a human colon carcinoma transplanted into nude mice, *Cancer Res.* 36:3978.

Cerottini, J. -C., and Brunner, K. T., 1974, Cell-mediated cytotoxicity, allograft rejection and tumor immunity, *Adv. Immunol.* **18**:67.

Dalen, H., and Burki, H. J., 1971, Some observations on the three-dimensional growth of L5178Y cell-colonies in soft agar culture, *Exp. Cell Res.* **65**:433.

Dethlefsen, L. A., Prewitt, J. M. S., and Mendelsohn, M. A., 1968, Analysis of tumor growth curves, *J. Natl. Cancer Inst.* **40**:389.

Folkman, J., 1974, Tumor angiogenesis, *Adv. Cancer Res.* **19**:331.

Folkman, J., and Hochberg, M., 1973, Self-regulation of growth in three dimensions, *J. Exp. Med.* **138**:745.

Gray, L. H., Conger, A. D., Ebert, M., Hornsey, S., and Scott, O. C. A., 1953, Concentration of oxygen dissolved in tissues at time of irradiation as factor in radiotherapy, *Br. J. Radiol.* **26**:638.

Haji-Karim, M., and Carlsson, J., 1978, Proliferation and viability in cellular spheroids of human origin, *Cancer Res.* **38**:1457.

Harris, J. W., 1976, The effect of tumor-like assay conditions, ionizing radiation, and hyperthermia on immune lysis of tumor cells by cytotoxic T-lymphocytes, *Cancer Res.* **36**: 2733.

Häyry, P., 1976, Problems and prospects in surgical immunology, *Med. Biol.* **54**:1.

Kaplan, H. S., 1974, On the relative importance of hypoxic cells for the radiotherapy of human tumors, *Eur. J. Cancer* **10**:275.

Lees, R. K., Bogenmann, E., Sordat, B., MacDonald, H. R., and Carrel, S., 1979, Growth of multicellular tumor spheroids of human origin, *Experientia* **35**:970.

Lord, E. M., 1979, Comparison of *in situ* and peripheral host immunity to syngeneic tumors employing the multicellular spheroid model, *Proc. 9th L. H. Gray Conf.*, in press.

Lord, E. M., Penney, D. P., Sutherland, R. M., and Cooper, R. A., 1979, Morphological and functional characteristics of cells infiltrating and destroying tumor multicellular spheroids *in vivo*, *Virchows Arch. B* **31**:103.

MacDonald, H. R., and Howell, R. L., 1978, The multicellular spheroid as a model tumor allograft. I. Quantitative assessment of spheroid destruction in alloimmune mice, *Transplantation* **25**:136.

MacDonald, H. R., Howell, R. L., and McFarlane, D. L., 1978, The multicellular spheroid as a model tumor allograft. II. Characterization of spheroid-infiltrating cytotoxic cells, *Transplantation* **25**:141.

MacDonald, H. R., Sutherland, R. M., Howell, R. L., and McCredie, J. A., 1976, Cytotoxic T lymphocyte function under conditions simulating the microenvironment of solid tumors, *Proc. Am. Assoc. Cancer Res.* **17**:221.

McAllister, R. M., Reed, G., and Huebner, R. J., 1967, Colonial growth in agar of cells derived from adenovirus-induced hamster tumors, *J. Natl. Cancer Inst.* **39**:43.

Medawar, P. B., 1944, Behaviour and fate of skin autografts and skin homografts in rabbits, *J. Anat.* **78**:176.

Roberts, P. J., and Häyry, P., 1977, Effector mechanisms in allograft rejection. II. Density, electrophoresis and size fractionation of allograft-infiltrating cells demonstrating several classes of killer cells, *Cell Immunol.* **30**:236.

Rockwell, S. C., Kallman, R. F., and Fajardo, L. F., 1972, Characteristics of a serially transplanted mouse mammary tumor and its tissue-culture-adapted derivative, *J. Natl. Cancer Inst.* **49**:735.

Ryser, J. -E., Sordat, B., Cerottini, J. -C., and Brunner, K. T., 1977, Mechanism of target cell lysis by cytolytic T lymphocytes. I. Characterization of specific lymphocyte-target cell conjugates separated by velocity sedimentation, *Eur. J. Immunol.* **7**:110.

Sanderson, C. J., 1976, Morphological studies of cell death by time-lapse microcinematography, *Proc. R. Soc. London, Ser. B* **192**:241.

Simonsen, M., Buemann, A., Gammeltaft, F., Jensen, F., and Jorgensen, K., 1953, Biological incompatibility in kidney transplantation in dogs. I. Experimental and morphological investigations, *Acta Pathol. Microbiol. Scand.* **32**:1.

Sordat, B., MacDonald, H. R., and Lees, R. K., 1980, The multicellular spheroid as a model tumor allograft. III. Morphological and kinetic analysis of spheroid infiltration and destruction, *Transplantation* **29**:103.

Strom, T. B., Tilney, N. L., Paradysz, J. M., Bancewicz, J., and Carpenter, C. B., 1977, Cellular components of allograft rejection: Identity, specificity, and cytotoxic function of cells infiltrating acutely rejecting allografts, *J. Immunol.* **118**:2020.

Sutherland, R. M., and Durand, R. E., 1976, Radiation response of multicell spheroids—An *in vitro* tumour model, *Curr. Top. Radiat. Res. Q.* **11**:87.

Sutherland, R. M., McCredie, J. A., and Inch, W. R., 1971, Growth of multicell spheroids in tissue culture as a model of nodular carcinomas, *J. Natl. Cancer Inst.* **46**:113.

Sutherland, R. M., MacDonald, H. R., and Howell, R. L., 1977, Multicellular spheroids: A new model target for *in vitro* studies of immunity to solid tumor allografts, *J. Natl. Cancer Inst.* **58**:1849.

Tannock, I. F., 1968, The relation between cell proliferation and the vascular system in a transplanted mouse mammary tumour, *Br. J. Cancer* **22**:258.

Thomlinson, R. H., and Gray, L. H., 1955, The histological structure of some human lung cancers and the possible implications for radiotherapy, *Br. J. Cancer* **9**:539.

Twentyman, P. R., 1978, The growth of the EMT6 tumour in the lungs of Balb C mice following intravenous inoculation of tumour cells from culture, *Cell Tissue Kinet.* **11**:57.

Watson, J. V., 1976, The cell proliferation kinetics of the EMT6/M/AC mouse tumour at four volumes during unperturbed growth *in vivo*, *Cell Tissue Kinet.* **9**:147.

Wiktorowicz, K., Roberts, P. J., and Häyry, P., 1978, Effector mechanisms in allograft rejection. IV. In contrast to late cytotoxic cells, the early killer cells infiltrating mouse sponge matrix allografts are predominantly T lymphocytes, *Cell. Immunol.* **38**:255.

Yuhas, J. M., Li, A. P., Martinez, A. O., and Ladman, A. J., 1977, A simplified method for production and growth of multicellular tumor spheroids, *Cancer Res.* **37**:3639.

Index